Down Syndrome

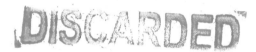

Down Syndrome
A Promising Future, Together

Edited by
Terry J. Hassold, Ph.D.
Department of Genetics
Case Western Reserve University
Cleveland, Ohio

and

David Patterson, Ph.D.
Eleanor Roosevelt Institute for Cancer Research
Denver, Colorado

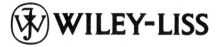

A JOHN WILEY & SONS, INC., PUBLICATION

NEW YORK • CHICHESTER • WEINHEIM • BRISBANE • SINGAPORE • TORONTO

Library of Congress Cataloging-in-Publication Data:

Down syndrome : a promising future, together / edited by Terry J.
  Hassold, David Patterson.
        p.   cm.
    Includes index,
    ISBN 0-471-29686-4 (cloth : alk. paper). — ISBN 0-471-29687-2
  (paper : alk. paper)
    1. Down syndrome   I. Hassold, Terry J.   II. Patterson, David,
    1944–
  RC571.D67   1998
  616.85′8842—dc21   98-3117

Printed in the United States of America.

10 9 8 7 6 5 4 3 2

Contents

VIII. TRANSITIONS TO ADULTHOOD

IX. THE ROLE OF THE FAMILY

X. PERSPECTIVES

Preface

This book grew out of a national conference on Down syndrome sponsored by the National Down Syndrome Society. The conference was intended to bring together a broad group of interested participants—people with Down syndrome, their families, health care professionals involved in the care of individuals with Down syndrome, and scientists engaged in research on Down syndrome—and to discuss clinical, educational, developmental, psychosocial and vocational issues relevant to people with Down syndrome. As the 500 participants can attest, a lot of material was presented in the four days of the conference, and this book represents an effort to summarize the highlights.

The book is divided into ten sections, beginning with a discussion of advocacy and the development of advocacy skills on behalf of people with Down syndrome. The next three sections are devoted to the genetics of Down syndrome and important health care issues. Included here are discussions of alternative and nonconventional therapies for Down syndrome, currently an extremely controversial and much-debated topic among parents and health care professionals alike. Additionally, this portion of the book includes Health Care Guidelines for Individuals with Down Syndrome: the Down Syndrome Preventative Medical Check List, edited by Dr. William Cohen on behalf of the Down Syndrome Medical Interest Group. These clinical guidelines were first introduced in the 1980s, and this represents their most recent update. A thoughtful composite of the input of many experts involved in the health care of people with Down syndrome, the Guidelines reflect current standards and practices of health care in the United States.

In the next five sections, the focus changes from clinical considerations to issues involving psychosocial development, communication, education and transitions to adulthood. Included her are chapters on behavioral issues and their management, strategies to improve reading skills, inclusion in the educational setting, and housing options for adults, among other topics. In the book's final two sections the focus changes again, to the family and to the individual—beginning with discussions of the role of the family in Down syndrome, and concluding with a series of perspectives written by individuals with Down syndrome.

This book should be valuable to several groups, including parents and relatives of individuals with Down syndrome, expectant parents of Down syndrome children, physicians who care for individuals with Down syndrome, and other health care professionals, including nursing personnel, physical and occupational therapists, speech-language workers, educators, and social workers. We hope the volume provides the reader with a sense of the excitement that has accompanied the many recent advances in the Down syndrome arena—from improvements in medical care and management to an understanding of the enormous potential of individuals with Down syndrome. Most importantly, of course, we hope that the information provided in the book will be useful in enriching the lives of people with Down syndrome.

Terry Hassold
David Patterson

Contributors

Lori Atkins
National Down Syndrome Society
666 Broadway, 8th Floor
New York, NY 10012-2317

Brenda Lynn Bargmann
6609 East Grandview
Scottsdale, AZ 85254

Michael Bérubé
1704 Henry Street
Champaign, IL 61821

Robin Bolduc
1546 Bradley Drive
Boulder, CO 80303

Chris Burke
3 Peter Cooper Road #5B
New York, NY 10010

George T. Capone
Kennedy Krieger Institute
Down Syndrome Clinic
707 North Broadway
Baltimore, MD 21205

Jane I. Carlson
17 Evergreen Road
Rocky Point, NY 11778

Mary Ann Carmody
6121 Nevada Avenue, NW
Washington, DC 20015

Brian A. Chicoine
Medical Director
The Adult Down Syndrome Center of
    Lutheran General Hospital
1255 N. Milwaukee Ave.
Glenview, IL 60025

William I. Cohen
Down Syndrome Center of Western
    Pennsylvania
Children's Hospital of Pittsburgh
One Children's Place
3705 Fifth Avenue
Pittsburgh, PA 15213-2583

Daniel B. Crimmins
Westchester Institute for Human
    Development
324 Cedarwood Hall
Valhalla, NY 10595-1689

Richard W. Fee
Director of Education
Idaho School for the Deaf and Blind
1450 Main Street
Gooding, ID 83330

Anne E. Fowler
66 Granby Drive
Madison, CT 06443

Marquita Grenot-Scheyer
California State University, Long Beach
College of Education
1250 Bellflower Boulevard
Long Beach, CA 90840-2201

Contributors

Terry J. Hassold
Department of Genetics
School of Medicine
Case Western Reserve University
10900 Euclid Avenue, Room E-645
Cleveland, OH 44106-4955

Judy S. Itzkowitz
Educational Consult
106 Talcott Ridge Road
South Windsor, CT 06074

Jason Kingsley
226 S. Greeley Ave.
Chappaqua, NY 10514

Libby Kumin
Professor and Department Chair
Dept. of Speech-Language
    Pathology/Audiology
Loyola College
4501 North Charles Street
Baltimore, MD 21210-2699

Mitchell Levitz
Capabilities Unlimited
2495 Erie Avenue
Cincinnati, OH 45208

Ira T. Lott
Department of Pediatrics
Bldg. 17
Irvine Medical Center, Rte. 81
101 City Drive South
Orange, CA 92668

Phil Mattheis
Medical Director
University of Montana Affiliated
    Program
University of Montana
52 Corbin Hall
Missoula, MT 59812

Kathleen H. McGinley
Assistant Director
The Arc Governmental Affairs Office
1730 K St. NW, Suite 1212
Washington, DC 20006

Dennis E. McGuire
Director of Psychological Services
The Adult Down Syndrome Center of
    Lutheran General Hospital
1255 N. Milwaukee Ave.
Glenview, IL 60025

Patricia Logan Oelwein
13110 North East 25th Place
Bellevue, WA 98005

Bonnie Patterson
Cincinnati Center for Developmental
    Disorders
University of Cincinnati
3333 Burnett
Cincinnati, OH 45229

David Patterson
President
Eleanor Roosevelt Institute for Cancer
    Research
1899 Gaylord Street
Denver, CO 80206

Mia Peterson
Capabilities Unlimited
2495 Erie Avenue
Cincinnati, OH 45208

Siegfried M. Pueschel
593 Eddy Street
Providence, RI 02903

Michael L. Remus
Kansas State Board of Education
Special Education Outcome
120 S.E. 10th Street
Topeka, KS 66612-1182

Nancy Roizen
5622 S. Woodlawn Avenue
Chicago, IL 60637

Christopher E. Smith
Program Coordinator
Developmental Disabilities Institute
Children's Residential Program
99 Hollywood Drive
Smithtown, NY 11787

Christi Todd
5250 East Sweetwater
Scottsdale, AZ 85254

Don C. Van Dyke
Associate Professor of Pediatrics
Division of Developmental Disabilities
University of Iowa Hospital & Clinic
Iowa City, IA 52242

Gloria Wolpert
49 Sprain Valley Road
Scarsdale, NY 10583

I. Advocacy Skills

If You Don't Like the Rules, Change Them!

Robin Bolduc

> To the old ones of my childhood who taught me the most important lesson of all: That I did not need to be perfect to be loved. That no one does.—Alice Walker, Introduction to *To Hell with Dying* (New York: Harcourt Brace Jovanich, 1967)

INDIVIDUAL ADVOCACY

"If you don't like the rules, change them" was the advice given to me as a young girl by my father. Little did I know how much I would rely on that advice upon becoming the parent of a child with Down syndrome. In 1987 I adopted a 4-year-old girl with Down syndrome. I, like most people, thought that there was a system in place to meet the very special needs of my daughter, and that the system would be responsive to my needs as her parent. It immediately became apparent that such was not the case. The county I lived in argued with the county that Tiffany previously resided in as to which county was responsible for her until the adoption was final. Having passed that first hurdle, I discovered that I was now eligible to receive respite services. In other words, I could send my brand new daughter away to a stranger's home for a period of time so I could "rest."

Shortly thereafter, a man from the school district came to my office to "help" me register my daughter for school. I thought it was very nice that he came all the way out to my office to have me sign "routine" papers. He assured me that the school district had a very nice program for children like mine. I soon discovered I had signed away my daughter's right to attend her local neighborhood school. She was sent to a school away from our neighborhood. She left for school before the neighborhood children left and returned home after they returned home. She went to school on a "special" bus that delivered her to a "special" door at the "special" wing of the school. She played in a "special" school yard and used a "special" bathroom. At lunchtime, she sat at a table reserved for her class. She responded by becoming a be-

Down Syndrome: A Promising Future, Together, Edited by Terry J. Hassold and David Patterson
ISBN 0-471-29686-4   Copyright © 1998 by Wiley-Liss, Inc.

havior problem. She climbed out the window of her "special" classroom and ran away to the playground where the other children were playing. At home, we noticed that she was having problems playing with the other children in our neighborhood. She was losing communication skills. We responded by working on weekends to make sure that she was an active part of our neighborhood. We made sure she had the best Barbie doll collection and enticed neighborhood children to play with her by offering pizza parties. It worked! One day, however, Tiffany asked, "How come I can't go to school with my friends and my brother?"

When we asked the school that same question, they responded, "We don't let kids like that in our kindergarten classes." So began my battle to change the rules of my school district and to enforce the rules of the U.S. Department of Education (among others). After two due process hearings, a brief encounter with the federal court system, a complaint with the Office of Civil Rights, two complaints with the Pennsylvania Department of Education, and the intervention of a U.S. Senator and the Governor's office, Tiffany walked to school with her brother and neighborhood friends. By now she was attending a regular first-grade classroom. Now the real work began! Now I had to work with the members of the Individual Education Plan (IEP) team that had so vehemently opposed my daughter's right to be educated in her local neighborhood school. I spent much time mending relationships with the people who would work with my daughter on a daily basis. In addition, I had to mend relationships with the parents of other children with disabilities. Many of them were threatened by the choice that I made for my daughter. They feared that if my daughter was successful in a regular classroom, the self-contained settings they wanted for their children would be closed. I am happy to say that as of 1996 when I left Pennsylvania, almost all of the children with disabilities were attending their local neighborhood schools and were spending at least part of their day supported in regular classrooms. As a result of the success of Tiffany, one by one parents requested similar educational settings for their children. As a result of one child's question and one parent's determination, the special educational services of a school district were changed to meet better meet the needs of all its students with disabilities.

I tell the story of Tiffany to illustrate that one person can indeed make a difference for large numbers of people. I know that her story has inspired other parents to change school district "rules" and even more people have become affected by her story. Individual advocacy is one way to change systemic rules that do not meet the needs of people with disabilities and/or their families.

Through the years, I have developed four simple strategies for successful individual advocacy. First, it is vital that you not only know your rights, but that you believe in your rights.

Step One is Research

Have a general understanding of your rights before you make a request or participate in a meeting. Know where to go and/or whom to ask for more detailed information as the need arises. For educational issues, every state has a federally funded parent information center. Call them, attend their training programs, read their materials. Every state has a federally funded protection and advocacy entity for people with disabilities. They can answer your questions and send you written materials concerning civil rights issues.

Step Two is to Prepare for Any Meeting.

A. Develop an agenda. This meeting is about your loved one. Your agenda should allow you to ask any questions concerning the issues of the meeting and allow you to ask for clarification of any issues discussed at the meeting.

B. Ask for any documents prior to the meeting so you have time to read them thoroughly. When the meeting concerns my daughter's Individual Education Plan (IEP), I ask for the *draft* IEP a week before the meeting. I explain that I do not want to waste anyone's time during the meeting while I read the document and develop my questions.

C. Invite a trusted friend to accompany you to a meeting. Your friend will hear things that you may not hear. I like to bring my mother with me. She is one of my daughter's best advocates. She knows nothing about special education law, but she does know and love my daughter. It is very hard to argue with a grandmother!

Step Three is about Conducting Successful Meetings

A. Start the meeting in a positive manner. If you called the meeting, take charge of the meeting by thanking everyone for coming. Ask people to introduce themselves.

B. Set your rules for the meeting. I have two rules for any meeting about my daughter. First, everyone must tell me one thing they like about her at the beginning of the meeting. Second, my daughter can only be discussed in terms of expanding her abilities and meeting her needs. I discovered that meetings that entail people telling me all the things my daughter cannot do were not very productive. These meetings were emotionally stressful for me and few of these meetings resulted in developing effective strategies to meet needs. For example, I remember being told, "Tiffany cannot button buttons and tie her shoes." The discussion seemed to end there. If I had been told, "Tiffany needs assistance in dressing," we could have discussed what assistance she needed. We could have talked about how we could meet her needs to put her coat on and tie her shoes while we were working on skill building so she could eventually complete these tasks independently.

C. Takes note at the meeting. It is effective to keep a notebook of all the meetings you attend with regard to your family member. If you have trouble taking notes, it is sometimes helpful to bring a tape recorder to the meeting. I would caution, however, that although you have the right to a tape recorder at educational meetings, it sometimes sets up an adversarial environment.

D. Be assertive, not aggressive. Start with the premise that everyone in the room is there with the best of intentions. Be clear, however, that there are issues you are willing to discuss and other issues on which you will stand firm. In my case, I wanted my daughter to attend our local neighborhood school. On this issue, I would not compromise. I would, however, allow her to spend some time in a resource room as long as it was productive time.

E. Take a "time out" if you are upset or angry. You can lose your credibility as an advocate if you lose your temper or become overly upset. It is, however, understandable that this may occur. This is a good time to take a break. Ask your friend to signal you when he/she believes it is time for a break.

F. Do not sign any documents until the next day. Give yourself time to go over your notes. Give yourself time to discuss the meeting and documents with trusted friends and family.

G. At the end of the meeting, confirm your understanding of the resolution of any issues. Confirm your understanding of what tasks need to be accomplished and who will be responsible for the completion of tasks. Set clear time lines.

Step Four is Perhaps the Most Important Advocacy Strategy: Effective Follow-up

A. Confirm all understandings in writing. Be proactive rather than responsive. A short letter outlining your understanding of the meeting is critical. End the letter by requesting that any misunderstanding is to be responded to quickly in writing.

B. If you are responsible for completing a task, make sure you do it within the time lines you established.

C. If a disagreement arises, take it to the next level in the "chain of command." Go as high as you need to go until the issue is resolved. Follow all the rules concerning the next steps in conflict resolution, if necessary.

SYSTEMIC ADVOCACY

> Never doubt that a small group of thoughtful, committed citizens can change the world: Indeed, it's the only thing that ever has."—Margaret Mead

Many people move from advocating for their individual family member to advocating on behalf of many people in similar situations. They may find that in order to meet the needs of their family member, they need to change rules at a level of decision making that will have an impact on a vast number of people. In order to change such rules, they need the support of many people experiencing the same difficulties. Some people are motivated to move to this systemic level of advocacy because they are outraged by the injustice they see in the way that their family member has been treated. They see others being treated the same way. They push for changes that will benefit all.

Today many organizations are involved in systemic advocacy. That is, they are working to change whole bureaucracies. I would caution anyone who becomes involved in this type of advocacy to remain involved in individual advocacy as well. Too often, I have seen people push for a change based on theory rather than respond to the issues of real life. For example, if you want to make changes in the special education system, make sure that you talk to parents of children in special education as well as to special education professionals. If you want to advocate for family support policies in your state, be sure to ask families what they want. If you are a family member, do not rely on your personal experience. Be sure that you have a broad-based knowledge of issues, based on the experience of many families.

Your first involvement in systemic advocacy may be through supporting the work of an advocacy group. Before heading off on your own, you will want to call groups in your state to find out if they are already working on your issue. They may have an advocacy strategy developed and would welcome your involvement. This can give you the opportunity to learn from experienced advocates. Unfortunately, there are far too many issues facing people with disabilities and far too few advocates working on their behalf, so you may find that you will need to take a leadership position.

Systemic advocacy is similar to individual advocacy in that the *first step* is to research your issues thoroughly. It is helpful to define your issue narrowly. It is important that you continually check that the issue does not become so broad that it is unmanageable or unclear to others.

A. Identify clearly the "rules" that are not working. Is it a rule that is not implemented or is it a rule that impedes a person from having his/her needs met? For example, for many children with disabilities, the educational placement option of a regular education classroom with support services is not always discussed at placement meetings. Therefore, a child may be placed in a more restrictive educational setting than is necessary. This is an example of a "rule," in this case a federal law, not being implemented. In some cases, there may be a "rule" missing. In the state of New Jersey, for example, there was no statewide policy driving family support services for families experiencing disability. A group of families and advocacy organizations worked together to pass family support legislation that allowed for a wide variety of family support services, tailored to the individual needs of each family. Find out whether the rule requires a legislative change or a regulatory change. Does the change need to happen at the local, state or national level? There are advocacy organizations in every state that can assist you in your research.

B. Research how change can occur. Many laws have a reauthorization period. At the end of such period there is usually time for public comment on whether a change needs to be made. Some regulations have an annual review period. Again, there is usually a public comment opportunity. Learn the legislative process. Your local League of Women Voters can assist you in learning how law is made in your state. You will be very surprised how simple it can be to have a bill introduced. When a current law is not being implemented, litigation can be instituted on behalf of an individual or many individuals (called a class action). Litigation is a lengthy and sometimes costly process. It should not be entered into without investigating the long-term effects of such an adversarial strategy.

Step two is to organize. Find others who are struggling with the same issue.

A. Problem-solve about what changes you want and what changes you do not want. When working with a group of parents regarding changing the social service system from one of service provider contract to one of consumer choice and control, I discovered that clarifying what we did not want was just as important as what we did want. Decide on what issues you can allow room for compromise and on what issues you will stand firm. Settle your differences behind closed doors. You may need to agree to disagree on certain issues. Continue to work together as long as you agree on the major issue.

B. Develop strategies for change. The following is a partial list of successful strategies: letter-writing campaigns, telephone call-in campaigns, demonstrations, meetings with key decision makers, editorials, finding a "gimmick." Finding a "gimmick" can make your work fun and keep people involved and motivated, as well as catch the eye of potential supporters. When working on family support legislation in New Jersey, we sent hundreds of Mother's Day cards to legislators asking them to "Give Mom the Best Mother's Day Ever, Support Family Support." When a seafood restaurant refused to install a ramp for wheelchair users, a member of one group dressed like a lobster and picketed the restaurant!

C. Identify potential friends and foes. Be as broad-minded as possible. Who will benefit from the change you are about to make other than people with disabilities? In the systemic move from institutionalization to supported living, durable medical goods suppliers may support this change because people leaving institutions may now be able to purchase the technology that will allow them greater independence in the community. Who can be harmed by the change you are about to make? Small business owners who made their living from providing services, such as nearby restaurants and gas stations, to employees of state institutions may oppose the closure of a state institution. Develop a strategy to address the concerns of foes, if possible.

D. Build coalitions. Invite all your potential "friends" to become involved in your change strategy. Remember to keep your issue narrowly and clearly defined. This will allow you to build larger and stronger coalitions. As they say, "politics makes strange bedfellows." I worked with a state teacher's union to oppose changes to special education with potential harm to students on one day, and on another day, I opposed the same teacher's union position on pupil discipline policies.

E. Develop a plan. Define roles of each member of your coalition. Assign tasks and keep time lines. Meet on a regular basis. Refine your plan. Celebrate each and every victory. Support each other during times of struggle.

Whether you are successful or not in making your change, know that you have educated many along the way. Know that you have done your best. Learn the lessons from your successes and your defeats. Change is difficult—the more broad reaching the change, the more difficult it can be to accomplish.

> . . . If there is no struggle, there is no progress. Those who profess to favor freedom, and yet depreciate agitation, are men who want crops without plowing up the ground. They want rain without thunder and lightening. They want the ocean without the awful roar of its many waters. . . .—Frederick Douglass, letter of an abolitionist associate, 1849

In closing, I would like to offer a word of caution. It is easy to be consumed by advocacy activities. As we offer our time and skills to work for positive change, more and more of our time and skills will be requested. We will hear people talk about typical or regular lives and full participation in community life for people with disabilities. We need to heed these words and apply them to ourselves. We need to take time to have a typical life, to leave disability issues behind. We need to be active participants in our communities by being involved in a broad range of activities.

Extra Efforts Needed For Extracurricular Inclusion

Lori Atkins

Many parents who have struggled with school boards or administrations to have their children included in typical classrooms may think that their battle is over. However, if your child is interested in any extracurricular activities—be it cross country or cheerleading—there's still work to be done.

Sally Lane of Greeley, Colorado, would like other parents to learn from her well-publicized campaign to allow her 20-year-old son with Down syndrome to play high school football. Her son, Gabe, had been practicing and conditioning with the high school football team throughout the summer, and was ready, willing, and able to begin the football season this past fall.

A college student who had helped condition Gabe for years of power lifting competition in the Special Olympics volunteered to attend every practice and game, to assist Gabe where needed. This college student, a flexible and progressive coach, and Gabe's extraordinarily supportive teammates helped fuel Gabe's growing enthusiasm for football. As summer training progressed, Gabe demonstrated noticeable improvement in motor and communication skills, cardiovascular health, and self esteem.

However, as football season was about to begin, the school was notified by the state's Athletic and Activities Association that Gabe would not be allowed to participate, owing to a regulation that limited participation to students up to 18 years of age. A one-year waiver could be requested for students who are 19, but an exception for a 20-year-old would not be considered.

The association, which develops regulations for all extracurricular activities and athletics in the state, would not even discuss the regulation, which was originally intended to prevent college-caliber football players from seriously injuring their adolescent teammates and opponents.

Armed with an attorney well-versed in the language of the Americans with Disabilities Act (ADA) and Individuals with Disabilities Education Act (IDEA), the

Down Syndrome: A Promising Future, Together, Edited by Terry J. Hassold and David Patterson
ISBN 0-471-29686-4   Copyright © 1998 by Wiley-Liss, Inc.

Lanes took their case to federal court, their state legislature, and the media. Appearances on every major television network and newspaper and wire stories resulted in overwhelming public support from all over the state. A state senator publicly threatened to dismantle the Activities and Athletics Association, and the Lanes convinced the school to include football in Gabe's IEP (Individualized Education Program).

"When Gabe started his education, special ed was confined to a small trailer behind the school. It took years for him to be able to attend assemblies, and by junior high he was walking in the front door with the other students," Mrs. Lane explained. "Now that Gabe had the teachers, the students, the coaches and his teammates on his side, I certainly was not going to let this association infringe on his right to be included."

Finally, the association agreed to consider the Lanes' request for a waiver, and through a tiresome 4-hour discussion, the Lanes successfully convinced a narrow majority of the 50-member panel that Gabe was not likely to injure other players, nor get injured himself.

This story has a happy ending: Gabe was able to participate in several games through the regular season, the team won the division championship, and the attention helped Gabe make more friends, meet the Denver Broncos, and even get elected homecoming king. However, Mrs. Lane explained that the fight "took over her life." "It got to the point where I couldn't go to work. I was constantly on two telephone calls at once. It consumed all my time and efforts."

What did Gabe have to say about this experience? "I love football. I hate rules." But, through it all, he was confident that things would work out in his favor. "We were right; they were wrong."

Gabe and his family may have paved the way for future students in Colorado to participate in extracurricular activities through their high school years, but parents in every state must be aware of their children's rights and their states' specific regulations.

Mrs. Lane and the National Down Syndrome Society have prepared some tips to help other students continue their activities until graduation, without quite the same fanfare.

If your child is interested in extracurricular activities, and is expected to be in high school beyond the age of 18:

1. As early as possible, include the extracurricular activity in your child's IEP. The benefits to your child's development should be apparent—consider self esteem, motor skills, speech, socialization, muscle tone, communication skills, and cardiovascular health. If the activity is in your child's IEP as early as freshman year, it is less likely to be questioned in later years.
2. Obtain a copy of your state's rules and regulations for public school activities and athletics. In most states, these activities are governed by an independent Association for Athletics and Activities. These regulations should be available through your school's athletic department, or through the state association, and there may be a small charge.

3. Check the regulations for restrictions placed on students' age, or the number of semesters a student is permitted to participate. Look for clauses that explain the process for applying for a waiver, or appealing the association's decision.

4. Find a classmate or friend who will volunteer to help the coach or activity director make any necessary adaptations. Local college students or Special Olympics coaches might be willing to volunteer. By proactively addressing the issue of special accommodations, you are diminishing the most obvious excuse for not including students with special needs in athletics or activities.

5. Begin your request for a waiver or appeals process as early as possible, before the situation becomes a crisis. Discuss the process with your child, and ask how comfortable your child might be with a high level of attention placed on his or her disability. Agree to call off the appeal if at any point your child is uncomfortable with the added attention.

6. Stay positive and keep each setback in perspective. You're likely to run into a few brick walls before you find an open door. If one avenue doesn't work, try another. You may have to appeal to the federal courts, the U.S. Department of Education, the governor, or your state legislature. Try to drum up some public support. Don't be afraid to talk to the media, but think carefully about how to word your statements.

II. Health and Clinical Care

Health Care Guidelines for Individuals with Down Syndrome: Down Syndrome Preventive Medical Checklist

Edited by William I. Cohen for the Down Syndrome Medical Interest Group*

Individuals with Down syndrome (DS) need the usual health care screening procedures provided to everyone. For example, children with DS need the usual immunizations and well child care procedures as recommended by the American Academy of Pediatrics.[†] (Immunization practices are continually evolving: be certain to use the most up-to-date protocols.) Similarly, adults with DS should have health evaluations using the standard accepted practices. However, children with DS have an increased risk of having certain congenital anomalies. Both children and adults may develop certain medical problems that occur in much higher frequency in individuals with DS. Described below is a checklist of additional tests and evaluations recommended for children and adults with DS. These recommendations should take into consideration available local expertise and referral patterns. They are based on our present level

These *Health Guidelines* are published in the journal *Down Syndrome Quarterly* (Vol 1, No 2, June, 1996) and are reprinted with the permission of the Editor. Information concerning publication policy or subscriptions may be obtained by contacting Dr. Samuel J. Thios, Editor, *Down Syndrome Quarterly,* Denison University, Granville OH 43023 (e-mail: Thios@Denison.edu).

*The *Down Syndrome Medical Interest Group* (*DSMIG*) was formed in early 1994, with the express purpose of serving as a forum for individuals addressing aspects of medical care of persons with Down syndrome. Bonnie Patterson M.D. and William I. Cohen M.D. serve as co-chairs. DSMIG wishes to promote the highest quality care for children and adults with DS (1) by fostering and providing professional and community education; (2) by disseminating tools for clinical care and professional support, such as these *Health Care Guidelines;* (3) and by engaging in collaborative clinical research regarding issues related to the care of individuals with Down syndrome. DSMIG schedules its meetings in conjunction with a variety of national organizations, such as the National Down Syndrome Congress (NDSC), the National Down Syndrome Society (NDSS), and the American Association on Mental Retardation. For more information on DSMIG, contact William I. Cohen, M.D., at Children's Hospital of Pittsburgh, 3705 Fifth Avenue, Pittsburgh, PA 15213, 412-692-7963 (e-mail: cohenb@chplink.chp.edu).

[†]American Academy of Pediatrics, *Guidelines for Health Supervision III,* Elk Grove, IL, 1997.

Down Syndrome: A Promising Future, Together, Edited by Terry J. Hassold and David Patterson
ISBN 0-471-29686-4   Copyright © 1998 by Wiley-Liss, Inc.

of knowledge and should be modified as new information becomes available. Modern primary health care includes educational and developmental concerns within its domain, and therefore we have included information and recommendations specific to these needs of individuals with DS.

These recommendations are a thoughtful composite of the input of many experts involved in the care of people with DS. They reflect current standards and practices of health care in the United States of America. They have been designed for a wide audience: for health care professionals who are providing primary care, such as pediatricians, family physicians, internists, and geneticists, as well as specialists, nursing personnel, and other allied health professionals, such as physical and occupational therapists, speech-language pathologists, and audiologists. In addition to educators and early intervention providers, these guidelines are designed for parents and other caregivers to use with the professionals who participate in the care of the individual with DS.

Certain recommendations are clearly supported by current scientific knowledge. This is the case for the recommendations to detect the presence of congenital heart disease, which occurs in some 50% of infants with DS. In other cases, the recommendations represent our educated guesses. Recognizing the increased frequency of thyroid dysfunction in children with DS, we continue to recommend yearly screening for hypothyroidism. However, we are uncertain as the appropriate periodicity and nature of the screening: how often, and what constitutes an adequate screening. Consequently, members of the *DSMIG* will be embarking on a prospective study of thyroid function screening to better be able to answer this question.

Be certain to use the specific DS growth charts in addition to regular charts to record height and weight (for children from birth to 18 years of age), and head circumference (for children birth to 36 months of age). If a child is below the third percentile, or if falling off the expected percentiles, consider congenital heart disease, endocrine disorders (thyroid or pituitary), or nutritional factors.

Immediately following the recommendations by age, you will find explanations for the specific medical recommendations listed below, descriptive information about other areas of interest to individuals interested in the needs of individuals with Down syndrome, and an updated bibliography.

ABOUT THESE HEALTH GUIDELINES (PREVENTIVE MEDICAL CHECKLIST)

These health guidelines continue the series begun in 1981 by Dr. Mary Coleman and published in *Down Syndrome Papers and Abstracts for Professionals* (*DSPAP*), the predecessor of *Down Syndrome Quarterly*. The previous version was prepared in June, 1992 by the members of the Ohio/Western PA Down Syndrome Network and published in *DSPAP* (Volume 15, Number 3, 1992, pages 1–9) and was based on the 1989 version prepared by Dr. Nancy Roizen, University of Chicago.

The preparation of this revision has been a cooperative effort. As editor, I have been particularly fortunate to have the expertise of the several members of Down Syndrome Medical Interest Group (DSMIG).*

---

*Special thanks to the following individuals: Bonnie Patterson M.D. (immunoglobulins); Kim McConnell M.D. (alternative therapies); George Capone M.D. (bibliography); Nancy Lanphear M.D. (atlantoaxial in-

With this edition, we have changed the title of the document to reflect its broader scope. No longer a list of screening procedures, this document has evolved over the last several versions into a comprehensive summary of current recommendations for medical, as well as developmental, social, and family needs for individuals with Down syndrome.

This is one of many such compilations. Please see the References, Section C, for a selected list of other protocols.

A Note about Flow Charts

These Health Guidelines were prepared with the goal of providing both depth and breadth to the topic of health promotion for individuals with Down syndrome. We trust that this will serve as a reference for families, educators, agencies, and, of course, health care providers. Nevertheless, we recognize the ease and simplicity of using a summary of these guidelines in a one-page graphic format. Such a summary can be placed in the front of a family's medical record book, and likewise, in the front of a medical chart for rapid consultation. Several members of DSMIG have developed such forms. In 1989, Dr. Allen Crocker prepared a "Healthwatch for Persons with Down Syndrome," which is reprinted in Dr. W. Carl Cooley's chapter in DC Van Dyke et al. (Eds.), *Medical and Surgical Care for Children with Down Syndrome.* Currently Dr. Cooley (Dartmouth-Hitchcock Medical Center) and Dr. Golder Wilson (University of Texas Southwestern Medical Center at Dallas) are preparing a compilation of similar preventive checklists for a variety of genetic disorders. They have prepared two one-page summaries for *children* with Down syndrome. Please contact Dr. Wilson at 214-648-8996 to obtain copies of this material/for more information. Dr. Brian Chicoine has prepared a variety of material for providing health care to *adults* with Down syndrome. These include history questionnaires, review of systems checklists, physical examination forms, and an assessment/plan form that includes screening information. You can contact him at the Adult Down Syndrome Clinic at Lutheran General Hospital, Park Ridge, Illinois at 847-318-2878 if you wish to obtain this material.

RECOMMENDATIONS BY AGE

Neonatal (Birth to 2 Months)

History. Review parental concerns. Was there a prenatal diagnosis of DS? With vomiting or absence of stools, check for gastrointestinal tract blockage (duodenal web or atresia or Hirschsprung disease); review feeding history to ensure adequate caloric intake. Are there concerns about hearing or vision? Inquire about family support.

Exam. Pay special attention to cardiac examination; check for cataracts (refer immediately to an ophthalmologist if the red reflex is not seen), otitis media, subjective

stability); Marilyn Bull M.D. (growth hormone position statement); Caryl Heaton D.O. (gynecology); Brian Chicoine M.D. (adult health care); Allen Crocker M.D., Golder Wilson M.D., Ph.D., W. Carl Cooley M.D., and Francis Hickey M.D. (flow charts); and Nancy Murray M.S., Robert Pary M.D., and Dennis McGuire Ph.D. (psychiatry/mental health).

assessment of hearing, and fontanelles (widely open posterior fontanelle may signify hypothyroidism).

Lab and Consults. Chromosomal karyotype; genetic counseling; thyroid function test (TSH and T_4): check on results of state-mandated screening; evaluation by a pediatric cardiologist including echocardiogram (even in the *absence* of a murmur); reinforce the need for subacute bacterial endocarditis (SBE) prophylaxis in susceptible children with cardiac disease; refer for auditory brainstem response (ABR) test or other objective assessment of hearing by 6 months of age, if not performed at birth. Refer to vision/ophthalmologic evaluation by 6–12 months of age for screening purposes. Refer immediately if there are any indications of nystagmus, strabismus, or poor vision. If feeding difficulties are noted, consultation with feeding specialist (occupational therapist or lactation nurse) is advised.

Developmental. Discuss early intervention and refer for enrollment in local program. Parents at this stage often ask for predictions of their child's abilities: "Can you tell how severe it is?" This is an opportunity to discuss the unfolding nature of their child's development, the importance of developmental programming, and our expectation of being better able to answer that question at closer to 2 years of age.

Recommendations. Referral to local DS parent group for family support, as indicated.

Infancy (2–12 Months)

History. Review parental concerns. Check for respiratory infections (especially otitis media); for constipation, use aggressive dietary management and consider Hirschsprung disease if resistant to dietary changes and stool softeners. Inquire about parental concerns regarding vision and hearing.

Exam. Perform general neurological, neuromotor, and musculoskeletal examination; visualize tympanic membranes or refer to ear, nose, and throat (ENT) specialist, especially if suspicious of otitis media.

Lab and Consults. Evaluation by a pediatric cardiologist including echocardiogram (if not done in newborn period): it is critical to consider progressive pulmonary hypertension in patients with DS with a ventricular or atrioventricular septal defect who are having few or no symptoms of heart failure in this age group; auditory brainstem response test (ABR) or other objective assessment of hearing by 6 months of age if not performed previously or if previous results are suspicious; pediatric ophthalmology evaluation by 6–12 months of age (earlier if nystagmus, strabismus, or indications of poor vision are present); thyroid function test (TSH and T_4), if not performed previously; evaluation by ENT specialist for recurrent otitis media.

Developmental. Discuss early intervention and refer for enrollment in local program (if not done during the neonatal period). This usually includes physical and occupational therapy evaluations and a developmental assessment.

Recommendations. Application for Supplemental Security Income (SSI) (depending on family income); consider estate planning and custody arrangements; continue family support; continue SBE prophylaxis for children with cardiac defects.

Childhood (1–12 Years)

History. Review parental concerns; current level of functioning; current programming (early intervention, preschool, school). Check for ear problems, sleep problems (snoring or restless sleep may indicate obstructive sleep apnea), constipation. Review audiologic and thyroid function tests; review ophthalmologic and dental care. Monitor for behavior problems.

Exam. General pediatric and neurological exam. Include a brief vulvar exam for girls.

Lab and Consults. Echocardiogram by a pediatric cardiologist if not done previously; thyroid function test (TSH and T_4) yearly; auditory testing (yearly for children 1–3 years old, every two years for children 3–13 years old). Continue regular eye exams every 2 years if normal, or more frequently as indicated. At 3 years and 12 years of age, lateral cervical spine X-rays (neutral view, flexion and extension) to rule out atlantoaxial instability: have radiologist measure the atlanto–dens distance. X-rays should be performed at an institution accustomed to taking and reading these x-rays. Initial dental evaluation at 2 years of age with follow-ups every 6 months.

Developmental. Enrollment in appropriate developmental or educational program; complete educational assessment yearly, as part of Individualized Family Service Plan (IFSP) for children from birth to 3 years of age, or Individualized Educational Plan (IEP) from age four until the end of formal schooling. Evaluation by a speech and language pathologist is strongly recommended to maximize language development and verbal communication. An individual with significant communication deficits may be a candidate for an augmentive communication device.

Recommendations. Twice daily teeth brushing. Total caloric intake should be below recommended daily allowance (RDA) for children of similar height and age. Monitor for well balanced, high fiber diet. Regular exercise and recreational programs should be established early. Continue speech therapy and physical therapy as needed. Continue SBE prophylaxis for children with cardiac defects. Monitor the family's need for respite care, supportive counseling, and behavior management techniques. Reinforce the importance of good self-care skills (grooming, dressing, money handling skills).

Adolescence (12–18 Years)

History. Review interval medical history, questioning specifically about the possibility of obstructive airway disease and sleep apnea; check sensory functioning (vision and hearing); assess for behavioral problems; address sexuality issues.

Exam. General physical and neurological examination (with reference to atlantoaxial dislocation). Monitor for obesity by plotting height for weight. Pelvic exam if sexually active, only. (See Consults, below).

Lab and Consults. Thyroid function testing (TSH and T_4) yearly. Hearing and vision evaluations every other year. Repeat cervical spine X-rays at 12 and 18 years in the asymptomatic individual. Echocardiogram for individuals *without* congenital heart disease once in early adulthood (18–20 years) to evaluate for valvular disease. Consult with adolescent medicine practitioner or a gynecologist experienced in working with individuals with special needs to address issues of sexuality and/or for pelvic examination for sexually active teenager.

Developmental. Repeat psychoeducational evaluations every year as part of Individualized Educational Plan (IEP). Monitor independent functioning. Continue speech/language therapy as needed. Health and sex education, including counseling regarding abuse prevention. Smoking, drug, and alcohol education.

Recommendations. Begin functional transition planning (age 16). Twice yearly dental exams. Consider enrollment for SSI depending on family income. SBE prophylaxis is needed for individuals with cardiac disease. Continue dietary and exercise recommendations (see **Childhood**, above). Update estate planning and custody arrangements. Encourage social and recreational programs with friends. Register for voting and selective service at age 18. Discuss plans for alternative long term living arrangements such as community living arrangements (CLA). Reinforce the importance of good self-care skills (grooming, dressing, money handling skills).

Adults (over 18 Years)

History. Review interval medical history. Ask about sleep apnea symptoms. Monitor for loss of independence in living skills, behavioral changes and/or mental health problems. Symptoms of dementia (decline in function, memory loss, ataxia, seizures, and incontinence of urine and/or stool).

Exam. General physical and neurological examination (with reference to atlantoaxial dislocation). Monitor for obesity by plotting height for weight. Sexually active women will need Pap smears every 1–3 years following the age of first intercourse. For women who are not sexually active, single-finger bimanual examination with finger-directed cytology exam. Screening pelvic ultrasound every 2–3 years for women who refuse or have inadequate follow-up bimanual examinations. This may require referral to a practitioner in adolescent medicine or a gynecologist with experience with individuals with special needs. Otherwise, pelvic ultrasound may be considered in place of pelvic examinations. Breast exam yearly by physician.

Lab and Consults. Annual thyroid screening (TSH and T_4). Ophthalmologic evaluation every 2 years (looking especially for keratoconus and cataracts). Continue auditory testing every 2 years. Repeat cervical spine X-rays once in adulthood in asymptomatic individual. Echocardiogram for individuals *without* congenital heart disease once in early adulthood (18–20 years) to evaluate for valvular disease. There are two different suggestions for mammography: Dr Heaton recommends yearly study after age 50; begin at age 40 for women with a first-degree relative with breast cancer. Dr Chicoine suggests a mammogram every other year beginning at 40, and yearly beginning at 50. Continue twice yearly dental visits. Mental health referral for individuals with emotional and behavioral changes.

Developmental. Continue speech and language therapy, as indicated. For individuals with poor expressive language skills, consider referral for augmentive communication device. Discuss plans for further programming/vocational opportunities at age 21 or when formal schooling ends. Be aware that accelerated aging may affect functional abilities of adults with DS, more so than Alzheimer disease.

Recommendations. Discuss plans for alternative long term living arrangements such as community living arrangements (CLA). SBE prophylaxis is needed for individuals with cardiac disease. Continue dietary and exercise recommendations (see childhood, above). Update estate planning and custody arrangements. Encourage social and recreational programs with friends. Register for voting and selective service at age 18. Reinforce the importance of good self-care skills (grooming, dressing, money handling skills). Bereavement counseling for individuals who have experienced the loss of an important person in their life, either via death or by other circumstances, for example, a sibling moving away after marriage or going off to college.

MEDICAL CONDITIONS AND INTERVENTIONS

An elaboration of the recommendations made above follows, as well as other information designed to promote optimal health care for individuals with Down syndrome.

Cardiac

Congenital heart disease is reported to occur in 30–60% of children with DS. Ventricular septal defects and complete atrioventricular septal defects are among the most common. A serious cardiac defect may be present in the absence of a murmur because of the increased tendency of children with DS to develop early increases in pulmonary vascular resistance which reduces the left to right intracardiac shunt, minimizes the heart murmur, and prevents symptoms of heart failure and respiratory problems. Children with DS with a significant cardiac defect who seem to be doing clinically well or getting better, especially during the first 8 months of life, may be developing serious pulmonary vascular changes. Timely surgery, frequently during the first 6 months of life, may be necessary to prevent serious complications. *Therefore, all infants and children need to have an evaluation by a pediatric cardiologist, preferably before 3 months of age, which should include an echocardiogram.* In some tertiary care centers, an echocardiogram alone is satisfactory if it will be evaluated by a pediatric cardiologist. If this is not available, a full evaluation by a pediatric cardiologist is mandatory. For the older child, who has never had a cardiac evaluation and who has no signs of cardiac disease, a screening echocardiogram is recommended. Adolescents and young adults with no known intracardiac disease can develop valve dysfunction and should be screened at age 18, especially prior to dental or surgical procedures. (See References, Section G, Geggel et al.)

Ear, Nose, and Throat and Audiology

Hearing loss is a significant area of concern for individuals with DS. Infants and children may have a sensorineural loss, a conductive loss (related to middle ear effusions) or both. All infants with DS should have an objective measure of hearing performed within the first 6 months of life. The most common method in widespread use is the measurement of auditory brainstem responses (ABR), also know as brainstem auditory evoked response (BAER). Two screening methods include ABR screening in the newborn nursery, and evoked otoacoustic emission testing. The typical behavioral audiology exam requires a developmental age of 7–8 months. Consequently, all children with DS need an objective measure when tested in the first 12 months. Subsequently, behavioral audiology may be appropriate. Audiologic evaluation for screening purposes should be performed on a yearly basis until three years of age and every other year thereafter.

Most children with DS have very small ear canals, making it difficult to examine them properly with the instruments found in the pediatrician's office. Consequently, it may be necessary to refer the child to an ear, nose, and throat physician to visualize the tympanic membranes using the microscopic otoscope. An ENT physician should evaluate all children with an abnormal hearing evaluation and/or tympanogram in order to aggressively manage treatable causes of hearing loss (using antibiotics and/or tympanostomy tubes as indicated). Fluid can accumulate as early as the neonatal period, and aggressive otologic care can minimize the effect of any hearing loss on language development.

Individuals with Down syndrome may begin to develop hearing loss in their second decade, which, if undetected, may lead to behavioral symptoms that could be misinterpreted as a psychiatric disorder.

Obstructive airway disease has been recognized as a significant problem for children and adults with DS. Symptoms include snoring, unusual sleeping positions (sitting up or bending forward at the waist with head on knees), fatiguability during the day, reappearance of napping in older children or behavior change. Individuals with these symptoms should be evaluated completely via detailed history (looking specifically for evidence of sleep apnea), physical examination with regard to tonsillar size, and prompt referral to an ENT physician for further evaluation (e.g., assessment of adenoidal size). In a number of children, hypotonicity and collapse of the airway leads to similar symptoms in the absence of obstruction caused by lymphoid tissue. Surgical intervention may be necessary to avoid hypoxemia and possible cor pulmonale. Sinusitis, manifested by purulent nasal discharge, occurs commonly and deserves aggressive management.

Infectious Disease/Immunology

Persons with DS who have serious recurrent respiratory and systemic infections are often evaluated for immune function. Consider measuring the IgG subclasses in such individuals. Total IgG level may not disclose any abnormality, although there may be a deficiency of IgG subclasses 2 and 4 and an increase of IgG subclasses 1 and 3. There is a significant correlation between the decreased IgG subclass 4 levels and bacterial infections. The mechanism is not known but theories include the possibility that this subclass plays a role in pulmonary host defense or possibly a deficiency of selenium. Intravenous gamma globulin replacement therapy should be a consideration in a person with DS who presents with serious recurrent bacterial infections and documented IgG subclass 4 deficiency.

The cellular immunity deficits described in individuals with DS have the greatest documented clinical impact on gingivitis and periodontal disease.

Children with chronic cardiac and respiratory disease are candidates for use of pneumococcal and influenza vaccines.

Eye/Vision

Congenital cataracts are a serious problem for infants with DS, leading to vision loss if not detected and treated. The absence of a red reflex is sufficient cause for immediate referral to a pediatric ophthalmologist, as are strabismus and nystagmus. Routine evaluations should begin at 6–12 months of age, and be performed every 1–2 years thereafter. Refractive errors are common and will be detected during these evaluations, as would serious, but rarer, conditions, such as keratoconus. Stenotic nasolacrimal ducts may lead to tearing in infancy. Blepharitis and conjunctivitis occur frequently.

Atlantoaxial Instability

Atlantoaxial instability (AAI) is a term used to describe increased mobility of the cervical spine at the level of the first and second vertebrae. This condition is found in approximately 14% of individuals with Down syndrome. The majority of individuals with AAI are asymptomatic, but approximately 10% of these individuals with AAI (representing 1% of individuals with Down syndrome) have symptoms, which occur when the spinal cord is compressed by the excessive mobility of the two vertebrae that form the atlantoaxial joint. Symptoms of spinal cord compression may include neck pain, unusual posturing of the head and neck (torticollis), change in gait, loss of upper body strength, abnormal neurological reflexes, and change in bowel/bladder functioning.

Routine radiographic screening for AAI of individuals with Down syndrome is controversial. In a recent review, the American Academy of Pediatrics Committee on Sports Medicine and Fitness concluded that screening radiographs are of "potential but unproven value" in detecting individuals at risk from sports injury. Close clinical scrutiny and further study of this issue was recommended. However, these studies continue to be required for participation in Special Olympics and community programs in horseback riding and gymnastics, for example.

Currently, DSMIG recommends screening individuals with lateral cervical radiographs in the neutral, flexed, and extended positions. The space between the posterior segment of the anterior arch of C1 and the anterior segment of the odontoid process of C2 should be measured. Measurements of less than 5 mm are normal; 5–7 mm indicates instability, and greater than 7 mm is grossly abnormal. The cervical canal width should also be measured. The interpretation of these studies should be performed by a radiologist experienced in this area. Individuals with Down syndrome who have not been screened may need to be evaluated prior to surgical procedures, especially those involving manipulation of the neck. These children should be managed cautiously by anesthesiology staff.

Because joint instability may change over time, individuals with normal evaluation should have periodic reevaluation as per the guidelines: 12 years, 18 years, and once in adulthood. Those with an abnormal screen should be reevaluated after 1 year.

Children with borderline findings or abnormal films should be evaluated with a careful neurological examination to rule out spinal cord compression. Neuro-imaging (CT scan or MRI) is probably indicated. Significant changes in a child's neurological status would necessitate evaluation and possible treatment (i.e., spinal fusion). Asymptomatic children with instability (5–7 mm) should be managed conservatively, with restriction only in those activities that pose a risk for cervical spine injury. Contact sports such as football, wrestling, rugby, boxing, and recreational activities such as trampolining, gymnastics (tumbling), and diving, which require significant flexion of the neck, would best be avoided. It is unnecessary to restrict all activities.

Physical/Occupational Therapy

Because infants with DS may have difficulty with feeding from birth, keep in mind that many centers have professionals (such as occupational therapists, speech pathologists, and feeding nurse specialists) who can provide expertise in this area. Some centers involve the occupational therapist or feeding specialist on a routine basis, and others assess the child's oral-motor function and refer as needed. In general, physical and occupational therapy services are included in most early intervention programs for infants, where positioning, feeding, and motor strengthening exercises are some of the services available.

Endocrine

The incidence of thyroid disease is significantly increased among individuals with DS of all ages. Normal thyroid hormone levels are necessary for growth and cognitive functioning. The signs of hypothyroidism may be subtle in individuals with DS and may be attributed to the DS itself. Therefore, screening is recommended on a yearly basis by monitoring TSH and T_4 levels. Because autoimmune conditions are common in individuals with DS, evaluation of suspected hypothyroidism in the school age child should include thyroid antibodies to look for thyroiditis. Some infants and young children have a condition known as idiopathic hyperthyrotropinemia, with borderline abnormal TSH with normal T_4. This may reflect a neuroregulatory defect of TSH, which, when studied by 24 hour sampling, varies between normal levels and very high levels. Therefore, some centers recommend repeating the TSH and T_4 every 6 months, withholding treatment unless the T_4 is low.

There has been some discussion about the use of human growth hormone in children with DS in response to a report that suggested that children with DS have an abnormality of growth hormone secretion. This issue has been addressed by members of the DSMIG and published in *Down Syndrome Quarterly* Volume 1, Number 1 (March, 1996), page 8: "On the basis of the available evidence, and until the recommended scientific studies are completed, the uncontrolled use of hormonal treatments such as growth hormone in children with Down syndrome is not supported by the Down Syndrome Medical Interest Group."

Genetics

A medical genetics consultation should be encouraged, in order to explain the genetic basis and risk of recurrence of DS. Such a consultation may be considered optional for children with Trisomy 21. However, in cases of translocation, the parents should be evaluated to determine whether one of them is a balanced carrier of the translocation, thereby increasing the likelihood that a subsequent children may have Down syndrome. This service should also be made available to individuals with DS, when appropriate.

Developmental, including Speech and Language

Early intervention programs (for infants 0-3 years old) are designed to monitor and enrich development comprehensively, focusing on feeding, gross and fine motor development, language, and personal/social development. Individuals with DS frequently understand spoken language better than they can express themselves verbally. Consequently, infants and children may be taught language using a total communication approach, which includes signing as well as spoken language. Signing permits these children to communicate more effectively at a time when their expressive language abilities may preclude the development of intelligible speech. Speech and language services should be considered throughout life, to maximize intelligibility. Additionally, some individuals may benefit from the use of augmentive (computer-based) communication devices.

Gynecology

Sexually active women should have a cytological screening (Pap smear) every 1–3 years, starting at the age of first intercourse. Those women who are not sexually active should have a single-finger "bimanual" examination with a finger-directed cytological screening every 1–3 years. Screening transabdominal pelvic ultrasound every 2–3 years is recommended for women who have a base-line bimanual examination but refuse to have or have inadequate follow-up bimanual examinations of adnexa and uterus. Yearly mammograms are recommended for women over 50 years of age. Begin yearly mammograms at age 40 for women with a first-degree relative with breast cancer. (Adapted from CJ Heaton, "Providing reproductive health services to persons with Down syndrome and other mental retardation." See References, Section Q, for full reference.)

Neurodevelopmental Issues

The frequency of *seizure disorders* in persons with Down syndrome is greater than that seen in the general population, but lower than in persons with mental retardation owing to other etiologies. Recent studies report an incidence of 5–10%. There appears to be a relationship between age and seizure prevalence in Down syndrome, with the peaks occurring in infancy and again in the fourth or fifth decade. There also appears to be a smaller peak in adolescence. *Infantile spasms* are the most common type of seizures seen in infancy and usually are well controlled with either steroids or other anticonvulsants. They generally have a favorable cognitive outcome, compared with the general population. Tonic–clonic seizures are most commonly seen in older persons with Down syndrome, and they respond well to anticonvulsant therapy in most cases. The increased incidence of seizures is not thought to be solely the result of abnormal brain development, but can be related to cardiac defects, infections, and irregularities of one or more neurotransmitters.

Attention deficit hyperactivity disorder (*ADHD*) occurs in individuals with Down syndrome in the same frequency as it does in the general population of individuals with mental retardation. In both cases, this is more frequent than in the general population. In general, children with Down syndrome respond well to stimulant therapy. There is no research to indicate that children with Down syndrome respond any differently to stimulant medication than children with other etiologies of mental retardation, who respond, in general, very well.

Autistic disorders appear to be more prevalent in children and adults with Down syndrome. Note that this is the case with individuals with mental retardation of other etiologies.

Psychiatric Disorders

Changes in behavior and decline in intellectual and functional capabilities usually leads the caregivers of persons with Down syndrome to consider the possibility of a psychiatric disorder. After excluding any medical reason(s) for the behavior, the individual should be evaluated by a clinician who is skilled in assessing individuals with mental retardation and psychiatric disorders. There are potential limitations in diagnosing psychiatric disorders in persons with Down syndrome. Individuals with moderate or severe mental retardation generally are unable to describe accurately their thoughts and perceptions. Persons with mild mental retardation, however, may be able to respond accurately to questions about feelings, perceptions, and thoughts.

This section focuses on affective disorders, adjustment disorders, dementia (including Alzheimer disease), anxiety disorders, and compulsive behavior. Attention deficit hyperactivity disorder and autistic disorders are discussed in the preceding section.

The presenting symptoms may include one of more of the following: "decreased self-care, loss of skills in activities of daily living, loss of verbal skills, loss of social skills, loss of job skills, withdrawal, slow down in activity level, paranoid features, increase in talking to themselves, aggressive behavior, self-abuse, change in sleep patterns, weight change, and/or persistent forgetfulness." (See Chicoine et al., page 103, in Section B of References.)

The major differential diagnosis is between depressive disorder and Alzheimer disease (dementia).

Dementia is a neuropsychiatric syndrome of memory loss that prevents new information from being learned and is characterized by a decline of intellectual skills that impairs social and/or occupational functioning. Alzheimer disease is a neurological disorder that is a progressive form of dementia having certain characteristic changes in the structure of the brain. It results in a total inability to care for oneself, and, eventually, in death. A careful history must be elicited from caregivers to look for evidence of potentially reversible conditions, such as depression.

The signs of depression in typical individuals usually consist of a sad, irritable mood, along with disturbances of appetite, sleep, and energy, and loss of interest in previously enjoyable activities. Persons with Down syndrome are more likely to present with skill and memory losses, significant activity slowdowns, and hallucinatory-like self-talk and more extreme withdrawal (psychotic features). Persons with Down syndrome often develop depressive disorders in reaction to loss; for example, death of a family member, change in a roommate, or retirement of a caregiver from a group home.

In general, the presentation of most psychiatric disorders tends to be more extreme, making the diagnosis more difficult. For example, an anxiety disorder may be manifested by self-injurious behavior or hyperactivity. Adjustment disorders to stressors may likewise include more severe or dramatic symptoms, such as self injury, reversal of sleep patterns, and anorexia.

Schizophrenia and psychotic disorders occur very infrequently in persons with Down syndrome in spite of the widespread use of anti-psychotic medication.

Self-talk is common and usually developmentally appropriate, given the cognitive levels of these individuals. Although obsessions are rare, compulsive behaviors occur quite commonly.

Treatment is available for most of these disorders, with the exception of Alzheimer disease. This treatment may consist of pharmacological agents, psychotherapy, and/or behavior therapies. It is important to stress that treatment should be under the direction of an individual who is skilled in addressing psychiatric disorders in individuals with mental retardation.

UNCONVENTIONAL AND CONTROVERSIAL ("ALTERNATIVE") THERAPIES

Over the years, a number of controversial treatments or therapies have been proposed for persons with Down syndrome. Sometimes such modalities are referred to as "alternative" therapies, meaning that they are outside the mainstream of traditional medicine. Often the claims made in support of such treatments are similar: that the treatment will result in improved intellectual function, alter physical or facial appearance, decrease infections, and generally improve the well-being of the child with Down syndrome.

Nutritional supplements including vitamins, minerals, amino acids, enzymes, and hormones in various combinations represent one form of therapy. There are a number of well-controlled scientific studies that have failed to show any benefit from megadoses of vitamins and minerals. Supplemental zinc and/or selenium may have an effect on immune function or susceptibility to infection, but studies thus far have been inconclusive. Sicca cell treatment (also called cell therapy) consists of injections of freeze-dried fetal animal cells, and has not been shown to be of any benefit. It also has potential side effects of allergic reactions and the risk of the transmission of slow virus infections.

There has been much interest generated in 1995 in the use of piracetam, a drug that is classified as a cerebral stimulant or nootropic. It has been tried in adults with Alzheimer disease without any benefit. It was shown to improve the reading abilities of typical boys with dyslexia. Piracetam is not approved by the Federal Drug Administration for use in the United States and there have been no scientific studies published reporting its use in children with Down syndrome. DSMIG has expressed concerns about its use in young children in the absence of studies demonstrating its safety. We are currently seeking to devise methods of discovering what value this drug may have. Further information in this area will be published in the "News from DSMIG" section of each issue of *Down Syndrome Quarterly*.

Facilitated communication is a technique whereby a person known as a "facilitator" assists a person by providing support to the hand or arm to enable them to communicate using some type of communication keyboard. Although there are claims of usefulness for persons with many types of disabilities, a number of carefully designed studies have not established this as a valid treatment.

Some parents choose to include chiropractic care in the spectrum of interventions for their children with Down syndrome. The scope of the chiropractic services offered to children includes musculoskeletal manipulations, recommendations for supplemental vitamins, and agents purported to improve immunologic function. The range of conditions claimed to be amenable to chiropractic treatment is broad and includes constipation, gastroesophageal reflux, and ear infections. Individuals with Down syndrome have ligamentous laxity and therefore may be at increased risk of injury from cervical-spinal manipulation. Parents should be very cautious when considering such treatment, especially if it is promoted in lieu of immunizations, antibiotics for infections, or hormone replacement for endocrine deficiency.

The treatments mentioned in this section are only a few of the approaches that have been tried or claimed to pose some benefit to children with Down syndrome. So far, there are no alternative medical therapies that have been scientifically documented to result in a significant improvement in the development and health of children with Down syndrome. Recently, members of DSMIG have received many anecdotal reports of significant and satisfying changes in a wide variety of functional areas (e.g., muscle tone, sleep, general health) following the institution of the use of nutritional supplements. We are carefully evaluating these reports in order to be able to formulate a thoughtful plan to address the questions voiced by the parents of children and adults with Down syndrome about the value of these supplements.

REFERENCES

A. Overview

Barclay A (Ed.) (1995): "Caring for Individuals with Down Syndrome and their Families," Report of the Third Ross Roundtable on Critical Issues in Family Medicine. Columbus, OH: Ross Products Division, Abbott Laboratories.

Cooley WC, Graham JM (1991): Down syndrome—an update and review for the primary care physician. Clin Pediatr 30(4):233–253.

Denholm CJ (ed.) (1991): "Adolescents with Down syndrome: International perspectives on research and program development." Victoria, BC: University of Victoria.

Giesinger C, for the Canadian Down Syndrome Society (no date): Annotated bibliography of journal articles on Down syndrome for parents and primary caregivers. Calgary, AB: CDSS (Telephone 403-270-8500).

Lott, IT, McCoy, EE (1992): Down syndrome: Advances in Medical Care." New York: Wiley-Liss.

Pueschel, SM (1992): The child with Down syndrome. In Levine MD, Carey WB, Crocker, AC (eds.) "Developmental-behavioral Pediatrics," 2nd ed. Philadelphia: WB Saunders.

Pueschel SM, Pueschel JK (1992): "Biomedical Concerns in Persons with Down Syndrome." Baltimore: Paul Brookes.

Rogers PT, Coleman M (1992): "Medical care in Down syndrome." New York: Marcel Dekker.

Van Dyke DC (1989): Medical problems in infants and young children with Down syndrome: Implications for early services. Inf Young Children 1(3):39–50.

B. Adult Health

Chicoine B, McGuire D, Hebein S, Gilly D (1994): Development of a clinic for adults with Down syndrome. Men Retard 32(2):100–106.

C. Other Checklists and Protocols

American Academy of Pediatrics Committee on Genetics (1994): Health Guidelines for Children with Down Syndrome. Pediatrics 93:855–859.

Chicoine B, McGuire D, Hebein S, Gilly D (1994): Development of a clinic for adults with Down syndrome. Men Retard 32(2):100–106.

Pueschel SM, Anneren G, Durlach R, Flores J, Sustrova M, Verma IC (1995): Guidelines for optimal medical care of person with Down Syndrome. International League of Societies for Persons with Mental Handicap (ILSMH). Acta Paediatr 84(7):823–827.

D. Specifically for Families

Kumin L (1994): "Communication Skills for Children with Down Syndrome: A Guide for Parents." Bethesda, MD: Woodbine House.

Van Dyke, DC Mattheis P, Eberly SS, Williams J (eds.) (1995): "Medical and Surgical Care for Children with Down Syndrome: A Guide for Parents." Bethesda: Woodbine House.

E. Anesthesia

DeLeon SY, Ilbawi MN, Egel RT, et al. (1991): Perioperative spinal canal narrowing in patients with Down's syndrome. Ann Thorac Surg 52(6):1325–1328.

Kobel M, Creighton RE, Steward DJ (1982): Anaesthetic considerations in Down's syndrome: Experience with 100 patients and a review of the literature. Can Anaesth Soc J 29:593–599.

Williams JP, Somerville GM, Miner ME, et al. (1987): Atlanto-axial subluxation and trisomy 21: another perioperative complication. Anesthesiology 67:253–254.

F. Audiology

Balkany TJ, Downs MP, Jafek BW, et al. (1979): Hearing loss in Down's syndrome. Clin Pediatr 18(2):116–118.

Buchanan LH (1990): Early onset of presbyacusis in Down syndrome. Scand Audiology 12(2):103–110.

Dahle AJ, McCollister FP (1998): Hearing and otologic disorders in children with Down syndrome. J Ment Def Res 32:333–336.

Diefendorf AO, Bull MJ, Casey-Harvey D, et al. (1995): Down syndrome: a multidisciplinary perspective. J Am Acad Audio 6(1):39–46.

Evenhuis et al. (1992): Hearing loss in middle-age persons with Down syndrome. Am J Ment Retard 97(1):47–56.

Glass RB, Yousefzadeh DK, Roizen NJ (1989): Mastoid abnormalities in Down syndrome. Pediatr Radiol 19(5):311–312.

Roizen NJ, Wolters C, Nicol T, Blondis T (1992): Hearing loss in children with Down syndrome. Pediatr 123:S9–12.

G. Cardiology

Baciewicz FA Jr, Melvin WS, Basilius D, Davis JT (1989): Congenital heart disease in Down's syndrome patients: a decade of surgical experience. Thorac Cardiovasc Surg 37(6):369–371.

Clapp SK, Perry BL, Farooki ZQ, et al. (1987): Surgical and medical results of complete atrioventricular canal surgery: a ten year review. Am J Cardiol 59:454–458.

Geggel RL, et al. (1993): Clinical and laboratory observations: development of valve dysfunction in adolescents and young adults with Down syndrome and no known congenital heart disease. J Pediatr 122(5):821–823.

Goldhaber SZ, Brown WD, St. John Sutton MG (1987): High frequency of mitral valve prolapse and aortic regurgitation among asymptomatic adults with Down's syndrome. JAMA 258:1793–1795.

Marino B, Pueschel SM (1996): "Heart Disease in Persons with Down Syndrome." Baltimore: Paul Brookes.

Martin GR. Rosenbaum KN, Sardegna KM (1989): Prevalence of heart disease in trisomy 21: an unbiased population. Pediatr Res 25:255A. Abstract.

Morris et al. (1992): Down syndrome affects results of surgical corrections of complete atrioventricular canal. Pediatr Cardiol 13(2):80–84.

Pueschel SM, Werner JC (1994): Mitral valve prolapse in persons with Down syndrome. Res Devel Disabilities 15(2):91–97.

Rizzioli E, et al. (1992): Does Down syndrome affect the results of surgically managed atrioventricular canal defects. J Thorac Cardiovasc Surg 104:945–953.

Rosenberg HC, Jung JH, Soltan HC, Li MD, Sheridan G (1994): Cardiac screening of children with Down's syndrome. Can J Cardiol 10(6):675–677.

H. Communication

Chapman RS, et al. (1991): Lanugage skills of children and adolescents with Down syndrome: I. Comprehension. J Speech Hearing Res 34:1106–1120.

Cooper SA, Collacott RA (1995): The effect of age on language in people with Down's syndrome. J Intell Disability Res 39(Part 3):197–200.

Gibbs ED, Springer AS, Cooley WC, et al. (1990): Total communication for children with Down syndrome. Annual Convention, American Speech-Language-Hearing Association, November. Abstract.

Kumin L (1986): A survey of speech and language pathology services for Down syndrome: state of the art. Appl Res Ment Retard 7:491–499.

Kumin L, Councill C, Goodman M (1994): A longitudinal study of the emergence of phonemes in children with Down syndrome. J Commun Disorders 27(4):293–303.

Marcell MM, Ridgeway MM, Sewell DH, Whelan ML (1995): Sentence imitation by adolescents and young adults with Down's syndrome and other intellectual disabilities. J Intellec Disability Res 39(pt 3):215–232.

Miller J (1987): Language and communication characteristics of children with Down syndrome. In Pueschel SM et al. (eds.): "New Perspectives in Down Syndrome." Baltimore, MD: Brookes Publishing.

Mundy P, Kasari C, Sigman M, Ruskin E (1995): Nonverbal communication and early language acquisition in children with Down syndrome and in normally developing children. J Speech Hearing Res 38(1):157–67.

I. Dental

Barnett ML, Press KP, Friedman D, et al. (1986): The prevalence of periodontitis and dental caries in a Down's syndrome population. J Peridontol 57(5):288–293.

Giannoni M, Mazza AM, Botta R, Marci T (1989): Dental problems in Down's syndrome. Overview and specific pathology. Dental Cadmos 57(12):70–80.

Modeer T, Barr M, Dahllof G (1990): Periodontal disease in children with Down's syndrome. Scand J Dental Res 98(3):228–234.

Randell et al. (1992): Preventive dental health practices of non-institutionalized Down syndrome children: a controlled study. J Clin Pediatr Dentistry 16(3):225–229.

Vittek J, Winik S, Winik A, Sioris C, Tarangelo AM, Chou M (1994): Analysis of orthodontic anomalies in mentally retarded developmentally disabled (MRDD) persons. Special Care Dentistry 14(5):198–202.

J. Development

Harris SR (1980): Transdisciplinary therapy model for the infant with Down's syndrome. Phys Ther 60:420–423.

Rogers MJ (1990): Functional management of gross motor development of children with Down syndrome. Dev Med Child Neurol 90:32(suppl 62):44–45.

K. Ear, Nose and Throat

Aboussouan LS, et al. (1993): Hypoplastic trachea in Down's syndrome. Am Rev Resp Dis 147:72–75.

Harley EH, Collings MD (1994): Neurological sequelae secondary to atlantoaxial instability in Down syndrome. Implications in otolaryngologic surgery. Arch Otolaryngol Head Neck Surg 120(2):159–165.

Kraus EM (1996): Down syndrome and the otolaryngologist: clinical characteristics and recommendations for management. In Hotaling AT and Stankiewicz JA, "Pediatric Otolaryngology for the General Otolaryngologist." Igaku-Shoin Medical.

Marcus CL, Keens TG, et al. (1991): Obstructive sleep apnea in children with Down syndrome. Pediatrics 88(1):132–139.

Roizen NJ, Martich V, Ben-Ami T, Shalowitz MU, Yousefzadeh DK (1994): Sclerosis of the mastoid air cells as an indicator of undiagnosed otitis media in children with Down's syndrome. Clin Pediatr 33(7):439–443.

Pappas DG, Flexer C, Shackelford L (1994): Otological and habilitative management of children with Down syndrome. Laryngoscope 104(9):1065–1070.

Southall DP, Stebbins VA, et al. (1987): Upper airway obstruction with hypoxaemia and sleep disruption in Down syndrome. Devel Med Child Neurol 29:734–742.

Stebbins VA, Dennis J, et al. (1991): Sleep related upper airway obstruction in a cohort with Down's syndrome. Arch Dis Childhood 66(11):1333–1338.

L. Education

Brown L, Long E, Udbari-Solner A, et al. (1989): The home school: why students with severe intellectual disabilities must attend the schools of their brothers, sisters, friends, and neighbors. J Assoc Persons Severe Handicaps 14(1):1–7.

Buswell BE, Venerls J (1989): "Building Integration with the IEP." Colorado Springs: PEAK Parent Center, Inc.

McDonnell JJ, Wilcox B, Hardman ML (1991): "Secondary Programs for Students with Developmental Disabilities." Boston: Allyn & Bacon.

Murray-Seegert C (1989): "Nasty Girls, Thugs, and Humans like Us: Social Relations between Severely Disabled and Nondisabled Students in High School." Baltimore: Paul Brookes.

Stainback W, Stainback S (1990): "Support Networks for Inclusive Schooling. Baltimore: Brookes.

Wilcox, B (1991): School restructuring and the re-thinking of "special education." Down Syndrome News (National Down Syndrome Congress) June:65–66.

M. Endocrinology

Cutler AT, Benezra-Obeiter R, Brink SJ (1986): Thyroid function in young children with Down syndrome. Am J Dis Child 140:479–483.

Fort P, Lifshitz F, et al. (1984): Abnormalities of thyroid functions in infants with Down syndrome. J Pediatr 104:545–549.

Mitchell C, Blachford J, Carlyle MJ, Clarson C (1994): Hypthyroidism in patients with Down syndrome. Arch Pediatr Adolescent Med 148(4):441–442.

Pueschel SM (1985): Thyroid dysfunction in Down syndrome. Am J Dis Child 139(6)636–639.

Rubello D, Pozzan GB, Casara D, et al. (1995): Natural course of subclinical hypothyroidism in Down's syndrome: prospective study results and therapeutic considerations. J Endocrinol Invest 18(1):35–40.

Selikowitz M (1993): A five-year longitudinal study of thyroid function in children with Down syndrome. Devel Med Child Neurol 35:396–401.

Stoll C, Alembik Y, Dott B, Finck S (1989): Anomalies in thyroid function in children with trisomy 21. J Genet Hum 37(4–5)389–393.

Zulke C, Thies U, Braulke I, Reis A, Schirren C (1994): Down syndrome and male fertility: PCR-derived fingerprinting, serological and andrological investigations. Clinic Genet 46(4):324–326.

N. Gastrointestinal

Hilhorst, MI, et al. (1993): Down syndrome and coeliac disease: five new cases with a review of the literature. Eur J Pediatr 152:884–887.

Knox GE, Bensel RW (1972): Gastrointestinal malformations in Down's syndrome. Minnesota Med 55:542–544.

Reddy VN, Aughton DJ, DeWitte DB, Harper CE (1994): Down syndrome and omphalocele: an underrecognized association. Pediatrics 93(3):514–515.

O. Genetics and Prenatal Screening

Cheng et al. (1993): A prospective evaluation of a second-trimester screening test for fetal Down syndrome using maternal serum alpha-fetoprotein, hCG, and unconjugated estriol. Obstet Gynecol 81(1):72–77.

Haddow et al. (1992): Prenatal screening for Down's syndrome with use of maternal serum makers. N Engl J Med 327(9):588–593.

Epstein C (ed.) "The Phenotypic Mapping of Down Syndrome and Other Aneuploid Conditions." Proceedings of a National Down Syndrome Conference. New York:Wiley-Liss.

Korenberg JR, Chen XN, Schipper R, et al. (1994): Down syndrome phenotypes: the consequences of chromosomal imbalance. Proc Natl Acad Sci USA 44(6):1039–1045.

Palomaki GE, et al. (1993): Maternal serum screening for fetal Down syndrome in the United States: a 1992 survey. Am J Obstet Gynecol 169(6):1558–1562.

Patterson D, Epstein C (eds.) (1989): "Molecular Genetics of Chromosome 21 and Down Syndrome." Proceedings of the Sixth Annual National Down Syndrome Society Symposium. New York:Wiley-Liss.

Pueschel, S. (1991): Ethical considerations relating to prenatal diagnosis of fetuses with Down syndrome. Ment Retard 29(4):185–190.

Tseng LH, Chuang SM, Lee TY, Ko TM (1994): Recurrent Down's syndrome due to maternal ovarian trisomy 21 mosaicism. Arch Gynecol Obstet 255(4):213–216.

P. Growth

Cronk C, Crocker AC, Pueschel SM, et al. (1988): Growth charts for children with Down syndrome: 1 month to 18 years of age. Pediatrics 81:102–110.

Palmer CG, et al. (1992): Head circumference of children with Down syndrome (0–36 months). Am J Med Genet 42:61–67.

Q. Gynecology

Bovicelli L, Orsini LF, et al. (1982): Reproduction in Down syndrome. Obstet Gynecol 59:135–165.

Edwards JP (1990): Sexuality, marriage, and parenting for persons with Down syndrome. In Pueschel SM (ed.): "The Young Person with Down Syndrome." Baltimore: Paul Brookes, pp. 187–204.

Edwards JP, Elkins TE (1988): "Just Between Us." Portland, OR: Ednick Communications.

Elkins TE (1987): Reproductive health concerns for the person with Down syndrome. J Ped Neurosci 3(1):28–36.

Elkins TE, Gafford S, Muram D (1986): A model clinic for reproductive health concerns of the mentally handicapped. Obstet Gynecol 68(2):185.

Elkins TE, McNeeley DG, Punch M, et al. (1990): Reproductive health concerns in Down syndrome. A report of eight cases. J Reprod Med 35(7):745–750.

Elkins TE, McNeeley DG, Rosen D, et al. (1988): A clinical observation of a program to accomplish pelvic exams in difficult-to-manage patients with mental retardation. Adolescent Pediatr Gynecol 1:195–198.

Evans AI, McKinlay IA (1988): Sexual maturation in girls with severe mental handicap. Child Care, Health Devel 14:59–69.

Goldstein H (1988): Menarche, menstruation, sexual relations and contraception of adolescent females with Down syndrome. Eur J Obstet Reprod Biol 27:343–349.

Heaton CJ (1995): Providing reproductive health services to persons with Down syndrome and other mental retardation. In "Caring for Individuals with Down Syndrome and their Families," Report of the Third Ross Roundtable on Critical Issues in Family Medicine, Columbus, OH: Ross Products Division, Abbott Laboratories.

McNeeley SC, Elkins TE (1989): Gynecologic surgery and surgical morbidity in mentally handicapped women. Obstet Gynecol 74:155.

Rosen DA, Rosen KR, Elkins TE, et al. (1991): Outpatient sedation: an essential addition to gynecologic care for persons with mental retardation. Am J Obstet Gynecol 164(3):825–828.

R. Hematology

Litz Ce, Davies S, Brunning RD, et al. (1995): Acute leukemia and the transient myeloproliferative disorder associated with Down syndrome: morphologic, immunophenotypic and cytogenetic manifestations. Leukemia 9(9):1432–1439.

Ribeiro RC, et al. (1993): Acute megakaryoblastic leukemia in children and adolescents: a retrospective analysis of 24 cases. Leukemia-Lymphoma 10(4–5):299–306.

Robinson LL, Nesbit ME, Sather HN, et al. (1988): Down syndrome and acute leukemia. A 10 year retrospective survey from Children's Cancer Study Group. J Pediatr 81:235–242.

Watson MS, et al. (1993): Trisomy 21 in childhood acute lymphoblastic leukemia: a pediatric oncology group study (8602). Blood 82(10):3098–3102.

Wong KY, Jones MM, Srivastava AK, et al. (1988): Transient myeloproliferative disorder and acute nonlymphoblastic leukemia in Down syndrome. J Pediatr 112:18–22.

S. Immunology

Nespoli L, et al. (1993): Immunological features of Down's syndrome: a review. J Intellec Disability Res 37:543–551.

Ugazio AG, et al. (1990): Immunological features of Down syndrome: a review. Am J Med Genet 7(suppl):204–212.

T. Longevity, Mortality, and Long-term Outcome

Baird PA, Sadovnik AD (1987): Life expectancy in Down syndrome. J Pediatr 110:849–854.

Carr J (1994): Long-term-outcome for people with Down syndrome [review]. J Child Psychol Psychiatr Allied Disciplines 34(3):425–439.

Thase ME (1982): Longevity and mortality in Down's syndrome. J Ment Defic Res 23:177–192.

U. Neurology (See X. Psychiatry, Neurology, and Developmental Biology, below.)

V. Ophthalmology

Caputo AR, Wagner R, Reynolds RD, et al. (1989): Down syndrome: clinical review of ocular features. Clin Pediatr 28:355–358.

Catalano RA, Simon JW (1990): Optic disc elevation in Down's syndrome. Am J Ophthalmol 110:28–32.

Courage ML, Adams, RJ, Reyno S, Kwa PG (1994): Visual acuity in infants and children with Down syndrome. Devel Med Child Neurol 36(7):586–593.

Perez-Carpinelli J, de Fez MD, Climent V (1994): Vision evaluation in people with Down's syndrome. Ophthalmic Physiol Optics 14(2):115–121.

Roizen NJ, Mets MB, Blondis TA (1994): Ophthalmic disorders in children with Down syndrome. Develop Med Child Neurol 36(7):594–600.

Shapiro MB, France TD (1985): The ocular features of Down syndrome. Am J Ophthalmol 99:659–663.

Wagner RS, Caputo AR, Reynolds RD (1990): Nystagmus in Down's syndrome. Ophthalmol 97(11):1439–1444.

W. Orthopedics

American Academy of Pediatrics Committee on Sports Medicine and Fitness (1995): Atlantoaxial instability in Down syndrome: subject review. Pediatrics 96(1 pt 1):151–154.

Davidson, RG (1988): Atlantoaxial instability in individuals with Down syndrome: a fresh look at the evidence. Pediatrics 81(6):857–865.

Diamond LS, Lynne D, Sigman B (1981): Orthopedic disorders in patients with Down syndrome. Ortho Clinics NA 12:57–71.

Mendez AA, Keret D, MacEwen GD (1988): Treatment of patellofemoral instability in Down's syndrome. Clin Ortho Related Res (234):148–158.

Morton RE, Khan MA, Murray-Leslie C, Elliott S (1995): Atlantoaxial instability in Down's syndrome: a five year follow-up study. Arch Dis Childhood 72(2):115–118; discussion 118–119.

Msall ME, Reese ME, et al. (1990): Symptomatic atlantoaxial instability associated with medical and rehabilitative procedures in children with Down syndrome. Pediatrics 85(3 pt 2):447–449.

National Down Syndrome Congress (1991): Atlanto-axial instability in persons with Down syndrome: guidelines for screening. Down Syndrome News June:61.

Parfenchuck TA, Betrand SL, Powers MJ, Drvaric DM, Pueschel SM, Roberts JM (1994): Posterior occipitoatlantal hypermobility in Down syndrome: an analysis of 199 patients. J Pediatr Orthopedics 14(3):304–308.

Pueschel SM, Scola FH (1987): Atlanto-axial instability in individuals with Down syndrome; epidemiologic, radiographic, and clinical studies. Pediatrics 80:555–560.

Pueschel SM, et al. (1990): Skeletal anomalies of the upper cervical spine in children with Down syndrome. J Pediatr Orthopaedics 10:607–611.

Pueschel SM, Scola FH, Pezzullo, JC (1992): A longitudinal study of atlanto-dens relationships in asymptomatic individuals with Down syndrome. Pediatrics 89(6):1194–1198.

White KS, et al. (1993): Evaluation of the craniocervical junction in Down syndrome: correlation of measurements obtained with radiography and MR imaging. Radiology 186:377–382.

X. Psychiatry, Neurology, and Developmental Biology

Brugge KL, et al. (1994): Cognitive impairment in adults with Down syndrome. Neurology 44:232–238.

Cooper SA, et al. (1993): Mania and Down syndrome. Br J Psychiatr 162:739–743.

Cooper SA, Collacott RA (1994): Clinical features and diagnostic criteria of depression in Down's syndrome. Br J Psychiatr 165(3):399–403.

Craddock N, Owen M (1994): Is there an inverse relationship between Down's syndrome and bipolar affective disorder? Literature review and genetic implications. J Intell Disability Res 38(pt 6):613–620.

Cuskelly M, et al. (19920: Behavioral problems in children with Down's syndrome and their siblings. J Child Psychol Psychiatr 33(4):749–761.

Dalton AJ, Crapper-McLachlan DR (1986): Clinical expression of Alzheimer's disease in Down syndrome. Psychiatr Clin North Am 9:659–70.

Evenhuis HM (1990): The natural history of dementia in Down syndrome. Arch Neurol 47:263–267.

Franceschi M, Comola M, Piattoni F, Gualandri W, Canal N (1990): Prevalence of dementia in adults patients with trisomy 21. Am J Med Genetics- Supplement 7:306–308.

Ghaziuddin M, et al. (1992): Autism in Down's syndrome: presentation and diagnosis. J Intellec Disability Res 36:449–456.

Haveman MJ, Maaskant MA, et al. (1994): Mental health problems in elderly people with and without Down's syndrome. J Intellec Disability Res 38(pt 3):341–355.

Howlin P, Wing L, Gould J (1995): The recognition of autism in children with Down syndrome—implications for intervention and some speculations about pathology. Devel Med Child Neurol 37(5):406–414.

Kesslak JP, Nagat SF, Lott I, Nalcioglu O (1994): Magnetic resonance imaging analysis of age-related changes in the brains of individuals with Down's syndrome. Neurology 14(3):304–308.

Lai F, Williams RS (1989): A prospective study of Alzheimer disease in Down syndrome. Arch Neurol 46(8):849–53.

Lund J, Munk-Jorgenson P (1988): Psychiatric aspects of Down syndrome. Acta Psychiatr Scand 78:369–374.

Myers BA, Pueschel SM (1991): Psychiatric disorders in persons with Down syndrome. J Nerv Ment Dis 179(10):609–613.

Nadel L, Epstein C (eds.) (1992): "Down Syndrome and Alzheimer Disease." New York: Wiley-Liss.

Nelson L, Lott I, Touchette P, Satz P, D'Elia L (1995): Detection of Alzheimer disease in individuals with Down syndrome. Am J Ment Retard 99(6):616–622.

Pueschel SM, Louis S, McKnight P (1991): Seizure disorders in Down syndrome. Arch Neurol 48(3):318–320.

Stafstron CE, Konkol RJ (1994): Infantile spasms in children with Down syndrome. Develop Med Child Neurol 36(7):576–585.

Strafstrom CE, Patxot OF, et al. (1991): Seizures in children with Down syndrome; etiology, characteristics, and outcome. Devel Med Child Neurol 33:191–200.

Stafstrom CE, et al. (1993): Epilepsy in Down syndrome: clinical aspects and possible mechanisms. Am J Ment Retard (suppl):12–26.

Wiesniewski KE, Miezejeski CM, Hill AL (1988): Neurological and psychological status of individuals with Down syndrome. In Nadel L (ed.): "Psychobiology of Down Syndrome." Cambridge: MIT Press, pp. 315–343.

What New Parents Need To Know:
Informing Families About Their Babies With Down Syndrome

Phillip Mattheis

Most babies with Down syndrome are born to families with no foreknowledge of their differences. Although the risk of trisomy is clearly elevated with advancing maternal age, most mothers of children with Down syndrome are well under 35 years of age at the time of the child's birth. Many or most have had little exposure to information about Down syndrome, and have not known anyone with the condition. Consequently there is often a need for new families to absorb a great deal of new information in the midst of a situation loaded with unexpected stresses.

Frequently, the information about the diagnosis is delivered in an atmosphere of shock; grieving for the lost "normal" child is often part of the process. Ideally, the surrounding professionals carry positive attitudes and accurate information to the child and family, in a setting that is physically and emotionally supportive. When the ideal is not realized, a sense of "gloom and doom" may pervade the nursery and intrude on the family's ability to adapt to their new reality.

THE INFORMING INTERVIEW

Receiving a new diagnosis of Down syndrome (or any one of many other life-affecting conditions) about a new baby is essentially a medical emergency for that child and family, and should get the same careful attention to detail given other emergencies.

Attempts have been made to define the optimal informing interview setting and sequence via surveys of families and professionals (Sharp et al., Cunningham et al., Buckman, Klein). A private setting early in the process, with both parents present, is the ideal. The informing professional should be knowledgeable, and ideally will already have a relationship with the family. When possible, the baby should be present to help focus attention on the child rather than upon the diagnosis. If physical features

Down Syndrome: A Promising Future, Together, Edited by Terry J. Hassold and David Patterson
ISBN 0-471-29686-4   Copyright © 1998 by Wiley-Liss, Inc.

are mentioned, their presence in the child should be demonstrated to avoid confusion and allow for questions. Referral to another family with a similar child should be one of the goals of the interview, for it is one of the features most often identified by families as part of a successful experience. Early access to family support networks has also been shown to be an important variable in achieving good long-term outcomes (Patterson and Blum, Santellini et al.).

The content of the interview should aim at addressing the variety of questions families bring with them, and should speak to their individual experiences and specific problems. Many parental concerns initially focus upon the specific medical complications in their child, but move on inevitably to consider potential long-term outcomes. Care should be taken to avoid saying "too much"; information overload is easily and often reached in the midst of emotion. Quiet pauses that allow reflection can help parents to find the words for their concerns. In the midst of the questions and answers, an essential goal should be to keep the baby in clear view.

All the players, including the professionals and the parents with their networks of extended family, friends, and acquaintances, carry attitudes and biases about people with disabling conditions. Information given must be accurate and must recognize those biases and opinions if the interview is to assist the family in their adjustments to the new reality of their child's diagnosis.

THE BABY WITH DOWN SYNDROME IS A BABY FIRST

For most families, and certainly for those delivering their first child, the most significant changes to their lives build from the presence of a new family member. Down syndrome as a diagnosis is an additional piece, but often not the most important one, among the many changes that accompany that child's birth. Not uncommonly, the family may be so overwhelmed by unexpected and unanswered questions that they may not be able to celebrate the birth of their child. A supportive and positive hospital and clinical environment can be essential as a base from which the family can begin to adapt.

THE CHILD WITH DOWN SYNDROME IS A CHILD FIRST

Similarly, children's lives are described by a series of childhood issues. To focus too much on the diagnosis risks setting artificial limits that become their own realities.

Children with Down syndrome are motivated by the same drives for friendship and growth as their "typical" peers and thrive in normal environments that recognize and assist with specific needs of every child.

CHILDREN WITH DOWN SYNDROME HAVE BROTHERS AND SISTERS

When siblings are joined by a new baby with a condition such as Down syndrome, the older children may sometimes become lost in the flurry of activity or may be neglected as the family attempts to cope with change. Early recognition of the needs of all family members as adjustments evolve is essential to limit the stresses upon individuals. A study of school-age siblings of children with disabilities found them as a group at risk for increased anxiety, and likely to spend less time with friends (Colbey,

1995). Increased use of respite care was recommended by the author as one way to decrease some of the risks.

A number of communities have developed sibling support groups to provide respite and common companionship. Many of the programs that work best simply treat the siblings as individuals with much in common, and downplay the conditions of the affected children.

Similarly, parents may find that their own roles and emotional needs shift as the adjustments occur. Active attention to each other's needs may be required to gain or keep stability.

CHILDREN WITH DOWN SYNDROME HAVE ABILITIES

This point may often be lost, for discussions with professionals tend to focus upon "disabilities," "defects," and "deficits." Most children with Down syndrome are social beings, and respond well to attention that plays to their strengths. Children with limited expressive language, for instance, are often very good at finding nonverbal ways to make their needs known. When those skills are recognized, communication happens. If the attempts are misread, frustration is a likely consequence, and behavior problems may follow.

CHILDREN WITH DOWN SYNDROME MAKE DEVELOPMENTAL PROGRESS

However, they do so at their own pace. Many families are uncertain about realistic expectations, and may focus unnecessarily upon milestone achievements. Down syndrome is not a condition that *prevents* development, but the rates and routes of development are often different from "typical." Children with Down syndrome should all learn to walk and to talk; they should have friendships, and most can learn to lead lives of some independence. They may require more help along the way, but at various times, so do we all.

DOWN SYNDROME IS NO ONE'S "FAULT"

"Why us?" is a common question with no real answer. But there is no good evidence that anything a parent did or didn't do "caused" the Down syndrome to occur. In a small number of cases the child inherits the condition from a parent who is a "normal" carrier. Most of the time the extra bits of chromosome appear for no known reason at all. A discussion of karyotypes and chromosomes may be useful, if only to give the family a basic grasp of the genetic mechanism and some images that might reduce some of the mystery.

Families of people with Down syndrome begin just like any other family; each is "special" in its own uniqueness. Those of us with relatives with Down syndrome are no more special or unique than others, at least in the beginning. Sometimes the presence of a disability in a family member can prompt significant shifts in perspective and expectations about children, life goals, and priorities. A new understanding of the definition and importance of normal" can help to shape those new perspectives and expectations and may bring increased tolerance and sensitivity to the differences in all of us.

BABIES WITH DOWN SYNDROME BELONG IN FAMILIES, NOT INSTITUTIONS

Only a generation ago, common advice to new families suggested that they consider placing their child in an institution. Occasionally that advice is still given, but the reality is that there are very few institutions in the United States that care for babies with disabilities. Many of the large state-run hospitals that used to fill this role have been shut down in the past 10–20 years. Those that remain are unlikely to care for babies.

The current equivalent to institutional placement might be the increasing number of adoptive homes that accept multiple individuals with Down syndrome and other disabilities. Although many remain family-focused, some have become so large that the resemblance to a family is lost, and the level of care begins to suggest the abandoned institutional model. In some homes, subsidies for the adoptions may total into many thousands of dollars, bringing into question the motivations of the operators.

FOSTER CARE AND ADOPTIVE HOMES ARE THE CHOICES FOR FAMILIES UNABLE TO CARE FOR NEW BABIES

For whatever reason, some families may be unable to take their child home with them. In the short term, most hospitals or social service agencies are able to arrange for foster care, in the home of a family screened for their ability to provide a safe and caring environment. The child can remain in the foster setting until the natural parents are able to assume care. If the decision is made to place the baby for adoption, the child usually stays in the same foster home until the adoptive family is found and the details of the placement are finalized.

Adoptive families for babies with Down syndrome are not hard to find. One agency that specializes in the placement of babies with Down syndrome, The Down Syndrome Adoption Exchange (of White Plains, New York), has been around for more than 10 years, and through much of that time has had a waiting list of families interested in such adoptions. Many or most babies can actually be placed locally, but agencies like the one mentioned are available when local options are not working.

Whatever their eventual decision, families that find themselves seriously considering placing their child may become very troubled by uncomfortable perceptions of themselves as parents. Sensitive counseling may be needed, to help with both the decision and the repercussions.

PARENTS OF CHILDREN WITH DOWN SYNDROME MUST BECOME EDUCATED CONSUMERS

As the child grows and faces a sequence of challenges, the family may work with a variety of professionals from several systems of services. Parents (and children) become expert at identifying bias and often have extensive experience to guide their judgment of current standards of care. Family networks represent a great deal of accumulated experience, with the behavior, attitude, and expertise of professionals as common topics of discussion. Parent support networks are very useful as resources for whom and what to avoid as families look into options to meet emerging needs.

No two children have the same sets of abilities and disabilities; most families differ in their needs for supportive services. The array of services available within any given community is frequently a shifting patchwork; few caseworkers or medical personnel can keep up with the changes and combinations as well as an active group of parent advocates.

Family-centered care models work best when they recognize the primary role of the family in prioritizing problems and services for young children with disabilities. The family-as-consumer is empowered by such models to review available services and providers critically in order to find the mix most likely to be beneficial (Hostler, 1991; McGonigal and Garland, 1988).

BABIES WITH DOWN SYNDROME HAVE INDIVIDUAL MEDICAL HISTORIES

Many medical conditions and incidental findings are more common in Down syndrome. Some require treatment and are so common as to require active search; others are of little relevance even if they appear. Putting balance to this discussion may be an important part to the informing interview and the sequence of interviews that follow with the child's growth. However, there is a high risk of information overload during these first visits. Comprehension and retention of information may be limited by the emotional stress of adapting to new realities. Discussion should focus on topics of immediate relevance to the child's health, while reserving topics of more distant potential for later opportunities.

In the immediate postnatal period, newborn care for babies with Down syndrome begins with standard nursery routine. Most potential problems reveal themselves through clinical signs or symptoms. Only a few important conditions are common enough to justify screening.

CARDIAC DEFECTS ARE COMMON AND SIGNIFICANT IN BABIES WITH DOWN SYNDROME

About 50% of people with Down syndrome have some defect of cardiac anatomy, and about half of those will require surgery. Families of new babies with Down syndrome will eventually become aware of these risks, and will want to have answers about their own baby's cardiac status. Many of those needing surgery do best if the procedure occurs at an early age (Tweddell et al., 1996), so early identification of problems is important.

In an unknown number, significant cardiac conditions can be present without clear clinical evidence. Absence of a murmur and a normal chest X-ray may not rule out defects, and present good health may not mean an undiagnosed condition is insignificant.

The high risk and incomplete clinical expression of cardiac conditions result in the need for careful investigation for occult problems in all individuals with Down syndrome. An echocardiogram is essential for reviewing anatomy, and is also a key part of following identified disease. Review by a cardiologist experienced in congenital defects is preferred when available. The exact timing of those investigations may vary depending upon availability of equipment or personnel; the degree of clinical suspicion and parental concern may also influence the schedule.

Children with Down syndrome and congenital cardiac conditions appear to be more prone to early development of pulmonary hypertension than "typical" peers, and require an elevated level of concern in the pre-repair stages of monitoring.

GASTROINTESTINAL PROBLEMS CAN OCCUR MORE FREQUENTLY IN BABIES WITH DOWN SYNDROME

Duodenal atresia is more common in newborns with DS, and it becomes obvious quickly as feeding fails. Other gastrointestinal problems may occur more often in the syndrome, and may be more difficult to identify, but these conditions are still rare and do not require any routine screening. Feeding problems related to low muscle tone are common in the first days and weeks after birth, but most infants with Down syndrome become successful oral feeders. Breast feeding may be more difficult, but is achieved by many families. Active supportive advice and demonstration by experienced nursery personnel may be pivotal in assisting early feeding success.

HEMATOLOGIC ABNORMALITIES MAY PRESENT AT BIRTH

The incidence of hematologic abnormalities is increased in babies with Down syndrome, but may not justify routine screening. If abnormalities are seen on routine testing, further evaluation can follow. Transient leukemia is a well-known occasional finding in babies with Down syndrome, and may be accompanied by other serum differences. Polycythemia or thrombocytopenia may occur independently of leukemia or other serious conditions and usually resolve without residual trouble.

The prospect of leukemia in a baby is understandably frightening to new families. Unless relevant, the topic can probably wait for later conversations. When the subject is discussed, emphasis should be placed on the high cure rate seen in most protocols for treatment of leukemia in Down syndrome (Lie et al., 1996)

SENSORY DEFICITS MAY APPEAR EARLY

Congenital cataracts are seen more frequently in Down syndrome, but may often be small and not require early action. Standard newborn care given to all babies should detect larger cataracts.

Hearing abnormalities are also more frequently found in children with Down syndrome. Hearing screening of newborns can identify congenital problems, and provides a base line for comparison if later problems are detected.

OTHER MEDICAL DISCUSSION CAN WAIT

The list of medical abnormalities and differences that can be associated with Down syndrome is long and complicated. Most individuals have some differences to their medical history, but none have all or even most of the possibilities on the list. The trick is to be aware of those possibilities without overstating the risks or creating unnecessary worries.

Part of a well-designed plan of anticipatory health care is an appropriate schedule of screening tests and questions that address those possibilities. The Health Guidelines of the Down Syndrome Medical Interest Group (Cohen, 1996) is one version of such a schedule. This evolving set of recommendations can serve as a good model for long-term health management by the local physician. There is also a growing variety of books that deal with medical issues in Down syndrome, targeting both parents and health providers (Pueschel and Pueschel, 1992; Rogers and Coleman, 1992; Vandyke et al., 1995).

Family and consumer education about health risks in Down syndrome is an ongoing process that adapts and adjusts to the changing needs of the individual and his/her family within their community. Development of a wide-ranging network of resources is an essential and normal part of every family's development, and no less important when a family member has a disability. The range of problems and necessary resources may increase substantially with many conditions that are potentially disabling.

ALTERNATIVE THERAPIES AND THEORIES ARE COMMON AND ATTRACTIVE

Disabling conditions in children drive families to search for solutions that will minimize the degree of disability. In many cases, "standard" solutions fall short. When there are no conventional answers for problems that demand attention, alternative or unconventional ideas may be explored.

Sometimes "standard" therapies have evolved from less accepted treatments by proving their worth over time. Much more often, alternative therapies prove to have no real value, and may represent additional risk, expense, or trouble for the family and child. Sorting out the balance of risks and possible benefits can be a very difficult and stressful occupation for families with limited amounts of energy, time, and financial resources.

A comfortable relationship with a professional who is able to help review objectively all available choices can be an invaluable help to the family trying to sort the many choices of standard and alternative approaches.

SUMMARY

Babies with Down syndrome may have one or more of many possible medical conditions, but they are babies first. New parents need to have accurate information, and they gain benefit from supporting networks of friends, family, and professionals who can help them to come to terms with the unexpected.

The first news of the diagnosis must be presented with care, and with both parents present whenever possible. The baby, not the diagnosis, should be the center of the discussion. Time and access must be made available for questions, with the certainty that many questions will emerge over the days and weeks that follow.

The specific medical problems likely to appear in the newborn period are limited, and fairly easy to identify. Most of the discussions about possible problems can wait until the family members have begun to adjust to their new realities, and are ready to plan for the future.

REFERENCES

Buckman, R (1992): Breaking bad news: A six-step protocol. In "How to Break Bad News: A Guide for Health Care Professionals." Baltimore, MD: Johns Hopkins Press, pp. 65–97.

Cohen, WI (1996): Health care guidelines for individuals with down syndrome. Down Syndrome Quart 1(2):1–10.

Colbey, M (1995): The school-aged siblings of children with disabilities. Dev Med Child Neurol 37(5):415–426.

Cunningham CC, Morgan PA, McGucken RB (1984): Down's syndrome: is dissatisfaction with disclosure of diagnosis inevitable? Dev Med Child Neurol 26(1):33–39.

Hostler SL (1991): Family-centered care. Pediatr Clin North Am 38:1545–1560.

Klein SD (1994): The challenge of communication with parents. In Darling RB, Peter MI (eds.): "Families, Physicians and Children with Special Health Needs: Collaborative Medical Education Models." Westport, CT: Auburn House, pp. 51–74.

Lie SO, Jonmundsson G, Mellander L, Siimes MA, Yssing M, Gustafsson G (1996): A population based study of 272 children with acute myeloid leukemia treated on two consecutive protocols with different intensity. Br J Haematol 94(1):82–88.

McGonigal M, Garland C (1988): The individualized family service plan and the early intervention team: Team and family issues and recommended practices. Infants Young Child 1:10–21.

Patterson J and Blum RW (1996): Risk and resilience among children and youth with disabilities. Arch Pediatr Adolesc Med 150:692–698.

Pueschel SM, Pueschel JK (1992): "Biomedical Concerns in Persons with Down Syndrome." Baltimore, MD: Paul H. Brookes.

Rogers PT, Coleman M (1992): "Medical Care in Down Syndrome." New York: Marcel Dekker.

Santellini B, Turnbull A, Lemur E, Marquis J (1993): Parent-to-parent programs. In "Coping Skills and Strategies for Family Interventions." Baltimore, MD: Paul H. Brookes, pp. 27–57.

Sharp MC, Straus RP, Lorch SC (1992): Communicating medical bad news: parent's experiences and preferences. J Pediatr 121(4):539–546.

Tweddell, JS, Litwin SB, Berger S, et al. (1996): Twenty-year experience with repair of complete atrioventricular septal defects. Ann Thor Surg 62(2):419–424.

Vandyke DC, Mattheis, PJ, Eberly SS, Williams, J (1995): "Medical and Surgical Care for Children with Down Syndrome." Bethesda, MD: Woodbine House.

Neurodevelopmental Disorders in Down Syndrome

William I. Cohen and Bonnie Patterson

One of the questions most frequently asked by parents of children with Down syndrome is if their child's behavior problems are caused by Down syndrome. It is often stated that pediatricians are always looking for one explanation for the problem at hand. Possibly the underlying simplicity of childhood health conditions make such a statement believable, when compared to the multisystem problems of adults who often have intercurrent illnesses galore. The fact that Down syndrome represents a chronic disorder that by nature is pervasive lends itself to the attribution of all ills to that extra chromosome 21.

This article will describes neurodevelopmental conditions that can occur in children with Down syndrome as well as the general population. We would like to provide physicians and parents with a way to make sense of their concerns regarding seizures, autism, and attention deficit hyperactivity disorder (ADHD).

EPILEPSY

The frequency of seizure disorders in persons with Down syndrome is greater than that seen in the general population, but lower than in persons with mental retardation due to other etiologies (20–50%). Recent studies report an incidence in Down syndrome of 5–10%.

A study by Stafstrom et al. in 1991 looked at a group of 737 children with Down syndrome and 47 (6.4%) had a history of seizures. Etiology of the seizures was known in 29 of the cases and included hypoxia secondary to cardiovascular disease, perinatal complications, infections, and trauma. In 18 of the cases the etiology for the seizure disorder was unknown. The age of onset of seizures in the cases with known etiology followed a bimodal distribution, with most occurring either prior to 3 years of age or after 13 years of age. Generalized tonic–clonic seizures occurred most often (>60%) and infantile spasms were seen in 13%. Febrile seizures were uncommon in

Down Syndrome: A Promising Future, Together, Edited by Terry J. Hassold and David Patterson
ISBN 0-471-29686-4 Copyright © 1998 by Wiley-Liss, Inc.

this population. Electroencephalographic (EEG) findings did not distinguish between seizures of known and unknown etiologies, but were useful in classification of seizures and following the clinical course. There are no characteristic EEG changes seen in individuals with Down syndrome and most have a normal EEG or nonspecific background slowing. Choice of anticonvulsant therapy was made by seizure type and patient tolerance. Most patients responded to single anticonvulsant therapy. Therapeutic serum levels and spectrum of side effects were similar to those seen in the general population.

Pueschel et al. in 1991 studied 405 individuals with Down syndrome ages 6 months to 45 years. Eight percent developed seizures and 40% occurred prior to 1 year of age. In this age group the most common seizure types were infantile spasms and tonic–clonic seizures with myoclonus. Another 40% of the seizures occurred in the third decade of life and were generally tonic-clonic or partial complex seizures. Seizure control was excellent in the younger age group and slightly less adequate in the older age group.

In 1994 Stafstrom and Konkel evaluated 17 children with Down syndrome and infantile spasms. They found that the developmental outcome was poorest in those with superimposed hypoxic insults and those who had an initial history of regression. Overall the prognosis was better than that seen in the general population. In a followup of 16 surviving patients 13 were seizure free for more than 1 year and only three had persistent seizures, but only one had an intractable seizure disorder.

The mechanism of increased seizure activity in Down syndrome is not known but may be related to some of the following factors:

1. Structural aspects including decreased brain weight, decreased neuronal packing density in the neocortex and hippocampus, malformed dendrite spines, and decreased number of dendrites.
2. Intrinsic neuronal membrane properties predisposing to hyperexcitability.
3. Neurotransmitter and neurochemical abnormalities.
4. Hypoxia, infections, and cardiovascular disease.

It is always important when evaluating a person with Down syndrome who develops seizures to search for an etiology and not just attribute the seizure to the fact that the person has Down syndrome. Recommended evaluations for a person presenting with a first seizure includes an EEG, neuro-imaging, cardiac evaluation, and search for infection.

AUTISM IN DOWN SYNDROME

In recent years, there has been an increasing awareness of the psychiatric and mental health needs of all persons with developmental disabilities. Whereas in the past, maladaptive behaviors were considered to be the result of the underlying cognitive deficits, it is now recognized that behavioral aberrations can be symptoms of neurological or psychiatric disorders. Individuals with Down syndrome represent one group in whom such changes in diagnosis are occurring. Children with Down syndrome can present with variable personality and temperament traits. There are an increasing number of reports of children with Down syndrome and pervasive developmental disorders/autism.

Autism is defined as a chronic and debilitating neurodevelopmental disorder related to central nervous system dysfunction, and is pervasive in the scope of developmental functions affected. It encompasses disorders of language, cognition, perception, and ability to relate socially. It is characterized by unusual responses to sensory stimuli, deviant attachment, disturbances of motility, and frequently self-stimulatory and self-injurious behaviors. Emotional responsiveness is often lacking or is inappropriate, and affected children may demonstrate an insistence on preservation of "sameness." Most children with autism test in the mental retardation range with regard to cognitive and adaptive abilities. The recently reported incidence of autism has increased to 13 in 10,000 population with a male to female predominance of 3 or 4 to 1. It occurs with similar frequency among various ethnic, racial, and socioeconomic groups. The etiology of autism is unknown, but there have been reports of a high incidence of autism in children with phenylketonuria, congenital rubella, and fragile X syndrome.

Recent reports by Ghaziuddin et al. (1992) and Howlin et al. (1995) describe a total of seven children with the dual diagnosis of Down syndrome and autism. No etiologic studies of the prevalence of autism spectrum disorders in a large population of children with Down syndrome have been done, but current evidence suggests it is in the region of 5–10%. The incidence for autism in a group of children with IQ's below 50 who did not have Down syndrome was 16% for Kanner's autism and 57% with other autistic spectrum disorders. On the basis of those figures, children with Down syndrome appear to have a higher incidence of autism spectrums than the general population, but a lower incidence than children with mental retardation of other etiologies. The diagnosis of autism in children with Down syndrome should be made on the basis of the *Diagnostic and Statistical Manual of Mental Disorders,* 4th edition (DSM-IV, American Psychiatric Association, 1994). The criteria include the following:

1. Qualitative impairment in social interaction.
2. Qualitative impairments in communication.
3. Restricted, repetitive, and stereotyped patterns of behavior, interests, and activities.

The possible etiologies for autism in Down syndrome are only speculative at this time and include cognitive delays, medical disorders such as seizures and hypoxic cardiac disease, and possible family history of psychiatric disorders. Recognition of autism in children with Down syndrome has important implications for the medical, social, and educational interventions offered to involved children and their families. Unfortunately, the diagnosis is often made later in children with Down syndrome and can have detrimental effects on their long-term outcome, particularly as related to school success. It is important for parents to have the opportunity to meet with professionals knowledgeable in the field of autism to help minimize the impact of obsessions and rituals and avoid secondary problems that may develop if the child's needs are not adequately understood.

ATTENTION DEFICIT HYPERACTIVITY DISORDER (ADHD)

Attention deficit hyperactivity disorder (ADHD) is one of the most commonly diagnosed disruptive disorders in childhood. The availability and efficacy of pharmacotherapy with stimulant medication has caused a furor in the national media related to concerns regarding overdiagnosis and treatment. Although medical management provides only symptomatic relief, few other childhood behavior disorders can make this claim. Unfortunately, the core symptoms of overactivity and distractibility/impulsivity occur in many other disorders: Children who are performing poorly in school frequently display these symptoms, and often ADHD is considered to be the reason for the poor performance. Consequently, many children who are inattentive may be diagnosed with ADHD, without discovering that cognitive deficits or specific learning disabilities, such as a language processing disorder, may underlie the difficulty. The same may be true for those children with anxiety disorders or agitated depression. The failure to respond to pharmacotherapy may be the clue that another, more fundamental explanation, has been overlooked.

The reverse condition seems to occur in the case of children with Down syndrome (DS). Because these children characteristically show cognitive impairments, generally functioning in the mild to moderate range of mental retardation, poor school performance is unlikely to be attributed to inattention or overactivity, even though teachers and parents may observe and report these symptoms. In general, health care providers often fail to diagnose a variety of conditions in children with DS that would be readily diagnosed in the typical child. These symptoms are frequently attributed to the more "obvious" disorder, DS itself. It was for this reason that physicians aware of this mistake in heuristics developed the Preventive Medical Checklist [currently called "Health Care Guidelines for Individuals with Down Syndrome" (Cohen, 1996)] in order to remind primary care and specialty physicians of the high incidence of treatable medical conditions, such as hypothyroidism, which occur more frequently in individuals with DS and whose symptoms can be mistaken for part of the syndrome itself.

Attention deficit hyperactivity disorder (ADHD) does occur in children with DS and it is indeed possible to distinguish those children with the disorder from the vast majority of children with DS who have appropriate attentional abilities and activity levels. The incidence of ADHD in the general population is estimated at approximately 3–5% (Barkley, 1990). A variety of studies has provided an incidence of ADHD in children with mental retardation ranging from 6 to 11% (Myers and Pueschcel, 1991; Barkley, 1990), which is two to three times the prevalence in the general population.

The current accepted definition of ADHD comes from the DSM-IV. These diagnostic criteria require six or more of the nine symptoms of *inattention;* and/or six or more of the nine symptoms of *hyperactivity/impulsivity.* These symptoms must be present for at least 6 months. Some of the symptoms must have been present before the age of seven years; there must be clear evidence of significant impairment in social and academic functioning (i.e., the symptoms must be present in more than one setting); and, the child must not have a pervasive developmental disorder. There should be no other mental disorder that would possibly account for these symptoms. It is important to note that these symptoms must be "maladaptive and inconsistent with developmental level" (American Psychiatric Association, 1994). This feature is most important: when considering a child with DS, we must modify the expectations to meet the developmental level of the child (Barkley, 1990).

There are few studies that look specifically at ADHD in children with Down syndrome. Green et al. (1989) studied a small group of children in England and found that there was a discrete subgroup of 4 of the 13 studied who had significant inattention. This group was found to be discontinuous from the rest of the sample, and they did not represent the extreme end of a continuous variable. Similarly, Myers and Pueschel (1991) found ADHD in 16 of 261 (6.1%) children with Down syndrome. They state that there appear to be no marked differences when children with DS are compared with children with other forms of mental retardation: the incidence appears the same. There is substantial literature confirming the validity of the diagnosis of ADHD in children with mental retardation and the efficacy of pharmacological treatment (Handen et al., 1990, 1992, 1994).

As in the case of typical children, the diagnosis of this disorder is based on the substantiation of the presence of symptoms in multiple settings: home, educational environment, and community. In addition, there must be a negative impact of the child's ability to function as compared to children on the *same developmental level*. Because children with DS are eligible for early intervention and preschool services, the clinician should have little difficulty in gathering this information. The use of standardized questionnaires and rating scales is of utmost importance. In the school-age child, the Achenbach Child Behavior Checklist and the Hyperactive Index of the Conners' Parent and Teacher Rating Scales are used. In the preschool child, we recommend the use of the Behar Preschool Behavior Questionnaire.

Differential Diagnosis

As in the case of typical children, the clinician must be sensitive to the mode of presentation of the problem. Some parents will complain that their child is unmanageable. Upon exploring the child's behavior in school, however, the physician may learn the educational personnel report no behavioral or attentional problems. The clinician must consider alternative hypotheses for the parents' complaint. For example, this may represent difficulty in establishing appropriate discipline, reflecting the confusion parents of children with disabilities often experience: "Poor Johnny, how can I say 'no' to him?" Parent–child interactional difficulties may be related to the issue of the child's disability, or reflect other factors that are more general in nature, and the absence of consistent ratings in all settings requires further investigation to determine alternative explanations for the parent's complaint.

As with typical children, the clinician is warned against misinterpreting observations of either "appropriate" or "overactive" behavior in the office without corroboration from the educational setting. This "snapshot" of behavior is notoriously inaccurate. In addition, the ability to watch a video or television program does not preclude consideration of the diagnosis.

One note of caution: children with DS commonly experience difficulty in expressive language skills, and we must be certain to evaluate the symptomatic behavior in light of the child's communication abilities; they may represent frustration resulting from the child's inability to respond verbally to his or her environment.

Treatment

The same treatment modalities used in the absence of Down syndrome are useful in children with DS and other developmental disabilities: behavioral interventions and pharmacotherapy. Behavioral intervention requires the development of a structured plan which analyzes the specific target behavior and provides contingencies for inappropriate behavior and reinforcement for the desired behavior. The goal of these interventions is to shape the behavior of this child in the desired way. As has been found in typically developing children with ADHD, these interventions often require enormous energy and often the changes do not generalize to other settings. Nevertheless, many experienced educators of children with developmental disabilities admirably provide a supportive and structured environment that can minimize attentional inefficiencies, disruptiveness, and off-task behavior.

On the other hand, pharmacological interventions are well-documented to provide rapid, relatively safe symptomatic relief. Handen et al. (1990, 1992, 1994) have demonstrated the efficacy of methylphenidate (Ritalin) in a population of school-age children with mild mental retardation. In addition to the use of stimulants, the use of clonidine, an alpha-2 adenoreceptor agonist, has been useful, especially in younger aggressive children. One finds a dramatic decrease in off-task behaviors, and often an improvement in participation in academic endeavors, based on the decreased impulsivity and distractibility. Behaviors on the school bus, at recess, and in the community at large (scouts, church, shopping at the mall) also generally improve. In general, children with Down syndrome respond well to stimulant therapy. There is no research to indicate that children with Down syndrome respond any differently to stimulant medication than children with other etiologies of mental retardation, who respond, in general, very well. Note, however, that often the most successful interventions combine behavior management, parental training, and pharmacotherapy.

Suggestions for Management

Skilled primary care physicians often may be comfortable making the diagnosis of ADHD and treating typical children. However, the specific pitfalls in detection, diagnosis, and management of ADHD symptoms in the child with DS or other developmental disability warrant consultation with a developmental-behavioral pediatrician, psychiatrist, or psychologist who has experience with these cases.

REFERENCES

American Psychiatric Association (1994): "Diagnostic and Statistical Manual of Mental Disorders," 4th ed. Washington DC.
Barkley A (1990): "Attention Deficit Hyperactivity Disorder." New York: Guilford Press.

Cohen W (Ed.) (1996): Health care guidelines for individuals with Down syndrome. Down Syndrome Quart 1(2):1–10.

Ghaziuddin M, Tsai L, Ghaziuddin N (1992): Autism in Downs' syndrome: presentation and diagnosis. J Intell Disability Res 36:449–456.

Green JM, Dennis J, Bennets, LA (1989): Attention disorder in a group of young Down's syndrome children. J Ment Defic Res 33:105–122.

Handen BM, Breaux AM, Gosling A, Ploof DL, Feldman H (1990): Efficacy of methylphenidate among mentally retarded children with attention deficit hyperactivity disorder. Pediatrics 86:922–930.

Handen BM, Breaux AM, Janosky J, McAuliffe S, Feldman H, Gosling A (1992): Effects and noneffects of methylphenidate in children with mental retardation and ADHD. J Am Acad Child Adolesc Psychiatry 31:455–461.

Handen BM, Janosky J, McAuliffe S, Breaux AM, Feldman H (1994): Predication of response to methylphenidate among children with ADHD and mental retardation. J Am Acad Child Adolesc Psychiatry 33:1185–1193.

Howlin P, Wing L, Gould J (1995): "The recognition of autism in children with Down syndrome-implications for intervention and some speculations about pathology." Devel Med Child Neurol 37:398–414.

Myers BA, Pueschel SM (1991): Psychiatric disorders in a population with Down syndrome. J Nervous Ment Dis 179:609–613.

Pueschel S, Louis S, McKnight P (1991): Seizure disorders in Down syndrome. Arch Neurol 48:318–320.

Stafstrom C (1993): Epilepsy in Down syndrome: Clinical aspects and possible mechanisms. Am J Ment Retard 98:12–26.

Stafstrom C, Omar F, Herbert E, Wisniewski K (1991): Seizures in children with Down syndrome: etiology, characteristics and outcome. Devel Med Child Neurol 33:191–200.

Stafstrom C, Konkol R (1994): Infantile spasms in children with Down syndrome. Devel Med Child Neurol 36:576–585.

Review of Clinical Research

Nancy Roizen

Two important and clinically relevant research findings include a review of the safety of growth hormone therapy and the finding of a lower resting metabolic rate in children with Down syndrome (DS) which is at least one factor in the high prevalence of obesity in individuals with Down syndrome. The findings of the research on metabolic rate in Down syndrome are presented by Roizen et al. (1995).

GROWTH HORMONE AND LEUKEMIA

In experimental protocols, children with Down syndrome have been treated with growth hormone (GH) to increase their height (Torrado et al., 1991). In 1988, reports of leukemia in children treated with GH raised concern about a possible association between GH therapy and a risk for leukemia (Watanabe et al., 1988). The laboratory finding that high concentrations of GH in a conditioned media induced a dose-dependent increase in the numbers of blast colonies of bone marrow cells from children with new or recurrent acute lymphocytic leukemia and acute myelocytic leukemia increased those concerns (Zadik et al., 1993). In a 1992 review of the worldwide cases of leukemia during GH therapy, a known risk factor for leukemia was present in at least 15 of the 32 reported cases including one child with DS (Stahnke, 1992). The number of remaining cases did not significantly exceed the number of new cases of leukemia that would be expected in the general population. In a recent review of the subject, Allen (1996) concluded that any increased occurrence of leukemia appears limited to those patients with known risk factors. The addition of these data is not conclusive but supports caution in the use of GH in children with DS who have prevalence of leukemia of 1:150 (Avet-Loiseau et al., 1995). Therefore, as recommended by the Lawson Wilkins Pediatric Endocrine Society (1993), there continues to be a need to assess the safety, efficacy, and ethical ramifications of GH treatment of children with DS.

MANAGED CARE

At this time, the monumental changes in the provision of medical care may have more of an effect on the quality of life of individuals with DS than many of the most re-

Down Syndrome: A Promising Future, Together, Edited by Terry J. Hassold and David Patterson
ISBN 0-471-29686-4   Copyright © 1998 by Wiley-Liss, Inc.

cent discoveries. Managed care has changed the practice of medicine by making the provision of medical care, more than ever before, a for-profit endeavor. Families and health care professionals are concerned that managed care programs will decrease access to needed subspecialty and supportive services in the process of controlling health care costs through limiting access, determining medical necessity prior to service, and establishing the most cost effective method of delivery (Ireys et al., 1996). Some of the possible problems and barriers related to the provision of proper medical care as described by Cohen (1996) include the following: (1) as primary care providers are expected to provide care to broader age groups, keeping current may be more difficult; (2) many of the medical problems that need regular monitoring such as thyroid dysfunction, vision, and hearing problems do not produce acute symptomatology and therefore require periodic reevaluations; and (3) the managed care plan may have only one consultant per subspecialty on the staff who is likely to be an adult specialist with limited training in the care of children and limited experience in the care of children with DS.

In response to the changes in the provisions of health care, parents need to know how to make sure that evaluation or monitoring is done accurately. What follows is a review of the disorders that must be evaluated and what constitutes doing it right with an emphasis on possible mistakes in management.

HEARING LOSS

Children with DS have an increased prevalence of multiple aberrations of their auditory system that can contribute to the development of conductive hearing losses (Coleman and Balkany, 1983). Structural differences include small external pinna (ear) length, small external meatus (ear opening), malformations and erosion of the middle ear bones, permanent fixation of the stapes (middle ear bone), abnormalities of the facial nerve, and aberrant length of the cochlear spiral. Functional differences include increased colds and ear infections, abnormal eustachian tube function, and pressure in the inner ear due to fibrous tissue.

Sixty-eight percent of children with DS have a hearing loss that is conductive, sensorineural, or both (Roizen et al., 1993). All children need an objective test of their hearing, which is an auditory brainstem response (ABR), or if no conductive loss is present an otoacoustic emission (OAE) test. These tests should be followed by behavioral audiometry that includes testing the lower frequencies. The ABR should be done in a facility accustomed to evaluating children. Behavioral testing does not allow for identification of unilateral losses, and 22% of children with DS have a unilateral loss. We have learned that unilateral losses do make a difference. Studies of typical children have shown that a unilateral loss of greater than 50 dB are more likely to repeat a grade in school and be functioning in the lower half of the class (Bess and Tharpe, 1984). In addition, behavioral testing does not allow for the differentiation of conductive from sensorineural losses.

After the child's base-line hearing status is objectively established with ABR testing, there are several possible follow-up evaluations needed.

1. If the child has no hearing loss, he/she needs behavioral auditory testing with tympanograms to identify a possible conductive hearing loss secondary to

fluid in the middle ear. These tests should be repeated every 6 months for at least the first 3 years of life and then yearly for the rest of their life (Joint Committee on Infant Hearing, 1995). Adults with DS may develop a high-frequency sensorineural loss.

2. If the child has a conductive loss due to middle ear fluid, the fluid must be treated medically or with pneumoeustachian (PE) tubes. After treatment, an objective hearing evaluation should reveal normal hearing. Some children have structural middle ear abnormalities that do not improve with PE tubes. These conductive losses are permanent.

3. Children with sensorineural hearing losses have irreversible hearing losses and may need hearing aids. They must have a hearing evaluation every 6 months until they are 3 years old, and then annually for their entire life (Joint Committee on Infant Hearing, 1995). The hearing evaluations are needed to identify any new conductive losses due to middle ear fluid, which may muffle the hearing that is preserved, to detect any progression in the sensorineural hearing loss, and to test the hearing in the lower frequencies not evaluated by an ABR.

Several things can be done to encourage optimal language development in children with DS with and without hearing loss. An environment rich in language with reading is essential. The background from the TV or the radio should be kept to a minimum and not be on unless someone is watching or listening. Signing is helpful to children who understand but have limited spoken language with which to communicate their needs. Hearing aids should be considered for children with hearing losses.

OPHTHALMIC DISORDERS

Sixty-percent of children with DS have an ophthalmic disorder that needs monitoring or treatment (Roizen at al., 1994). The most common disorders are refractive errors (nearsightedness and farsightedness), which occur in 35% of children and increase in frequency with age. Refractive errors occur commonly in the general population but severe refractive errors occur much more frequently in the population of individuals with DS than in the general population. Other disorders found in a survey of children with DS include strabismus (27%), nystagmus (20%), spasmus nutans (3%), congenital cataracts (4%), acquired cataracts (1%), congenital glaucoma (1%), ptosis (5%), congenital stationary night blindness (1%), choreoretinal coloboma (1%), and retinal detachment (1%) (Roizen et al., 1994). Thirty-five percent who have a normal physical exam when evaluated by a pediatrician have a disorder when evaluated by a pediatric ophthalmologist (Roizen et al., 1994). Therefore, all children with DS should have an evaluation by a pediatric ophthalmologist within the first 6 months of life with follow-ups as indicated or every 1 or at most 2 years if there are no ophthalmic disorders identified. Possible problems related to evaluation for ophthalmic problems include the following: (1) referral to an ophthalmologist who does not specialize in children and therefore is not trained to evaluate children who are frequently uncooperative and who have a different spectrum of ophthalmic disorders from adults; (2) no follow-up after the initial evaluation as children, which may delay the identification of myopia (nearsightedness) and hyperopia (farsightedness) in the early years and keratoconus and lens opacities in the teen-age years and later; (3) a lack of rigorous treatment and follow-up of strabismus (lazy eye) resulting in loss of vision in the lazy eye.

THYROID DYSFUNCTION

Thyroid dysfunction is a treatable cause of problems in behavior, attention, and cognitive development. Thyroid dysfunction is easily identified by blood tests although the child may not have symptoms that are apparent except in retrospect for months or years. Fortunately, all children are evaluated at birth for thyroid dysfunction. Thereafter, in children with DS, thyroid function tests should be done yearly so that thyroid dysfunction can be identified and treated early in the development of the disease.

OBESITY

Early in infancy, children with Down syndrome (DS) frequently have problems with weight gain. As toddlers, 18–27% of the children with DS have problems with textured foods, chewing table foods, and preferring special food groups (Pipes and Holm, 1980). Then, over time, children with DS tend to gain more weight percentiles compared to height percentiles. The result is the development of obesity in 50% of 3-year-old girls with DS and the majority of boys by early childhood (Cronk et al., 1988). This is in contrast to between 5 and 25% both of children and adolescents in the general population and of children and adolescents with mental retardation being obese (Dietz, 1983; Burkart et al., 1985; Gortmaker et al., 1987).

To develop an intervention plan to prevent obesity, careful monitoring of the relationship of weight to height over time is imperative. To monitor growth in children with DS intelligently, gender-specific growth charts for both typically developing children (Hamill et al., 1979) and children with DS (Cronk et al., 1988) must be used. Calculation of percent ideal body weight is especially helpful in monitoring growth changes. To calculate this ratio, plot the height of the child on the growth chart for typically developing children and determine the height age or the age for which this height is at the 50th percentile. Then determine the weight at the 50th percentile for this height. Divide the actual weight of the child by this weight, which would be the expected average weight for a typically developing child of the same height as the child with DS. This ratio multiplied by 100 gives the percent ideal body weight (IBW).

The goal for all of us is to maintain a percent IBW between 90 and 110%. A percent IBW of 110–120% is considered overweight while a ratio of >120% is considered obese. Children with DS tend to have an IBW ratio of 80–100% in the first 2 years of life. Although each child has an individual growth curve, the children with DS tend to increase their IBW ratio over time and become obese.

Obesity is associated with both social and health problems. Social problems include obese children being less sought after as playmates and limited motor performance (Malina, 1980). Health problems include an increased risk for hypertension, diabetes, surgery risk, and pulmonary problems (Bray, 1976; Kannel and Gordon, 1979; Van Itallie, 1979). The specific impact of obesity in the child and adolescent with DS has not been studied.

In a study of obesity in school-age, prepubertal children with DS, Luke et al. (1994) discovered that children with DS have a resting metabolic rate of 10–15% lower than age- and size-matched controls. The children with DS had activity levels that were comparable to controls. There was an inverse relationship between body fat and physical activity; that is, the more active children had a lower percentage of body fat. The children with DS had a good dietary distribution of carbohydrates, fats, and proteins, with fat representing 30% of the daily caloric intake (Luke et al., 1996). However, the leaner children with DS with lower food intakes were especially at risk for dietary deficiencies of vitamins and minerals.

The problem of obesity is best managed with preventive actions in relation to activity, diet, and behavior. As soon as the children are able to walk, regular daily physical activity such as walk should become part of their regimen. Activities that can be continued through life such as bike riding, skiing, swimming, and tennis should be encouraged. Starting at 2 years of age, twice a year the diet should be reviewed and if the child's weight per height ratio is increasing substitutions of lower calorie items should be made. In addition (Luke et al., 1994) recommended a multivitamin supplement. Behavior modifications in the form of limiting eating to the dinner table and restricting eating in front of the TV, not rewarding with food, and using smaller plates reduces unnecessary food intake.

CONCLUSION

In the present medical climate, the parents of a child with DS need to be aware and vigilant. They need to understand why a specific evaluation should be performed and to think about whether the evaluation has answered the question asked. The parents should maintain a file on their child's evaluations. After each evaluation, the parents should request that a copy of the evaluation be sent to themselves as well as involved professionals and that the recommendations include the appropriate time for follow-up. They need to be careful observers of their child and immediately bring changes in the child's functioning to the attention of the pediatrician. If parents and professionals work together, they can remove barriers to appropriate care for all individuals with special needs.

REFERENCES

Allen DB (1996): Safety of human growth hormone therapy: current topics. J Pediatr 128:S8–13.

Avet-Loiseau H, Mechinaud R, Harousseau J-L (1995): Clonal hematologic disorders in Down syndrome: a review. J Pediatr Hematol Oncol 17:19–24.

Bess FM, Tharpe AM (1984): Unilateral hearing impairment in children. Pediatrics 74:206–216.

Bray GA (1976): "The Obese Patient." Philadelphia: Saunders.

Burkart JE, Fox RA, Rotatori AF (1985): Obesity of mentally retarded individuals: prevalence, characteristics, and intervention. Am J Ment Defic 90:303–321.

Cohen WI (1996): Health care guidelines for individuals with Down syndrome (Down Syndrome preventive medical check list). Down Syndrome Quart 1:1–10.

Coleman M, Balkany TJ (1983): Abnormalities of the ear in Down syndrome. Down Syndrome Papers Abstr Professionals 6:1–2.

Cronk CR, Crocker AC, Pueschel SM, et al. (1988): Growth charts for children with Down syndrome: 1 month to 18 years of age. Pediatrics 81:102–110.

Dietz WH (1983): Childhood obesity: susceptibility, cause and management. J Pediatr 103:676–686.

Gortmaker SL, Dietz WH, Sobel AM, Wehler FA (1987): Increasing pediatric obesity in the United States. Am J Dis Child 141:535–540.

Hamill PVV, Drizd TA, Johnson CL, et al. (1979): Physical growth: National Center for Health Statistics percentiles. Am J Clin Nutr 32:609–610.

Ireys HT, Grason HA, Guyer B (1996): Assuring quality of care for children with special needs in managed care organizations: roles for pediatricians. Pediatrics 98:178–185.

Joint Committee on Infant Hearing (1995): 1994 Committee statement. Pediatrics 95:152–156.

Kannel WB, Gordon T (1979): Physiological and medical concomitants of obesity: the Framingham study. In Bray GA (ed.): "Obesity in America" (NIH Publication No. 79-359). Washington DC: Department of Health, Education and Welfare, pp. 125–163.

Lawson Wilkins Pediatric Endocrine Society Board of Directors and Drug and Therapeutics Committee (1993): Growth hormone for children with Down syndrome. J Pediatr 123:742–743.

Luke AH, Roizen NJ, Sutton M, Schoeller DA (1994): Energy expenditure in Down syndrome. J Pediatr 125:829–836.

Luke A, Sutton M, Schoeller DA, Roizen NJ (1996): Nutrient intake and obesity in prepubescent children with Down syndrome. J AM Diet Assoc 96(12):1262–1267.

Malina RM (1980): Growth, strength and physical performance. In Stull GA (ed.): "Encyclopedia of Physical Education, Fitness and Sports." Salt Lake City: Brighton.

Pipes P, Holm VA (1980): Food and children with Down syndrome. J Am Diet Assoc 77:277–281.

Roizen NJ, Luke A, Sutton M, Schoeller DA (1995): Obesity and nutrition in children with Down syndrome. In Nadel L and Rosethal D (eds.): "Down Syndrome. Living and Learning in the Community." New York: Wiley-Liss, pp. 213–215.

Roizen NJ, Mets MB, Blondis TA (1994): Ophthalmic disorders in children with Down syndrome. Devel Med Child Neurol 36:594–600.

Roizen NJ, Wolters CA, Nicol TG, Blodis TA (1993): Auditory brain stem evoked response in children with Down syndrome. J Pediatr 123: S9–12.

Stahnke N (1992): Leukemia in growth-hormone treated patients: an update. Hormone Res 38(suppl 1):56–62.

Torrado C, Bastian W, Wisniewski KE, Castells S (1991): Treatment of children with Down syndrome and growth retardation with recombinant human growth hormone. J Pediatr 119:478–483.

Van Itallie TB (1979): Obesity: adverse effects on health and longevity. Am J Clin Nutr Suppl:2723–2733.

Watanabe S, Tsunematsu Y, Fujumoto J, Komiyama A (1988): Leukemia in patients treated with growth hormone (letter). Lancet 21:1159–1160.

Zadik A, Estrov A, Karov Y, Hahn T, Barak Y (1993): The effect of growth hormone and IGF-I on clonogenic growth of hematopoietic cells in leukemia patients during active disease and during remission. J Pediatr Endocrinol 6:79–83.

Cervical Spine Abnormalities in Persons with Down Syndrome

Siegfried M. Pueschel

The earliest report of a cervical spine abnormality dates back nearly 5000 years. The Edwin Smith Papyrus describes a person's displacement of a cervical vertebra in an ancient Egyptian man (Power D'Arcy, 1933).

During the nineteenth century numerous reports of cervical spine disorders were published (Aung, 1973; Lazzaretto, 1813). Whereas these early reports of cervical spine abnormalities were primarily noted in the general population, atlantoaxial instability in persons with Down syndrome was first reported by Spitzer et al. (1961). Since then, many case reports have been published describing patients with Down syndrome and atlantoaxial instability (Andrews, 1981; Aung, 1973; Beltran, 1970; Curtis et al., 1968; Dzenitis, 1966; Finerman et al., 1976; Grobovschek and Strohecker, 1985; Herring, 1982; Martel and Tishler, 1966; Nordt and Stauffer, 1981; Pandya, 1972; Sherk and Nicholson, 1969; Shield et al., 1981; Tishler and Martel, 1965; Whaley and Gray, 1980). Although the vast majority of these papers discuss atlantoaxial instability in persons with Down syndrome, other cervical spine disorders such as atlantooccipital instability, degenerative changes, and skeletal anomalies of the upper cervical spine have also been reported in the literature.

ATLANTOAXIAL INSTABILITY

Atlantoaxial instability is considered to be present when the atlanto–dens interval is 5 mm or greater. Atlantoaxial instability in individuals with Down syndrome is primarily due to ligamentous laxity of the transverse ligaments that ordinarily hold the odontoid process close to the anterior arch of the atlas. It has been estimated that the frequency of atlantoaxial instability is between 9 and 30% (Alverez and Rubin, 1986; Martel and Tishler, 1966; Pueschel and Scola, 1987; Semine et al., 1978; Spitzer et al., 1971; Tishler and Martel, 1965).

Down Syndrome: A Promising Future, Together, Edited by Terry J. Hassold and David Patterson
ISBN 0-471-29686-4   Copyright © 1998 by Wiley-Liss, Inc.

When Pueschel et al. (1981) studied a large population with Down syndrome they observed that the atlanto–dens interval in these individuals was significantly wider than in children who did not have this chromosomal abnormality. In a subsequent study, Pueschel and Scola (1987) compared various neck positions (flexion, neutral, and extension) and found that the measurements of atlanto–dens intervals obtained in flexion were significantly greater than those in extension or in neutral position. In addition, 59 (14.6%) of 404 persons with Down syndrome displayed atlantoaxial instability; 53 (13.1%) had asymptomatic atlantoaxial instability; and 6 patients (1.5%) had symptomatic atlantoaxial instability.

Individuals with Down syndrome who have asymptomatic atlantoaxial instability, that is, with radiological evidence of this disorder but no neurological involvement, need close follow-up. These children are usually not allowed to participate in certain sports activities during Special Olympic games including training or competition in gymnastics, diving start in swimming, butterfly stroke in swimming, high jump, pentathlon, soccer, and alpine skiing. Whereas most of these individuals continue to be asymptomatic, some of them may sustain an injury to the neck and become symptomatic (Pueschel et al., 1984).

In order to identify those who are at high risk of becoming symptomatic, Pueschel et al. (1987) carried out a study that included roentgenographic, neurological, and somatosensory investigations. Twenty-seven persons with Down syndrome who did not have atlantoaxial instability were compared with an age-matched and sex-matched group of 27 persons who had atlantoaxial instability. No significant differences in mean composite neurological scores and somatosensory evoked responses were observed. However, when a subsample of those individuals with high and low latencies were compared with radiological findings, there was a high correspondence between somatosensory evoked potentials and atlanto–dens interval measurements. Therefore the authors concluded that a combined approach using computerized tomographic scans, radiological assessments, and neurological and neurophysiological investigations will provide information on the risk status of persons with Down syndrome and atlantoaxial instability.

In 1992, Pueschel et al. reported a longitudinal study designed to investigate the natural history of atlantoaxial instability in individuals with Down syndrome. There was no significant change in C1–C2 relationship over time and the vast majority of persons with Down syndrome had only minor changes of atlanto–dens interval measurements comparing various examinations. In only 11 persons (8%) were marked changes observed. None of the individuals with marked changes of the atlanto–dens intervals, however, displayed clinical symptoms on physical examinations and all functioned neurologically within normal limits.

If persons with Down syndrome are diagnosed to have symptomatic atlantoaxial instability, surgical intervention is often recommended. Reviewing the world literature on this subject, it was found that about 126 persons with Down syndrome have been reported with symptomatic atlantoaxial instability. These individuals usually exhibit a variety of neurological symptoms including brisk deep tendon reflexes, extensor plantar responses, ankle clonus, muscle weakness, gait abnormalities, sensory impairments, and local symptoms such as limited neck mobility, neck pain, and head tilt. The main goal of the surgical intervention is to reduce the atlantoaxial subluxation as much as possible and to stabilize the upper segment of the cervical spine by applying wires to the upper cervical vertebrae and bone graft posteriorly. Pueschel et al. (1984) observed that those individuals with long-standing symptoms and marked neurological involvement show little or no improvement postoperatively; however, those with more recent onset of this disorder usually make an excellent recovery. Because symptomatic atlantoaxial instability can be a serious debilitating disorder with long time neurological involvement, it is paramount that individuals with Down syndrome who are at risk to develop this condition be identified as early as possible.

ATLANTO-OCCIPITAL INSTABILITY

There have been numerous reports in the literature relating to atlanto-occipital instability in persons with Down syndrome (Brooke et al., 1987; Collacott et al., 1989; EL-Khoury et al., 1986; Holmes and Hall, 1978; Hungerford et al., 1981; Rosenbaum et al., 1986; Tredwell et al., 1990). When our group (Parfenchuck et al., 1994) examined radiographs of 199 individuals with Down syndrome and compared them with those of 102 normal individuals, 8.5% of them were found to have posterior occipitoatlantal hypermobility. Although standardized radiographic criteria for the evaluation of the atlanto-occipital joint has not been developed, our group found that the Powers ratio is the most reliable radiographic parameter for assessment of atlanto-occipital instability because it yields very consistent values in "normal" persons regardless of neck position and, in addition, it is unaffected by radiographic magnifications. Atlanto-occipital instability may become of great significance in patients with Down syndrome who will undergo surgery under general anesthesia. Increased extension of the neck during intubation and vigorous manipulations of head and neck during anesthesia may cause injury to the spinal cord. Therefore, special precautions should be taken during anesthesia. It is important that radiographs of the cervical spine be obtained prior to surgery.

SKELETAL ANOMALIES OF THE UPPER CERVICAL SPINE

Pueschel et al. (1990) found that a significant number of children with Down syndrome and atlantoaxial instability have cervical spine anomalies when compared with an age-matched and sex-matched control group. This study suggested that cervical spine anomalies may be a contributing factor in the pathogenesis of atlantoaxial instability. There have also been other investigators reporting abnormalities of the odontoid process and other skeletal structures of the C1–C2 region in persons with Down syndrome (Dawson and Smith, 1979; Fielding and Griffin, 1974; Finerman et al., 1976; Martel and Tishler, 1966; Roach et al., 1984; Semine et al., 1978).

DEGENERATIVE CHANGES

In 1986, Fidone reported that 16 of 42 persons with Down syndrome had various degrees of degenerative arthritis of the cervical vertebrae and intervertebral discs. The degenerative changes included osteophyte formation, subarticular sclerosis, cystic changes, fusion, and disc narrowing. Miller et al. (1986) reported a high prevalence of degenerative changes in the C2–C3 and C3–C4 cervical spine interspaces. Four of these individuals demonstrated cervical spine subluxation at interspaces other than C1–C2 and six had congenital fusion of either vertebral bodies or facets in the cervical spine region.

RADIOLOGICAL SCREENING RECOMMENDATIONS

Because of the above described increased prevalence of atlantoaxial and atlantooccipital instability, skeletal anomalies of the cervical spine, and degenerative changes in persons with Down syndrome which ultimately could lead to spinal cord injury, it is important that persons with Down syndrome undergo cervical spine examinations. We recommend that children with Down syndrome have radiological examinations of the cervical spine at about 3 years of age and before entering Special Olympics sports activities at about 8 years. Some professionals also reexamine the cervical spine radiologically during adolescence.

The American Academy of Pediatrics statement (1994), however, mentions that radiological screening of the cervical spine in persons with Down syndrome is not indicated and that "good medical histories and physical and neurologic examinations" would be more important than X-rays. We favor radiological examination of the cervical spine, because if one waits until significant neurological symptoms become evident, then spinal cord damage might already have occurred and may be irreversible. Moreover, the prevalent motor dysfunction and broad-based gait in many individuals with Down syndrome may conceal significant neurological concerns. Also, a number of individuals with Down syndrome are not able to verbalize specific complaints relating to neck discomfort and neuromotor difficulties. Others may not cooperate during physical and neurological examinations. For these reasons and because symptomatic atlantoaxial instability and other cervical spine conditions in persons with Down syndrome can be severely debilitating and impair their quality of life, it is recommended that children undergo radiographic examination of the lateral cervical spine in hyperflexion and hyperextension as well as have regular physical and neurological evaluations. It is important to identify high risk children as early as possible in order to avoid the serious consequences of symptomatic atlantoaxial instability and other cervical spine disorders.

There is a need for controlled studies that investigate the evolution from asymptomatic to symptomatic atlantoaxial instability in order to find those individuals who are at an increased risk of developing neurological symptoms. Moreover, forthcoming research should focus on the relationship between asymptomatic atlantoaxial instability and subsequent injury leading to neurological signs and symptoms. The efficiency of preventive measures as promulgated by Special Olympics Inc. (1983) should also be studied. Until such investigations have been carried out and results are obtained that can properly be interpreted and translated into guidelines to be followed by practitioners, it is paramount that children with Down syndrome and atlantoaxial instability be protected from cervical spine injury and be provided with close surveillance. If individuals with Down syndrome receive optimal medical care including radiological examination of the cervical spine, their quality of life can be enhanced significantly.

REFERENCES

Alvarez N, Rubin L (1986): Atlantoaxial instability in adults with Down syndrome: a clinical and radiological survey. Appl Res Ment Retard 7:67–68.

American Academy of Pediatrics (1994): Atlantoaxial instability in Down syndrome: subject review. Pediatrics 96:151–154.

Andrews, LG (1981): Myelopathy due to atlanto-axial dislocation in a patient with Down's syndrome and rheumatoid arthritis. Dev Med Child Neural 23(3):356–360.

Aung MH (1973): Atlanto-axial dislocation in Down's syndrome: report of a case with spinal cord compression and review of the literature. Bull Los Angeles Neurol Soc 38:197–210.

Beltran P (1970): La dislocation atlanto-axiodienne (Atlantoaxial dislocation). Sandoz de Mexico.

Brooke DC, Burkus JK, Benson DR (1987): Asymptomatic occipitoatlantal instability in Down syndrome (trisomy 21): report of two cases in children. J Bone Joint Surg 69:239–295.

Collacott RA, Ellison D, Harper W, Newland C, Ray-Chaudhurt K (1989): Atlanto-occipital instability in Down's syndrome: case report. J Ment Defic Res 33:499–505.

Curtis BH, Blank S, Fisher RL (1968): Atlanto-axial dislocation in Down's syndrome: report of two patients requiring surgical correction. J Am Med Assoc 205:212–213.

Dawson EG, Smith L (1979): Atlanto-axial subluxation in children due to vertebral anomalies. J Bone Joint Surg 61:582–587.

Dzenitis AJ (1966): Spontaneous atlanto-axial dislocation in a mongoloid child with spinal cord compression: case report. J Neurosurg 25:458–460.

El-Khoury GY, Clark CR, Dietz ER, Harre RG, Tozzi JE, Kathol MH (1986): Posterior atlantooccipital subluxation in Down syndrome. Radiology 15:507–509.

Fidone GS (1986): Degeneratice cervical arthritis and Down syndrome. New Engl J Med 314:320.

Fielding JW, Griffin PR (1974): Os odontoideum: An acquired lesion. J Bone Joint Surg 56:187–190.

Finerman GAM, Sakai D, Weingarten S (1976): Atlanto-axial dislocation with spinal cord compression in a mongoloid child: a case report. J Bone Joint Surg 58:408–409.

Grobovschek M, Strohecker J (1985): Congenital atlanto-axial subluxation in Down's syndrome. Neuroradiology 27:186–192.

Herring JA (1982): Cervical instability in Down's syndrome and juvenile rheumatoid arthritis. J Pediatr Orthoped 2:205–207.

Holmes JA, Hall JE (1978): Fusion for instability and potential instability of the cervical spine in children and adolescents. Orthoped Clinics North Am 9:923–943.

Hungerford GD, AKkaraju V, Rawe SE, Young GF (1981): Atlanto-occipital and atlanto-axial dislocations with spinal cord compression in Down syndrome: a case report and review of the literature. Brit J Radiol 54:758–761.

Lazzaretto E (1813): A remarkable case of dislocation of the atlas. Edinburgh Med Surg J 9:165–167.

Martel W, Tishler JM (1966): Observations on the spine in mongolism. Am J Roentgenol Radium Therap Nucl M 94:630–638.

Miller JD, Capusten BM, Lampard R (1986): Changes at the base of skull and cervical spine in Down syndrome. Can Assoc Radiol J 37(2):85–89.

Nordt JD, Stauffer ES (1981): Sequelae of atlanto-axial stabilization in two patients with Down syndrome. Spine 6:437–448.

Pandya SK (1972): Atlantoaxial dislocations. Neurol India 20:13–48.

Parfenchuck TA, Bertrand SL, Powers MJ, Drvaric DM, Pueschel SM, Roberts JM (1994): Posterior occipitoatlantal hypermobility in Down syndrome: an analysis of 199 patients. J Pediatr Orthopedics 14:304–308.

Power D'Arcy L (1933): Some early surgical cases—The Edwin Smith Papyrus. Brit J Surg 21:1–6.

Powers B, Miller MD, Dramer RS, Martinez S, Gehweiler JA (1979): Traumatic atlantooccipital dislocation. Neurosurgery 4:12–17.

Pueschel SM, Findley TW, Furia J, Gallagher PL, Scola FH, Pezzullo JC (1987): Atlantoaxial instability in Down syndrome: Roentgenographic, neurologic, and somatosensory evoked potential studies. J Pediatr 110:515–521.

Pueschel SM, Herndon JH, Gelch MM, Senft KE, Scola FH, Goldberg MJ (1984). Symptomatic atlantoaxial subluxation in persons with Down syndrome. J Pediatr Orthoped 4:682–688.

Pueschel SM, Scola FH (1987): Atlantoaxial instability in individuals with Down syndrome: Epidemiologic, radiographic, and clinical studies. Pediatrics 80: 555–688.

Pueschel SM, Scola FH, Perry CD, Pezzullo JC (1981): Atlantoaxial instability in children with Down syndrome. Pediatr Radiol 10:129–132.

Pueschel SM, Scola FH, Pezzullo JC (1992): A longitudinal study of atlantoaxial instability in individuals with Down syndrome. Pediatrics 89:1194–1198.

Pueschel SM, Scola FH, Tupper TB, Pezzullo JC (1990): Skeletal anomalies of the upper cervical spine in children with Down syndrome. J Pediatr Orthoped 10:607–611.

Roach JW, Duncan D, Wenger DR, Maravilla A, Maravilla K (1984): Atlanto-axial instability and spinal cord compression in children—Diagnosis by computerized tomography. J Bone Joint Surg 66:708–714.

Rosenbaum DM, Blumhagen JD, King HA (1986): Atlantooccipital instability in Down Syndrome. Am J Roentgenol 146:1269–1272.

Semine AA, Ertel AN, Goldberg MJ, Bull MJ (1978): Cervical spine instability in children with Down syndrome (trisomy 21). J Bone Joint Surg 60:649–652.

Sherk HH, Nicholson AT (1969): Rotatory atlanto-axial dislocation associated with ossiculum terminale and mongolism. J Bone Joint Surg 51:957–964.

Shield LK, Dickens DRV, Jensen F (1981): Atlanto-axial dislocation with spinal cord compression in Down syndrome. Austral Pediatr J 17:114–116.

Special Olympics Bulletin (1983): Participation by individuals with Down syndrome who suffer from atlantoaxial dislocation condition. Washington DC: Special Olympics Inc.

Spitzer R, Rabinowitch JY, Wybar KC (1961): A study of abnormalities of the skull, teeth, and lenses in mongolism. Can Med Assoc J 84:567–572.

Tishler JM, Martel W (1965): Dislocation of the atlas in mongolism: preliminary report. Radiology 84:904–908.

Tredwell SJ, Newman DW, Lockitch G (1990): Instability of the upper cervical spine in Down syndrome. J Pediatr Orthoped 10:602–606.

Whaley WJ, Gray WD (1980): Atlanto-axial dislocation in Down's syndrome. Can Med Assoc J 123:35–37.

III. Genetics

The Incidence and Origin of Human Trisomies

Terry J. Hassold

An additional chromosome 21, or trisomy 21, is the most commonly identified chromosome abnormality in liveborns, occurring in approximately 1/600 to 1/800 newborn babies. Because of the clinical importance of the resulting syndrome (Down syndrome), it is sometimes assumed that trisomy 21 is the only chromosome abnormality that occurs in humans. In fact, nothing could be further from the truth, for at least 5% of all human pregnancies involve a fetus with an extra chromosome. In this chapter, we consider three questions related to the incidence and etiology of human trisomies, and summarize recent molecular information relevant to these questions.

1. What is the frequency of trisomy in humans?
2. How do trisomies usually originate?
3. What factors predispose to the occurrence of trisomy?

WHAT IS THE INCIDENCE OF TRISOMY IN HUMANS?

The answer to this question is more complicated than it seems, because it depends on the type of population being considered. That is, as can be seen from Figure 1, not all human pregnancies come to term. Hormonal studies indicate that a large proportion miscarry very early, even before the pregnancy is recognized. Such pregnancies are referred to as "biochemical pregnancies" or "subclinical miscarriages," and although we know nothing about the chromosomal status of the fetuses in these pregnancies, it is generally thought that a large proportion are trisomic.

Much more is known about the incidence of trisomy in clinically recognized pregnancies, that is, in those situations in which it is clear that a pregnancy has occurred. Such pregnancies are generally divided into three categories, those 15–20% of cases in which the fetus is spontaneously aborted (a miscarriage), those 1% of cases in which a stillborn infant is delivered, and the remaining 80–85% of cases that result in a liveborn infant. The frequency of trisomy is lowest for the last category, as approximately 1/300

Down Syndrome: A Promising Future, Together, Edited by Terry J. Hassold and David Patterson
ISBN 0-471-29686-4   Copyright © 1998 by Wiley-Liss, Inc.

CATEGORIES OF PREGNANCY OUTCOME

Week of pregnancy	Outcome of pregnancy	% of clinically recognized pregnancies
0 (conception)		
	Sub-clinical loss	?
6-8 (clinical recognition)		
	Spontaneous abortion	15-20
20-28		
	Stillbirth	1
40 (term delivery)	Livebirth	80-85

Fig. 1. Approximate frequencies of different categories of pregnancy outcome.

newborns have an additional chromosome (Table 1). Most commonly, the additional chromosome is chromosome 21, although trisomies for an additional chromosome 13, 18, or sex chromosome (the X or Y chromosome) also are occasionally identified.

The frequency of trisomy is much higher among those fetuses that are lost either as stillbirths or spontaneous abortions. Among stillbirths, the incidence of trisomy is approximately 4%, and consists largely of trisomies 13, 18, and 21. Among spontaneous abortions the frequency is even higher, for no less than 25% of all such pregnancies involve a trisomic fetus. Trisomies identified in spontaneous abortions also include types that are never seen among liveborn individuals. For example, trisomy 16 is responsible for approximately 7–8% of all spontaneous abortions, making it the most common of all human trisomies. Trisomies 2, 14, 15, and 22 are also quite common and, together with trisomy 16, account for more than one-half of all trisomies identified in spontaneous abortions. None of these abnormalities is associated with live birth, presumably because the fetal malformations are too severe to permit survival to term.

By considering the frequency of trisomy in newborns, stillbirths, and spontaneous abortions and taking into account the frequency with which each of these outcomes occurs among all clinically recognized pregnancies, we can estimate the overall incidence of trisomy in humans. This value is approximately 5%, meaning that about 1 in 20 of all human pregnancies involves a trisomic fetus. Furthermore, this is clearly an underestimate, because it does not take into account those "subclinical" spontaneous

Table 1. Incidence and Types of Trisomies in Different Types of Clinically Recognized Pregnancies

Pregnancy Outcome	Overall Frequency of Trisomy	Most Commonly Occurring Trisomies
Live born infant	1/300	Trisomies 21, 18, 13; sex chromosome trisomies (47,XXY; 47,XXX; 47,XYY)
Stillborn infant	1/25	Trisomies 21, 18, 13
Spontaneous abortion	1/4	Trisomies 16, 22, 21, 15, 14, 2

abortions, some proportion of which must be trisomic. Indeed, chromosome studies of sperm and eggs suggest that as many 20% of all human pregnancies may have an extra or missing chromosome. Thus it is clear that trisomy is the most common, and clinically the most important, of all human genetic disorders.

HOW DOES THE EXTRA CHROMOSOME ORIGINATE?

To answer this question, we must first review the behavior of chromosomes during the development of human eggs and sperm. A cell destined to become a mature egg or sperm contains 46 chromosomes, consisting of 23 pairs of "homologous" chromosomes. For example, the cell has two chromosomes 21, one of which is maternally inherited and one paternally inherited; it also has two copies of all other chromosomes numbered 1–22, and has two sex chromosomes as well.

Because normal fertilization consists of the union of an egg and sperm, it is important that this number be reduced from 46 to 23 in the mature gametes—otherwise the number of chromosomes would double with each generation. This reduction is accomplished by two successive rounds of cell division, known as the first and second meiotic divisions (Fig. 2). In meiosis I, each member of a homologous pair of chromosomes seeks out its partner so that all 23 pairs become aligned. Subsequently material is exchanged, or "recombined" between the members of an homologous pair, in a process that appears to be important in properly orienting the chromosomes. After this recombination process is completed, each member of an homologous pair goes to opposite daughter cells, thus ending the first meiotic division. The second meiotic division occurs immediately after meiosis I and is much more straightforward. Each chromosome simply divides longitudinally, with one-half (a "chromatid") going to one daughter cell and one sister chromatid to the opposite daughter cell. Thus, prior to the initiation of meiosis I the "pre-sperm" or "pre-egg" consists of 46 chromosomes, each with two chromatids; following completion of meiosis II, the mature sperm or egg consists of 23 chromosomes, each with one chromatid.

Theoretically, errors in chromosome movement ("nondisjunction") at meiosis I or II could lead to the presence of an extra chromosome in either the sperm or egg. It is, of course, impractical to study nondisjunction directly in human sperm or eggs, for this

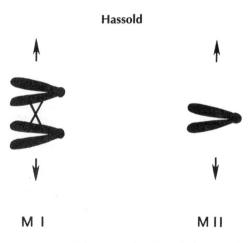

M I   M II

Fig. 2. Schematic representation of the normal meiotic behavior of a single homologous pair of chromosomes. In meiosis I (MI), the two members of the pair (1) align with one another, (2) recombine with one another (this involves a physical exchange of genetic material between the two chromosomes and is indicated by the "X") and (3), following the recombination process, separate from one another, with the two chromosome going in opposite directions to different daughter cells (indicated by the arrows).

In meiosis II (MII), the chromosome divides in half, with each chromosome half (a chromatid) going in opposite directions (indicated by the arrows). Note that in this example, only one of the two chromosomes from the previous MI is depicted; the other should behave in exactly the same way.

would require obtaining testicular or ovarian tissue. However, by using molecular techniques to study trisomic individuals and their parents, it is possible to determine the gamete and meiotic stage of origin of the extra chromosome. This is done by studying regions of chromosomes that vary among individuals, much in the same way that fingerprints vary among individuals. An example of this approach is shown in Figure 3.

This approach, known as DNA polymorphism analysis, has been used to study the origin of the extra chromosome in several hundred trisomic fetuses and liveborn individuals (Table 2). The results indicate that most human trisomy originates from nondisjunction at maternal meiosis I. This is perhaps not surprising, because this stage of development of the egg is quite unusual: it begins before birth in the fetal ovary, but is arrested until the onset of puberty, at which time one egg per ovulatory cycle (on average) completes meiosis I and proceeds to meiosis II. This process continues each month until the oocytes are depleted with the onset of menopause.

Although most trisomic conditions derive from maternal meiotic errors, it is clear that paternal nondisjunction also contributes significantly. Thus, depending on the chromosome, approximately 5–20% of cases appear to be due to an error in the sperm. Furthermore, for the 47, XXY condition this frequency is even higher, with approximately 50% of cases being attributable to paternal nondisjunction.

DNA polymorphism analysis has also been useful in studying the underlying molecular mechanisms associated with chromosome nondisjunction. For example, by studying multiple variable regions that span the entire chromosome, it is possible to

a

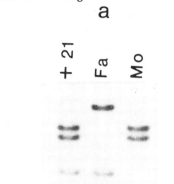

Fig. 3. Use of DNA polymorphisms to determine the origin of the additional chromosome in trisomy 21. In this example, molecular analysis is used to study a variable region on chromosome 21; the variation is detected by the location of the dark bands or "fragments." In this case, the trisomic individual (+21) has three fragments, representing the three chromosomes 21. Because two of the three come from the mother (mo), the additional chromosome must have arisen in the oocyte.

Table 2. Molecular Studies of Parental and Meiotic Stage of Origin in Autosomal and Sex Chromosome Trisomies

Trisomy	No Informative Cases	Paternal			Maternal			% Maternal
		I	II	I or II	I	II	I or II	
2–12	16			3			13	81
13–15	54	1	4	2	12	8	27	87
16	62				51	1	10	100
18	101			9	16	35	41	90
21[a]	776	17	27		556	176		94
22	19			2	6		11	89
XXY	133	58			40	13	22	56
XXX	46		2		24	10	10	94

[a]For trisomy 21, we have presented only those cases having information on both parent and meiotic stage of origin of trisomy.

determine where, and how frequently, recombination occurs between homologous chromosomes during meiosis I. These kinds of studies are in their infancy but they have already led to a surprising conclusion; namely, that abnormalities in meiotic recombination are associated with a large proportion, if not a majority, of trisomies. In general, it appears that a reduction in recombination at meiosis I predisposes to trisomy, but there is also evidence that the occurrence of recombination at the wrong location may increase the chance of nondisjunction. An understanding of the relationship between recombination abnormalities and trisomy is now one of the most active areas of study in human chromosome research.

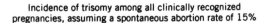

Incidence of trisomy among all clinically recognized
pregnancies, assuming a spontaneous abortion rate of 15%

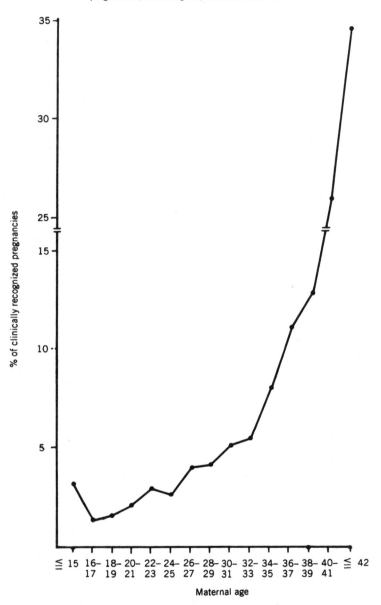

Fig. 4. The relationship between increasing maternal age and trisomy. The graph shows estimates of the overall frequency of trisomy, by maternal age, among all clinically recognized pregnancies (i.e., spontaneous abortions + stillbirths + live births).

WHAT FACTORS PREDISPOSE TO TRISOMY?

Much has been written about factors that increase the likelihood of having a trisomic offspring. For example, there have been reports of associations between trisomy and occupational or environmental exposures (e.g., exposure to pesticides, heavy metals, toxic waste, and electromagnetic fields), medical exposures (e.g., X-rays and anesthetics), reproductive "drugs" (e.g., oral contraceptives, spermicides, and fertility drugs), habituating agents (e.g., tobacco, alcohol, and caffeine-containing drinks) and intrinsic predispositions (e.g., age of the father, parental consanguinity, thyroid autoimmunity, or presence of chromosomal variants such as double nucleolar organizing regions). However, it is important to stress that none of these factors has ever been proved to be associated with trisomy. Indeed, despite exhaustive study there remains only one factor that is incontrovertibly linked to trisomy, namely increasing age of the woman.

The association between maternal age and trisomy is a remarkable one, as indicated by Figure 4. For women in their early twenties, the likelihood of having a clinically recognized pregnancy involving a trisomic fetus is approximately 2–3%, but for women in their mid-forties this value approaches 35%. The association between age and trisomy is observed for almost all human chromosomes and, because the vast majority of such trisomic fetuses perish in utero, this means that the primary effect of age is to increase the frequency of miscarriages. Nevertheless, an age effect is also observed for those trisomies compatible with live birth (i.e., trisomies 13, 18, 21, and the sex chromosome trisomies), thus providing the rationale for offering prenatal diagnosis to older women. It is also important to note that the age effect is observed regardless of race, socioeconomic status, or geographic location, and appears to be part of the normal aging process in females.

Despite a wealth of information characterizing the association between increasing maternal age and trisomy, we remain surprisingly ignorant of the reason for the age effect. Indeed, until recently, we did not even know if the effect was attributable to age-related abnormalities in the egg, or alternatively to an inability of the older uterus to recognize and spontaneously abort an abnormal fetus. This question, at least, seems finally to be resolved, because molecular studies have shown that increased maternal age is correlated with trisomies of maternal, but not paternal, origin. Thus the effect of age is due to something "altered" in the egg itself. However, what this process is and when it occurs are mysteries that remain to be solved.

SUMMARY

As a class, trisomies are the most common genetic disorder in humans, occurring in at least 5% of all human pregnancies. The most common mechanism of origin of trisomy is nondisjunction at maternal meiosis I, although paternal errors are a significant contributor as well. Presently, there is little evidence that race, socioeconomic status, geographic location, or exposure to suspected etiological agents increases the likelihood of trisomy; indeed, the only known factor linked to trisomy is increasing age of the woman.

SUGGESTED READING

Bond DJ, Chandley AC (1983): "Aneuploidy." New York: Oxford University Press.

Hassold T, Abruzzo M, Adkins K, et al. (1996): Human aneuploidy: incidence, origin and etiology. Envir Molec Mut 28:167–175.

Thompson M, McInnes R, Willard HF (1991): "Genetics in Medicine," 5th edition (chapters 9–10). Philadelphia: WB Saunders Co.

Understanding the Importance of Genes on Chromosome 21

David Patterson

Down syndrome affects one in approximately 700 live births. It is therefore the most common genetic cause of significant mental retardation in the human population. Individuals with Down syndrome also have increased risk for health problems such as congenital heart disease, leukemia, and Alzheimer disease. Down syndrome has been recognized as a specific condition for more than 100 years, and the hypothesis that it might be due to chromosomal nondisjunction and the resulting presence of three copies of some human chromosome (trisomy) instead of the normal two, was put forward in the 1930s. Nonetheless, the nature of the genetic alteration remained unknown until 1959 when the cause of the syndrome was shown to be the presence of an extra copy, or trisomy, of chromosome 21, the smallest human chromosome (Lejeune et al., 1959; Jacobs et al., 1959). Study of chromosome 21 and Down syndrome has been at the forefront of human medical genetics research ever since this seminal discovery.

Chromosomes are the structures in the cells of our bodies that contain our genes, the units of heredity that transmit inherited characteristics from parents to offspring. Genes control how we develop from a single cell, the fertilized egg, into a human being. Each of our cells contains 23 pairs of chromosomes, 22 pairs of chromosomes that we number from 1 to 22, plus one pair of sex chromosomes. One chromosome of each pair comes from the mother and one from the father. This is how characteristics of each parent are transmitted from generation to generation.

Each of us has about 100,000 genes that are strung like beads along the chromosomes. The same set of genes is always on the same chromosome, so that every chromosome 21 contains the same set of genes as every other chromosome 21. In addition, the order of the genes on the chromosomes is always the same, except in rare cases in which some sort of rearrangement of genes or chromosomes has occurred.

Chromosome 21 is estimated to contain about 500–1000 genes. People with Down syndrome have three doses of the set of genes on chromosome 21 instead of the two

Down Syndrome: A Promising Future, Together, Edited by Terry J. Hassold and David Patterson
ISBN 0-471-29686-4   Copyright © 1998 by Wiley-Liss, Inc.

doses present in people without Down syndrome. This means that the features of Down syndrome ultimately result from having three copies, instead of two, of these genes. The challenge is to identify these genes, to determine which of them contributes to particular features of Down syndrome, and to attempt to counteract the effects of having three copies of these genes instead of two.

GENE IDENTIFICATION

It is not likely that there is a single gene on chromosome 21 which, when present in three copies, leads to all of the features of Down syndrome. If this were true we would expect to see individuals with Down syndrome and no extra chromosome 21 material, simply by mutation or duplication of the responsible gene.

Most of the time, individuals with Down syndrome have an extra copy of all of chromosome 21. Rarely, however, individuals with Down syndrome have an extra copy of only part of the chromosome. Careful study of the clinical features of these individuals has led to the realization that it is possible to correlate the presence of particular regions of the chromosome with the presence of particular aspects of Down syndrome, for example, congenital heart defects. Conversely, it is possible to eliminate certain chromosomal regions, and therefore the genes in these regions, as causes of some of the characteristics of Down syndrome, because the appearance of these features is not affected by the presence or absence of an extra copy of these regions of the chromosome. This has led to the concept of a correlation between particular regions of the chromosome, the genotype, and particular features of Down syndrome, the phenotype. As we gain more detailed knowledge of the precise location of genes on the chromosome and of the nature of the specific features present in Down syndrome, more meaningful and specific genotype/phenotype correlations will be possible. The importance of this is that it will allow more rapid identification of specific genes responsible for specific aspects of Down syndrome. This information will enhance our ability to design and test possible therapies to mitigate specific aspects of the syndrome.

One of the most challenging, and also most important, aspects of Down syndrome is that of cognitive function. So far, the analysis of partial trisomies has led to the conclusion that there must be several genes on chromosome 21, located in different regions of the chromosome, which can, when present in an extra copy, lead to learning difficulties.

This is not an unexpected result. Human learning is a complex process comprising many components. Therefore, it seems likely that many genes might be involved. This would make it unlikely that there would be a single gene that is solely responsible for the learning difficulties affecting people with Down syndrome. However, it may be that specific genes could be correlated with more highly defined learning weaknesses. Therefore, an important step in analyzing the genetics of the learning difficulties affecting people with Down syndrome is a detailed dissection of these learning strengths and weaknesses. This same principle has been applied successfully to other human conditions, including dyslexia and Williams syndrome (Pennington, 1997). The more precisely and narrowly we can define the learning deficits, the more informed will be our choices of candidate genes that might affect these.

Currently, more than 300 genes and gene fragments from chromosome 21 have been identified. Genes consist of the chemical DNA, which is a linear molecule capable of carrying information in its structure. The information defining the genes on chromosome 21 consists of roughly 40 million bits of linear code. As a part of the Human Genome Project, an international consortium of investigators has been established to decode completely the 40 million bits of information contained on chromosome 21. Already more than 20% of this information is known and is freely available to medical scientists throughout the world. This is particularly important because the time has come when this information, appropriately interpreted and utilized, promises to lead to therapies for certain aspects of Down syndrome.

GENE FUNCTION: ANIMAL MODELS

Characterization of genes includes understanding the role each gene might play in the development of Down syndrome and why an extra copy of this gene could cause some of its features. Often, but by no means always, it is possible to make hypotheses regarding how a particular gene might lead to a particular aspect of Down syndrome. In a significant number of these cases, it is also possible to design a potential chemical treatment approach based on this information.

Before these can be tried in human clinical studies, it is important to test them in animal models, both for effectiveness and for lack of harmful side effects. The best animal models currently available are mice in which regions of chromosome 21 or the equivalent mouse chromosome regions are present in extra copies. Clearly, many aspects of Down syndrome cannot be tested in mice; however, it is possible to test mice for functionality of many of the same body systems, including regions of the brain, which appear to pose special problems for individuals with Down syndrome.

The first mouse model useful for the study of Down syndrome was the trisomy 16 mouse (Gropp et al., 1975). This mouse is useful because perhaps as many as 65% of the genes located on human chromosome 21 are located on mouse chromosome 16. This mouse has many features reminiscent of Down syndrome, but has two very serious disadvantages. It does not survive birth, and it is trisomic for genes not on human chromosome 21 and is not trisomic for all genes that are on human chromosome 21. Therefore developmental events that occur after birth cannot be studied in this mouse model and it is hard to be sure that the developmental problems seen in the mice are actually caused by genes that are located on chromosome 21 in humans.

Recently, this situation has changed dramatically. Dr. Muriel Davisson has developed a mouse that eliminates many of the problems seen with the trisomy 16 mouse (Davisson et al., 1990). This mouse, called the Ts65Dn mouse, is trisomic only for the region of mouse chromosome 16, which contains the same genes as human chromosome 21; it survives well into adulthood; and it has behavioral and learning features reminiscent of those seen in individuals with Down syndrome. This mouse model amply verifies the approach of creating partial trisomy mice with characteristics that reflect aspects of human learning and behavior.

A second approach to creation of mouse models to study aspects of Down syndrome is purposely to introduce specific human genes or groups of genes into mice and to examine the effect of the presence of the extra copy of these genes on the mice. These mice, called transgenic mice because human *genes* have been *trans*mitted into the mice, have begun to serve a valuable role in the study of Down syndrome. Indeed, mice with very defined small regions of human chromosome 21 and even single human genes located on human chromosome 21 have been constructed having some features reminiscent of Down syndrome.

CLINICAL RELEVANCE

With the identification of genes contributing to the phenotype of Down syndrome, we will be able to consider methods of treatment. There are two general treatment possibilities. As discussed earlier, if the genes have a known function, it may be possible to manipulate these functions pharmacologically or by diet. On the other hand, if no information on a specific gene's function is available, or if there is no known way safely to influence the function of the gene, it may still be possible to intervene. This is because the problem in Down syndrome is that the important genes are present in three copies instead of two. In general, it appears that this leads to the gene function roughly proportional to the number of copies of the gene, that is, 150% of the level in individuals with only two copies of the gene. Therefore, if we could "turn down" the gene function by one-third, we might mitigate its harmful effects. Methods have been developed that promise to allow this and currently are being tested for effectiveness in cells in culture with promising results.

CONCLUSIONS

Within the next few years it seems certain that all of the genetic information on chromosome 21 will be obtained. Fortunately, mouse models are being developed as this genetic information is being obtained which seem to have the promise of serving as guides toward understanding the medical and learning problems encountered by individuals with Down syndrome. The combination of these two major medical research endeavors should allow for the rapid development and testing of possible therapies to aid in dealing with these difficulties. In this way, the human medical genetics research for Down syndrome which has been ongoing for the past decades should truly contribute to assuring a promising future, together.

REFERENCES

Davisson MT, Schmidt C, Akeson EC (1990): Segmental trisomy of murine chromosome 16: a new model system for studying Down syndrome. In Patterson D, Epstein CJ (eds.): "Molecular Genetics of Chromosome 21 and Down Syndrome." Progress in Clinical and Biological Research, Volume 360. New York: John Wiley & Sons, pp. 263–280.

Gropp A, Kolbus U, Giers D (1975): Systematic approach to the study of trisomy in the mouse II. Cytogenet Cell Genet 14:42–62.

Jacobs P, Baikie A, Court-Brown W, Strong J (1959): The somatic chromosomes in mongolism. Lancet I:710–711.

Lejeune J, Gauthier M, Turpin R (1959): Etudes des chromosomes somatiques de neau enfants mongliens. CR Acad Sci (Paris) 248:1721–1722.

Pennington BF (1997): Using genetics to dissect cognition. Am J Hum Genet 60:13–16.

IV. Alternative and Nonconventional Therapies

Pharmacological Therapies for Down Syndrome: Current Information

George T. Capone

The past two decades have witnessed unprecedented growth and development in the neurosciences. Although there is still much to be learned about the neurochemistry of Down syndrome, several lines of research suggest that certain neurotransmitter systems are vulnerable to impairment in persons with this condition. Pharmacological therapies are being used increasingly for a variety of neurobehavioral conditions which sometimes coexist with Down syndrome. Together with behavioral and educational treatments, medications may be helpful in reducing disturbances of mood, affect, attention, and certain maladaptive behaviors that can interfere with the quality of life. The prospect of pharmacological treatment for cognitive impairment is continually being discussed and sought after by many families.

Pharmacological strategies for cognitive enhancement are still in the development stage; recommendations for drug intervention are premature and cannot be routinely prescribed for persons with Down syndrome at this time. As new "cognitive medicines" are developed it is imperative that they be thoroughly and carefully tested to ensure safety and efficacy. The need for clinical neurobiologic research on behalf of persons with Down syndrome is emphasized in this chapter. Within this context, the philosophy and design of conducting clinical research trials are discussed. Patient and parents' rights are emphasized.

Several topics regarding pharmacological treatments used in persons with Down syndrome are presented here: The first part focuses on neurobehavioral disorders associated with Down syndrome and their treatment, specifically, attention deficit hyperactivity disorder (ADHD) and depression. The second part addresses the prospect of cognitive medications and their use in persons with Down syndrome. Finally, the rationale, design, and implementation of clinical research trials when testing new pharmacologic therapies for Down syndrome are discussed.

Down Syndrome: A Promising Future, Together, Edited by Terry J. Hassold and David Patterson
ISBN 0-471-29686-4   Copyright © 1998 by Wiley-Liss, Inc.

NEUROBEHAVIORAL DISORDERS

What do we know about neurobehavioral disorders in Down syndrome? More is known about prevalence and diagnostic criteria than pharmacological treatments at this point. In fact, there are very few studies that address any of these issues specifically within the setting of Down syndrome. During the past 5 years, several studies have appeared in the literature which look at the prevalence and diagnostic criteria for depression and dementia in Down syndrome. Regarding several of the other neurobehavioral disorders, we depend mostly upon isolated case reports. Almost nothing has been published regarding the use of psychoactive medications and whether there are differences in the way persons with Down syndrome respond to specific classes of medication. Based upon the combined clinical experience of people working in the field, there is no obvious reason to believe that persons with Down syndrome respond differently from other persons with a cognitive disability. Remember, however, that response to any medication can show significant individual variation.

Presentation

Often a neurobehavioral disorder is first suspected by parents, teachers, or other individuals who work closely with the child. It is not unusual for parents to be given very different interpretations of this behavior by teachers, relatives, or well-meaning friends; typically this information is often conflicting. Probably the most common piece of information that is given to parents by professionals is that the behavior is "a part of the Down syndrome." Clinical experience, however, indicates that this is not always the case and that a separate neurobehavioral diagnosis is often warranted.

When a neurobehavioral disorder is suspected, parents usually ask:

How common is the disorder?
How is it diagnosed?
How is it treated?
What are the goals of the treatment?

Professionals seeing these children need to be attentive to these concerns expressed by the family. It is important that the child be evaluated by someone with experience with children with Down syndrome or at least other children with developmental and cognitive disabilities with neurobehavioral problems. Additional factors that professionals need to consider when evaluating a child for a neurobehavioral disorder include the following: (1) specific medical conditions that may have a behavioral presentation; (2) the degree of cognitive and language impairment; (3) the age and gender of the individual, because certain disorders are more common at various times in the life cycle; and perhaps most importantly, (4) psychosocial and environmental stressors that may precipitate or exacerbate many different kinds of behaviors.

Dual Diagnosis

Sometimes the term "dual diagnosis" is used to describe persons with mental retardation and a psychiatric illness. Criteria used for diagnosing a psychiatric illness are based on a standardized set of criteria that have been developed over the past several decades by the American Psychiatric Association (*Diagnostic and Statistical Manual of Mental Disorders,* DSM-IV, 1994). Although many of the criteria given are helpful in conceptualizing the broad variety of symptoms that can be classified under a single disorder, there are certain limits inherent to the use of DSM-IV. Specifically, many of the criteria developed apply to individuals of average intelligence and are not specific to individuals with cognitive impairments. Again, the need for evaluation by a psychiatrist, developmental pediatrician, or child neurologist who is familiar with seeing individuals with developmental disabilities and dual diagnoses is emphasized. Many of the criteria used to arrive at a formal diagnosis are based on a careful history of the development of symptoms over time. Typically, this history is best obtained from parents, teachers, and other caretakers who are intimately familiar with the day-to-day routines and behavior of the individuals. There are several limitations inherent in evaluating persons with cognitive impairments; in particular (1) the diminished ability for self-reporting of symptoms; (2) misinterpretation of symptoms based upon the level of social skill development and social integration experienced by that individual; (3) extreme environmental stress or medical illness that may further diminish speech and cognitive processing and/or lead to the development of maladaptive behaviors that may be misinterpreted as "psychotic behaviors." This is particularly true in the setting of major depression.

Attention Deficit Hyperactivity Disorder

Prevalence. One study by Meyers and Pueschel (1991), estimates the frequency of ADHD in children with Down syndrome (< 20 years) at about 6–8%; in adults (> 20 years), it is seen in about 2–3% of their outpatient population. Overall this is similar to the frequency of ADHD in children in the general population (2–10%). Compared to non-Down syndrome, cognitively impaired groups from other studies, the frequency of ADHD in children with Down syndrome may be decreased. Such studies have indicated an 8–15% frequency of ADHD in children with unclassified cognitive impairment.

Diagnostic Criteria. The diagnostic criteria used to define ADHD include (1) short attention span, (2) distractibility, (3) poor impulse control, (4) motor hyperactivity, (5) fidgeting, and (6) low frustration tolerance. These six features represent the most commonly observed features of the disorder. However, disorganization, failure to complete tasks, frequent interruptions or intrusions, moodiness, sleep disturbances, and poor sense of danger may also be seen.

To make the diagnosis of ADHD with confidence, symptoms must be present to such a degree as to cause impairment in academic or social function. Their duration must be of at least 6 months or greater with onset prior to 7 years of age. It is also important that the clinician evaluating the child be assured that these symptoms are more frequent or severe than in the majority of children with Down syndrome of the same mental age. It is usually clear to most clinicians working with Down syndrome that DS/ADHD children are a different group, readily distinguishable from their peers with Down syndrome without ADHD.

Associated Problems. Some of the associated problems seen with ADHD include (1) an increased risk of accident or injury, (2) difficulty with participating in an academic or therapeutic program, (3) social rejection by peers, and (4) behavioral disorders, most commonly, noncompliance, oppositional defiance, and aggressive behaviors. It is usually these associated problems that first bring ADHD to the attention of clinicians.

Professionals evaluating children with Down syndrome for suspected ADHD need to consider (1) the cognitive level of the child, (2) the degree of expressive speech impairment (and associated behaviors), (3) medical conditions (hearing loss, hypo- or hyperthyroidism, lead toxicity, obstructive sleep apnea with hypoxemia, and medication effects, especially caffeine, antihistamines, or bronchodilators). In addition, other psychiatric disorders may mimic ADHD, especially anxiety disorder, post-traumatic stress disorders, conduct or oppositional disorders, stereotypical movement disorder, and the autistic-spectrum disorders. As always, a thorough family, school, or workplace history must be obtained to explore for stressful life events that may precipitate some of these symptoms.

Treatment. Treatments for ADHD include (1) educational and environmental interventions, (2) behavioral management, and (3) medications. Typically, educational and environmental interventions and/or behavioral management are tried for a 3–6 month period. If the individual shows no appreciable change or benefit from these therapies, then a trial of medication is often warranted. The targets of pharmacotherapy for ADHD are the dopaminergic and noradrenergic neurotransmitter systems of the brain. Dopamine plays a role in reward, attention, and executive function whereas norepinephrine plays a role in arousal and anxiety.

First-line medications for ADHD include stimulant medications that augment dopamine and norepinephrine neurotransmission. Typically, methylphenidate (Ritalin), dextroamphetamine (Dexedrine), or pemoline (Cylert) would be used. Side effects may include insomnia, loss of appetite, growth suppression, or tics. The alpha-adrenergic agent clonidine (Catapres) is often used as second line therapy. Side effects may include sedation, dry mouth, or low blood pressure. Antidepressants, particularly the tricyclic compounds, have been used for ADHD, in particular imipramine (Tofranil). The tricyclics may cause anticholinergic side effects such as dry mouth, blurry vision, urinary retention, constipation, or drowsiness; however, many of these effects can be minimized at the low doses used.

The basic principles to follow when initiating a medication trial in children should be observed. Start with a low dose, advance to a higher dose as tolerated, and continuously monitor for target symptoms and side effects.

Depression

Prevalence. A study of the frequency of major depression in persons with Down syndrome by Meyer and Pueschel shows this to be relatively uncommon in children (< 20 years). However, an increase in the frequency of depression is noted in adults with Down syndrome (> 20 years). Meyers noted a (5–12%) incidence of major depression. Other studies have shown that major depression disproportionately affects females by a ratio of about 3:1. This frequency of depression in adults with Down syndrome appears to be increased compared to adults in the general population (2–5%) as well as non-Down syndrome, cognitively impaired control groups (4%) from other studies. Persons with Down syndrome may be vulnerable to developing depression, owing to a combination of neurobiologic, psychological, and medical factors.

Diagnostic Criteria. Diagnostic criteria for major depression according to DSM-IV include at least five of the following: (1) depressed mood, (2) decreased interest in previously pleasurable activities, (3) weight loss or gain, (4) sleep disturbance, (5) fatigue, (6) agitation, (7) psychomotor slowing, (8) impaired concentration, and (9) feelings of guilt or worthlessness.

To arrive at the diagnosis, symptoms must be present to such a degree as to cause significant impairment in social or occupational function. Duration of symptoms must be at least 2 weeks and should not be attributable to medications, concurrent medical conditions, or another psychiatric disorder. Common medical problems that may manifest with depressive symptomatology include hypothyroidism, cardiac failure, visual or hearing loss, vitamin B12 deficiency, seizures, leukemia, and dementia. It is critical for physicians evaluating persons with Down syndrome for suspected depression to rule out any other treatable medical conditions prior to arriving at this diagnosis. It is also important to emphasize that depressive symptoms may present with something of a "psychotic flavor" in persons with cognitive impairment. The incidence of psychoses in persons with Down syndrome is actually quite low, although bipolar (manic–depressive) illness is sometimes seen.

A study by Cooper and Collacott examined a population of 378 adults with Down syndrome living in the United Kingdom. Of these, 42 (11.1%) were identified as having had at least one depressive episode. The average age of onset of depression was 29.5 years. Interestingly, only 50% of subjects met DSM criteria for major depression and only 50% responded to antidepressant medication. The most common symptoms observed (greater than 50% of cases) included (1) decreased interest or pleasure, (2) depressed mood, (3) psychomotor retardation, (4) frequent crying, (5) fatigue, and (6) weight loss or gain. Symptoms observed in fewer than 50% of cases included sleep disturbance, aggression/tantrums, frequent physical complaints, reduced speech, anxiety, poor concentration, irritability, or labile mood. Mood congruent delusions were seen in about 5% of persons, and a history of mania was seen in about 11%. It is noteworthy that feelings of guilt/worthlessness or recurrent thoughts of death were not observed in individuals with Down syndrome, although these symptoms are common in depression in the general population.

This study emphasizes a number of important and interesting points: (1) the high prevalence of neurovegetative signs in persons with Down syndrome and depression; (2) the absence of suicidal ideation; and (3) some of the inherent difficulties with pharmacological treatment in this population. Clearly, additional studies are required to elaborate on the finding of treatment-resistant depression, particularly as it relates to the issue of dementia. It is also imperative for clinicians to collect clinical data and report on their experiences in treating Down syndrome subjects with selective serotonin reuptake inhibitors (SSRIs) and the newer combination serotonin/norepineph-rine reuptake inhibitor (SNRIs) medications.

Treatment. Treatment for major depression is multifaceted and includes (1) medication, (2) stress reduction, (3) re-socialization, (4) counseling for the individual and family when indicated, and (5) education for the family and staff. Typically, all five approaches are introduced over several visits in a way that does not overburden the family. It is particularly important to identify and alleviate any sources of ongoing stress in the lives of the individual either at home or in the workplace. It is not unusual for depressed persons with Down syndrome to be with-drawn from their school or workplace environment only to spend many long, un-structured hours in the care of family members. In such circumstances, the individual needs may need to be reintroduced into the social milieu via recreational or group activities as tolerated. Medications are particularly helpful in treating the neurovegetative symptoms of depression and getting the individual "jump started" on the road to recovery.

The targets of pharmacotherapy for major depression include the serotonergic and noradrenergic neurotransmitter systems. Serotonin plays a prominent role in mood, aggression, appetite and the sleep–wake cycle. Norepinephrine, as previously mentioned, has been implicated in arousal and anxiety states.

First-line antidepressant medications usually include the SSRIs, such as fluoxe-tine (Prozac), paroxetine (Paxil), or sertraline (Zoloft). More recently, the SNRIs have been introduced and include the drugs venlafaxine (Effexor) and nefazadone (Serazone). Tricyclic antidepressants may also be useful and include imipramine (Tofranil), desipramine (Norpramin), and nortriptyline (Pamelor). Side effects asso-ciated with the SSRIs and SNRIs may include insomnia, jitteriness, headache, or gastrointestinal distress. Overall, the SSRIs and SNRIs are usually well tolerated, particularly in comparison to the tricyclic antidepressant compounds. Several of these antidepressant medications have also been shown to be helpful in treating anx-iety, agitation, and obsessive–compulsive symptomatology which may occur either in isolation or within the setting of major depression.

PROSPECTS FOR COGNITIVE THERAPIES

The character of Scarecrow in the 1939 classic "The Wizard of Oz" is remembered as an individual who went to great lengths on a dare from a wizard who promised to increase his mental capacity. Consider, though, that Scarecrow was really quite capa-ble in his own right of performing many clever feats of mental acumen when pre-sented with the proper challenge, motivation, and team support. *He didn't need a wizard* to make him shine. He had this strength all along. In many ways, this reminds me of children with Down syndrome who have the capacity to learn, think, and par-ticipate meaningfully in educational and social activities. The message is that cogni-tive medicines used to help individuals overcome a limitation should never be intended to replace the early intervention or educational programs that continue to benefit children with Down syndrome. It is likely that in the not too distant future, some combination of pharmacotherapy designed to enhance or preserve neuronal function will be used with greater frequency in combination with the educational programs already in place.

History of Biomedical Interventions for Down Syndrome

The modern history of biomedical treatments for persons with Down syndrome goes back at least several decades. A number of these treatments have been advocated by professionals within the medical community. Many of these agents were recommended based upon an apparently sound scientific rationale, others, not. Various hormones including thyroid hormone, steroid hormone, and growth hormone occasionally have been recommended by practitioners, as well as various combinations of vitamins, enzymes, minerals, amino acids, and other nutritional supplements. A number of these therapies have been tested in double-blind, placebo-controlled studies. In other cases, these therapies have been recommended on the basis of theoretical benefits. By currently accepted medical standards, none of these agents given either singly or in combination has ever been shown to improve cognitive performance or change any of the phenotypic features of Down syndrome. The only exception is thyroid hormone for the treatment of hypothyroidism, which may be associated with some degree of reversible cognitive dysfunction.

Cognitive-Enhancing Medications

Ideally, a cognitive enhancing medication would be specific in its action and have a low incidence of side effects. Its effects should also be dose-dependent and reversible, without long-term negative consequences. In Down syndrome such medications would be useful for several different purposes: (1) to enhance the neural substrate for cognitive processes during early development; (2) to enhance the storage and retrieval of newly learned information throughout childhood and adulthood; and (3) to prevent the premature demise in cognitive function that so often occurs with aging. For children and young adults enhancement in learning and memory function may translate into improvements in vocabulary and language use, problem solving skills, regulation of attention, social adaptive function, and perhaps even behavior. There is as yet no precedent for enhancement of these functions during childhood.

Recently, the notion of cognitive-enhancing medications has become something more than just talk. The pharmaceutical industry is very interested in and actively pursuing the development of cognitive enhancing compounds because of the "favorable demographics" of Alzheimer disease (AD) in the general population. Currently, about four million people in the United States suffer from Alzheimer disease, at a cost of 60–90 billion dollars per year, and an untold amount in human suffering. By the year 2040 an estimated 14 million persons in the United States will be affected by AD. The premise that we may be able to enhance or preserve cognitive function is based on the concept that neuronal function can be enhanced or preserved. To do this, a significant foundation of basic science research needs to be established, specifically regarding the pharmacological regulation of neuronal function. Broadly speaking, there are two approaches for enhancing cognition in humans which have special relevance for individuals with Down syndrome. One approach is to enhance electrochemical neurotransmission in the brain. This approach is generally considered to be of "short-term" benefit based upon enhancement of existing synaptic function. Current strategies have targeted the cholinergic and glutamatergic neurotransmitter systems that serve an important role in learning, memory, and synaptic development. Medications such as physostigmine, tacrine, donepezil, aniracetam, and piracetam have been used with some success for this purpose in adults with dementia. A second approach attempts to protect neurons from premature dysfunction and/or degeneration. A variety of biologically active agents including neurotrophins, antioxidant compounds, anti-inflammatories, and anti-amyloid agents are currently under development by pharmaceutical companies for therapeutic use in humans. It is important to emphasize that virtually none of these compounds has been tested in individuals with Down syndrome for either safety or efficacy. In the absence of carefully conducted clinical research trials, none of these agents can be routinely prescribed at this time.

Neurochemistry of Memory and Learning

Cholinergic neurons, located in the basal forebrain region at the base of the brain, send axons upward to provide diffuse innervation to the hippocampus and cerebral cortex. The neurotransmitter acetylcholine synchronizes cortical and hippocampal neurons and readies the cortex to receive incoming sensory information. Inputs into the hippocampus from the various cortical subregions process information from the modalities of vision, hearing, touch, smell, and motion. Neurons from these cortical regions send their connections into the amygdala and hippocampus, which serve as a way station for new memory. These neurons use the neurotransmitter glutamate to provide the signal that actually encodes memory in neurons. Sensory information arriving to the amygdala and hippocampus in the form of electrochemical signals is usually stored as an unstable "short-term memory" for a brief period of time. If this "memory trace" is reinforced by concurrent electrochemical signals from other sensory modalities, then it is more likely that it will survive to become a "long-term memory." It is well known that memories that have a significant emotional content are more likely to be remembered than those that are deemed emotionally neutral. Long-term memories are stored in modality specific cortical association regions distributed throughout the neocortex. For these reasons, pharmaceutical companies have targeted the cholinergic and glutamatergic systems as areas of intervention for enhancing memory and new learning in humans.

TESTING COGNITIVE-ENHANCING MEDICATIONS: CLINICAL DRUG TRIALS

When testing a medication in any medically vulnerable population, questions of safety should outweigh those of efficacy initially. In the initial phase of testing, new medications are usually given to a large number of healthy, adult volunteers to determine the type and frequency of unwanted side effects. Less often new medications are tested in healthy children. Drug efficacy designed to alleviate specific target symptoms then becomes the focus of the second and third phases of drug testing.

Clinical Research Design

Research studies must be designed around specific questions or hypotheses that test the proposed effect of a medication on one or more target-symptoms. Targeting cognitive impairment can be a difficult undertaking because of difficulties in measuring intelligence against the background of neurodevelopmental change. Such studies must be carefully designed with well-defined outcome measures, systematic data collection, and analysis using appropriate statistical methods. It is challenging to design well-controlled studies in children with cognitive impairments because of problems in identifying meaningful outcome measures. Simply measuring IQ, for instance, is fraught with difficulties including the fact that IQ represents a very global measurement of overall function. In order to avoid unwanted bias or uninterpretable data, rigorous experimental design is of utmost importance. This usually entails *random subject selection* with assignment to either treatment or nontreatment groups. The use of a *placebo control* is often quite helpful in discerning true medication effects from those perceived to occur because of increased anticipation. A *triple-blind* design is one in which parents, subjects, and investigators are blinded as to whether the subject is receiving an active compounds or placebo. Finally, a *cross-over* in treatment which allows each subject to receive both placebo and active medication for a period of time allows each child to serve as his or her own control and increases the statistical certainty of finding subtle, individual treatment effects. It also ensures that each individual subject will have the opportunity to receive a trial of active compound.

Controversial or Untested Treatments

In researching untested drug therapies, it should be obvious that anecdotal observation, although important, does not exclude the need for controlled clinical-scientific studies; no matter how convincing the treatment effect appears to be or how high the frustration associated with the lack of effective treatments. Furthermore, the research findings must be evaluated based upon the proper design, conduct, and statistical interpretation of the measured results, not upon the reputation or opinion of the investigator or institution they represent.

Patient and Parental Rights

Patient and parental rights need to be observed during the period of clinical testing and consist of a number of essential elements including (1) informed *written consent* with a complete explanation given of anticipated risks and benefits; (2) an explanation of *costs,* if any; (3) a review of any medically acceptable *alternatives,* other than the study treatment; and (4) the preservation of the parents' right to *decline* or *withdraw* from the study, without penalty, and the right to ask questions. Any human research conducted within a university, hospital, or other medical facility must be reviewed and approved by an institutional review board for consideration of human safety and ethically acceptable research practice. Parents who allow their children to receive untested therapies do so at their own risk because issues of safety and efficacy remain essentially unaddressed. Parents are discouraged from allowing their children to participate in any research study or untested therapy not respectful of these rights.

MEDICAL SCIENCE: A SOCIAL ENDEAVOR

Assuming that the pharmaceutical industry will continue to research and develop potential cognitive-enhancing compounds, we in the Down syndrome community need to determine our responsibility and level of interest in using such medications. Medical professionals need to become familiar with data that support safety and efficacy prior to prescribing such medications for their patients.

Cognitive-enhancing medications that are both safe and efficacious will be of great interest to families of children with Down syndrome. However, this will also place additional burdens on parents as decision makers who must then decide whether or not to use pharmacologically active compounds in an effort to enhance cognitive development. As medical professionals it will be important to educate and guide families through the often complex maze of decision-making, and urge them always to consider the potential for risks and benefits inherent in any medically invasive therapy. Ultimately, these decisions will rest on the shoulders of parents to decide what is right for their child.

There will always be ethical and economic considerations inherent in any new biomedical treatment particularly those that appear to hold the promise of cognitive enhancement. Parents, family members, health professionals, and persons with Down syndrome will need to embrace certain basic questions. Is cognitive enhancement a worthwhile goal for children with Down syndrome? To what degree do we value and want to explore clinical neuropharmacological research in children with Down syndrome, and who should pay for it? What does this say about the value we place on cognitive ability and the intrinsic worth of each individual in our society? These are trying questions, with no clear right or wrong answer, only risks, benefits, and costs. The benefit of embracing these questions as a united front of parents and professionals is that we will learn together, and establish clear guidelines for safety and efficacy in developing innovative biomedical treatments for Down syndrome. The risks of failing to address these questions as partners is a continuing dearth of real solutions, a lack of research direction, and divisiveness within the Down syndrome community. I propose that a coherent system for selecting and evaluating new therapeutic agents, for safety and efficacy, be established for children with Down syndrome so that advances in therapy may occur in a timely fashion both today and in the decades to come.

I close with this quotation from the seventeenth century philosopher, Francis Bacon, who helped establish the scientific method of inquiry.

> It would be an unsound fancy and self-contradictory to expect that things which have never yet been done can be done except by means which have never yet been tried.—Francis Bacon, *Novum Organum* (1620), Aphorism VI

REFERENCES

American Psychiatric Association (1994): "Diagnostic and Statistical Manual of Mental Disorders," 4th ed. Washington, DC: p. 886.

Cooper SA, Collacott RA (1994): Clinical features and diagnostic criteria of depression in Down's Syndrome. Brit J Psychiatr 165:399–403.

Green JM, Dennis J, Bennets LA (1989): Attention disorder in a group of young Down's syndrome children. J Ment Defic Res 33:105–122.

Johnston MV (1992): Cognitive disorders. In: "Principles of Drug Therapy in Neurology." Philadelphia: F.A. Davis Co., pp. 226–267.

Kumar V, Cantillon M (1996): Update on the development of medication for memory and cognition in Alzheimer's disease. Psychiatr Ann 26(5):280–284.

Marx J (1996): Searching for drugs that combat Alzheimer's. Science 273(July 5):50–53.

Mercugliano M (1993): Psychopharmacology in children with developmental disorders, in The child with developmental disabilities. Pediatr Clin N Am 40(3):593–616.

Meyers BA, Pueschel SM (1991): Psychiatric disorders in persons with Down Syndrome. J Nervous Ment Dis 179:609–613.

Van Dyke DC (1995): Alternative and unconventional therapies in children with Down Syndrome. In: "Medical and Surgical Care for Children with Down Syndrome: A Parent's Guide. Bethesda, MD: Woodbine House, pp. 277–302.

Alternative Therapies: From a Parent's Perspective

Philip Mattheis

Children with Down syndrome (or other disabilities), may have a variety of problems or needs. Some of these issues can be easily managed using available "standard" therapies or services. Resolution of other problems may require more effort or a combination of resources. In some cases there are no "standard" or conventional solutions that seem to satisfy the need or question. In such cases, uncommon approaches may be required or explored in the hope of achieving some level of success.

Although medical therapies and processes are commonly accepted as "the standards" for addressing matters of health and illness, this has been the case only for the past century or so. Even within that time frame, for many conditions medicine has only recently had truly effective therapies to offer. For a wide variety of conditions, medical options have been only part of the choices available.

When there are a lot of answers to a particular problem, it signifies that either the problem is easy to fix, or none of the solutions is really effective. Solutions that provide part of the answer are further developed, whereas options of less proven value fade from use. When one or a few treatment approaches become well established as effective, the emergence or promotion of alternatives tends to fade as well.

People with disabilities often have problems or conditions that do not respond well to standard therapies. Consequently, for many conditions there are many proposed alternatives from which to choose. Many times the choices are made for very individual reasons that have little to do with medicine, with no real evidence that the therapy might be effective.

ALTERNATIVE TO WHAT?

Conventional Medical Systems

The diagnosis of Down syndrome is usually an unexpected piece of information, delivered by a representative of the medical system, to a family often unprepared for

Down Syndrome: A Promising Future, Together, Edited by Terry J. Hassold and David Patterson
ISBN 0-471-29686-4   Copyright © 1998 by Wiley-Liss, Inc.

the long series of adjustments that follow. Frequently, that medical system is the setting for many of those adjustments. When everything works well, the informing is handled sensitively, and the family and child are helped into a good start.

Unfortunately, the tone in which the baby's diagnosis is shared with the family is often dominated by a sense of gloom that hangs over what should be a joyful transition, as the family comes to know their newest member. Occasionally, the medical information is inaccurate, outdated, or loaded with bias. In either situation, the conventional medical system fails to support the family adequately at a critical point of need.

If problems appear, and no easy answers follow, that conventional medical system may again have little help to offer. Certainly, previous experience may direct the family to look elsewhere.

Nothing

Some families return home with their new baby to a home and community that offer little or no support. Again, misinformation and low expectations make for a void of choices.

Early Intervention and Education Supports

Although there may be as much variety in style of operation or attitudes of professionals as in medicine, early intervention and educational systems provide additional sets of conventional offerings to children with Down syndrome and their families.

When the supports are directed individually at needs identified for the child, and are designed and provided with respect for the family's input, early intervention and educational services very often play key roles in promoting the child's development.

However, if educational services are provided based upon a general category or diagnosis ("All children with Down syndrome go to this program"), and do not reflect an understanding of the specific needs of that child, there is a increased likelihood that the child and family will again be failed by a conventional system, and will look for alternatives.

WHY SEEK ALTERNATIVES?

A Need for Options

When problems occur for a child, and none of the conventional supports or networks provide any effective resolutions, families may feel forced to turn elsewhere.

The Family Already Uses a Variety of Treatment Types

A large percentage of families who choose alternative therapies for their child with a disability have made similar use of nonstandard therapies for themselves, as part of their own health care choices. For this group of people, the "standards" are shifted.

In fact, most of us have our own uniquely developed standards for our own health care, which may include a varied mix of ethnic or "folk remedies" (some very effective), superstition, "conventional service," and professional or semiprofessional services less likely to be considered "conventional" (such as chiropracty, accupuncture, and massage therapy).

Alternative Theories Suggest New Potentials for Treatment

When the standard notions leave little room for hope, the attraction of new ideas may be irresistible. Friends and other family members may hear of the alternatives and add their voices, again responding to the attraction of the positive reinterpretation of possibilities.

"New" theories may simply challenge common misconceptions. For example, many children with Down syndrome have learned to read. Most traditional educational systems have not recognized this potential, and have not gained the result. In this case, the "old theory" states that most people with Down syndrome can't read because they are mentally retarded owing to Down syndrome. The "new theory" maintains that most people with Down syndrome can't read because expectations have been too low, and they haven't been taught the necessary skills.

Some theories present alternative notions of why people with Down syndrome are different, and then propose treatments that follow those notions. If the treatments work, the theories gain attention. If other explanations for the success can't be found, the alternative explanations may gain acceptance.

Alternative Therapies May Work

Most "standard therapies" begin life as alternatives to some other method or procedure, and become "standard" exactly by the increasing use that goes with success.

Alternative Therapy Proponents Provide Strong Support Networks

When traditional networks have failed, contact with a unified group of advocates may provide an important substitute. With attention to educational interventions and increased expectations in addition to the specific therapies, the child may well show marked improvements. The family's coping success may also increase dramatically.

WHAT ARE THE POTENTIAL BENEFITS?

Improvement in the Target Problem

The goal of any therapy should be aimed at a particular problem, with the hope that treatment will improve the outcome more than it causes new trouble. Children with disabilities frequently have health or illness issues that do not respond to the standards. More often, the child's function is delayed from normal, and is not very responsive to whatever services are being provided from conventional sources.

When the problem has no apparent mainstream solution, alternatives may offer the only possibilities of effective change.

Savings in Time, Energy, or Money

If an alternative approach to a problem is cheap, easily available, and/or fits the family's and child's life-style better than the conventional answer, the balance may preserve family resources.

Early Access to the Next Standard of Care

As mentioned above, current standards had to start somewhere. Getting on board early as new solutions are discovered avoids wasting effort or losing time on less effective treatments.

Peace of Mind

Whether or not a therapy works, if the problem has no other solution, there is benefit in looking at all the options to be sure no potential answers will be missed.

Avoidance of the Medical System

Sometimes a family may have such a painful history of interactions with physicians, hospitals, and other parts of the medical system that any alternative seems preferable. At other times, the alternative may be tried in addition to medical visits as a less intrusive way to address some of the issues.

Many conventional medical solutions carry well-known risks and side effects. An alternative that has less risk while providing the same or better outcome is an obvious choice.

WHAT ARE THE POTENTIAL RISKS?
Cost in Time, Energy, or Money

Part of the balancing that goes into decisions about treatment choices has to measure the costs in comparison to the potential risks. If the therapy chosen does not work, those resources are lost to other possible choices. Few families have all the money, time, or energy that they need; for most, at least some of those resources are severly limited.

Delay in Essential "Conventional" Medical Care

When a large investment of time, energy, and/or money has been directed at alternative methods, other immediate needs may be put off. This balancing of priorities sometimes can put the child's health at real risk. A 1-year-old child with a serious cardiac defect, for example, should not have surgery postponed to allow the family to travel cross country to attend extended sessions of neuromotor patterning. Medical stability is an essential priority of any child's health management plan.

Side Effects of the Therapy Are Often Not Well Known or Described

Many alternative approaches have not been completely studied to define the risks, and advocates often downplay the possibility of problems. Safety should be the first priority of every decision made regarding therapies (conventional or alternative).

Alternative Theories May Be Wrong

If the new notion of cause or possibilities changes the family's view of their child, but is later shown to be incorrect, the family may be left with confusion and distress as they attempt to make sense of the change.

A current alternative theory presents Down syndrome as a progressive condition that begins after birth of an essentially normal child. The proponents claim that their treatment protocol will protect babies and children from those progressive effects. If a family accepts that theory, but finds that the treatment does not seem to be preventing differences in appearance or function, they may assume that their child is doomed to long-term failure.

In reality, most babies with Down syndrome have similar characteristic facial differences which are present at birth (even in very premature infants). In most children, that appearance shifts a bit as they get older. There is no evidence that anything short of surgery will really change the bone and skin relationships.

Alienation from Existing Support Networks

Some proponents of alternative therapies work aggressively to undermine existing parent groups that do not accept the alternative theory or therapy. In several recent examples, this kind of challenge has become a dominant intrusion into the support organization's agenda, and left the membership fragmented by anger and confusion. If the alternative supports do not replace all the resources damaged in the process, the net outcome is a loss for all involved.

HOW DO YOU CHOOSE?—"RED FLAGS" TO WATCH FOR IN EVALUATING ALTERNATIVES

The style of promotion can often be very helpful in trying to sort out the claims made by advocates for a therapy or theory. Separating the style issues from the substance of the claims being made can be very difficult. The following "red flags" should prompt some suspicion about the claims being made.

"Pseudo-Science," Claims and Theories Presented as Science, That Are Not Supported by Research

Some advocates commonly mention "many studies" that support the claims being made, but the studies are never described or referenced in a way that the original works can be reviewed. The research in question may have been badly done or have little to do with the subject, or may not even exist.

Good research is difficult to do. Many studies are not well done, or may give only limited information on the subject. An open scientific debate demands that any claims being made be backed up by specific citations that allow for discussion of those supporting papers. When advocates refuse to provide references to support their claims, it is difficult to debate the value of those supports.

In some cases, details about research into a therapy may be offered only as part of the package that is purchased, often at high cost. After a large investment has been made, it may be impossible to keep an open mind about the information presented.

Refusal to Collaborate in Objective Research

Too often, advocates refuse to be part of research studies that could verify their claims of results. They may be so certain of their program that they consider it unethical to withhold the treatment even for the duration of a study trial. In reality, if a program works that well, it should be easy to prove. Refusing to engage in meaningful research then delays scientific acceptance, and deprives many more children of quick access to the treatment.

"There Are No Side Effects to Worry About"

Every effective therapy known has some side effects, in some people. Very effective therapies are more likely to cause problems. Advocates of a therapy should want to know about potential problems, and should be actively looking for that information. If no adverse effects are reported, either the therapy does not really work, or the effects are being missed or hidden. Accurate information about potential problems is essential to sorting out the balance of risks versus benefits.

Time Passes and No New Information Appears

Again, if a treatment works well, it should be easy to prove. Often the only changes to a promotion are changes in the product name, or dose, with no new evidence to show that the product or therapy is effective. The passage of time should also give more information about side effect risks.

Avoidance of Open Debate

When information is presented only in closed meetings, or questions are not allowed or are ignored, one has to wonder why. Attempts by questioners to find a neutral ground for debate may be ignored or attacked, or may be met with offers of very stacked settings that can't provide balance.

Aggressive Personal Attacks on Critics

Again, the content of discussion should be on the claims and supporting information. If advocates shift to the offensive when questioned, it may be that they may have no answers.

The Use of Guilt or Fear in Promotion

Statements such as "If you don't do this, you will never forgive yourself, and your child will never catch up" have no place in discussion of therapies, proven or otherwise.

The Therapy Program Is Expensive

Many good things cost a lot of money; others are cheap. If an alternative therapy is very expensive, and works, it may well be worth the expense. On the other hand, someone may be making a lot of money promoting a questionable product. When the costs are low, the odds are that the advocates are really in it because they believe in their cause. If the costs are high, the dollars may be part of the motive, and should bring the claims more into question.

"Before" and "After" Photographs Are Presented as Support

Each of us have pictures of ourselves or our children that we like, and others we dislike. For our children with Down syndrome, the pictures we dislike are easy to identify. Others may show the child as we prefer to see them, as happy playful members of the family. There may be very little of "the look" of Down syndrome in the second group. This variability in images makes the use of "before" and "after" therapy pictures equivalent to commercial diet plan advertising.

WHEN DO ALTERNATIVES MAKE THE MOST (AND LEAST) SENSE?

There are usually no easy answers to most of the questions raised here. When a child has an obvious problem for which there are no standard answers, there are both the need for options and the possibility of monitoring real change. On the other hand, if a child is doing well, is healthy, and is meeting reasonable expectations at the start of a therapy, how will the family know if they have gained a good result (and how will they know when to stop)?

WHO CAN HELP SORT ALL OF THIS OUT?
Existing Support Networks

Most local support groups include families who have tried alternatives, and others who decided not to do so. Group discussions that share those experiences can help new families to work their way through the issues. Other families who have "been there" are almost always the best resource for someone facing a new problem

National organizations (NDSS, NDSC, ARC, etc.) have certainly been confronted with questions many times about alternative therapies. On that topic, most take positions that support the need to consider all options, and call for careful research from the scientific community to provide more information.

Physicians and Other Professionals

Because children with Down syndrome often have very real medical needs, it is important to involve the child's physician in any decisions about alternatives. Physicians may be able to access information resources that can help, and certainly should be aware of any changes the family chooses that might effect the child's health.

Similarly, teachers and therapists may have useful information about options. They also may want to know about therapies that could affect their interactions with the child.

Both groups of professionals include people who have long experience in the field of disabilities, and who care about their patients, clients, and students. A strong relationship with such a professional may be a big help to a family confronted with difficult choices.

SUMMARY

For a wide variety of reasons, many families consider or choose "alternative therapies" to help with medical, educational, or other problems. Families of children with Down syndrome are no different in that respect, and may be more likely to face problems that have few dependable or proven solutions.

Conventional systems and professionals may be seen to offer no acceptable answers, and the tone of discussion may be so negative as to drive the family to seek more positive perspectives.

A wide variety of alternative therapies have been offered to families of children with Down syndrome, and continue to be developed. Some may go on to become new standards of treatment, but most will prove of little use, and some may be shown to be dangerous or fraudulent.

Sorting out the value of the choices can be a major challenge to a family already coping with heavy stress, and requires attention to the style and credibility of the advocates, as well as consideration of input from all available resources. Potential benefits must be balanced against cost (in energy and time as well as dollars) and potential risks of injury. Medical and educational needs should not be lost in the pursuit of alternatives.

Alternative and Unconventional Therapies in Down Syndrome

Don C. Van Dyke and Philip Mattheis

A number of terms may be used to describe alternative therapies: alternative, complementary, unconventional, unorthodox medicine; nonstandard therapy; and controversial therapies (Kunzi, 1994; Van Dyke, 1995; Roberts et al., 1995). Regardless of how these treatments are described, their popularity is increasing. More than 61 million Americans are currently using alternative therapies, and an estimated 425 million visits were made in the United States to providers of unconventional therapies in 1990 (Eisenberg et al., 1993; Roberts et al., 1995). Studies have suggested that as many as 11% of children have received some form of alternative health care (Spigelbaltt et al., 1994). The annual cost of alternative and unconventional therapies has been estimated at 13.7 billion dollars (Eisenberg et al., 1993).

The motivations and rationales for individuals and families seeking alternative and unconventional therapies are powerful, multiple, and complex (Golden, 1984; Roberts et al., 1995; Nickel, 1966). Parents who do so may view such treatments as more humane, easier for families to control, and more likely to lead to cure or functional improvement (Barlow, 1992). Parents may regard alternative therapies as less invasive than traditional medical procedures; this may not, however, always be the case. A general dissatisfaction with conventional medicine, often based on prior contacts with the health care system, may motivate a family to choose an alternative therapy. Most parents, however, are not looking for alternative therapies to replace traditional medicine but rather for something to supplement it and "help their child" (Roberts et al., 1995). The advent of electronic information sources has increased individual and family access to alternative health care information, as have frequent television and print media coverage of such topics.

The rise in the popularity of alternative health care has prompted efforts at legislation. Stimulated by increasing public and political awareness of alternative health care, the federal government established the Office of Alternative Medicine (OAM) in 1992.

Down Syndrome: A Promising Future, Together, Edited by Terry J. Hassold and David Patterson
ISBN 0-471-29686-4   Copyright © 1998 by Wiley-Liss, Inc.

Table 1. Alternative Therapies in Down Syndrome

Medical
Vitamins
   Megavitamins
   U-series
   Vitamin and mineral supplements with and without piracetam
   Specific mineral supplements, e.g., zinc, selenium
Thyroid hormone/extract
Dimethyl sulfoxide (DMSO)
Sicca cell/cell therapy: animal fetal cells, human fetal cells
Human growth hormone
Dehydroepiandrosterone
Neuropharmacology
   Piracetam
   Tacrine
   Fluoxetine
   Glutamic acid
   5-Hydroxytryptophan

Surgical
Plastic surgery of the face
Tongue reduction

Physical Therapies
Patterning
Craniosacral therapy
Massage
Sensory-motor integration

Educational/Communication Therapy
Facilitated communication
Auditory integration therapy

Since its establishment, the OAM annual budget has more than doubled to its 1995 figure of $5.4 billion (OAM Public Information Center, 1995). This agency has participated in reviewing alternative medicine practices and supporting research in alternative medicine (OAM Public Information Center, 1995). Insurance companies in a few states are now covering the cost of alternative therapies. In 1994, Blue Cross developed separate insurance plans in Alaska and Washington to provide coverage of alternative therapies such as homeopathy, naturopathy, and acupuncture (Roberts et al., 1995).

Although they are continuing to increase in popularity, alternative therapies are still viewed with caution by many practitioners of traditional health care. Unlike many but certainly not all treatments employed by traditional health care practitioners, alternative therapies often do not undergo statistical analysis and study, or standard scientific testing that includes rigorous assessment of safety, effectiveness, and side effects (Van Dyke et al., 1990a, b; Brown, 1979; Golden, 1987; Golden, 1992; Nickel, 1996). Such therapies may in some cases be based on individual beliefs, anecdotal reports, and the experiences of a small group of individuals who have chosen the therapy (Van Dyke et al., 1990b; Starrett, 1996). Although many of these therapies are obviously controversial, and not necessarily harmful, their efficacy and safety may frequently be in doubt. Whereas some alternative and unconventional therapies have a scientific and medical basis, others are derived from superstitions and are promoted via exaggerated claims and for financial motivations.

Alternative therapies fall into four general categories: medical, physical, surgical, and educational (Van Dyke et al., 1995) (Table 1). Alternative medical therapies used in Down syndrome have included sicca cell injections, vitamin and mineral therapy, pituitary extract, dimethyl sulfoxide, glutamic acid, 5-hydroxytryptophan, and thyroid hormone (Foreman and Ward, 1986; Golden, 1987; Golden, 1992; Van Dyke et al., 1995; Starrett, 1996). Alternative surgical therapies include cosmetic procedures to alter the facial appearance of Down syndrome, reduction of tongue size, enlargement of nose and chin, and changes to the eyes and face (Hohler, 1977; Lemperle and Radu, 1980; Rozner, 1983; Feurstein, 1985; Lefebvine, 1987; Van Dyke, 1990b; Van Dyke et al., 1995). Reported physical therapies include patterning (Sparrow and Zigler, 1978; Harris, 1981; Van Dyke, 1995). Infant massage and craniosacral therapies may also be involved in the treatment of Down syndrome, but their use has not been reported in the literature. Education and communication therapies include facilitative communication and auditory integration therapy (Hostler, 1996; Rimland and Edelson, 1994, 1995). Other alternative therapies reported but not noted specifically for the treatment of Down syndrome include Rolfing, aromatic therapy, herbal therapy, reflexology, therapeutic touch, radionics, gems, crystals, spiritual healing, antifungal agents, special diets, intravenous gammaglobulin (IVIG), and melatonin (Roberts et al., 1995; Nickel, 1996).

MEGAVITAMIN THERAPY

Vitamin and mineral therapy as an alternative, supplemental, or traditional medical therapy has existed for many years. The use of vitamins as medical therapy has a long history in general medical care going back as far as the 1700s. Its use can be divided into three historical eras: the prevention of disease related to vitamin deficiency, the treatment of vitamin-responsive inborn errors of metabolism, and orthomolecular megadose vitamin therapy (Blumbalo, 1964; Turkel, 1975; Karp, 1983; Pruess et al., 1989; Rudman and Williams, 1985; Nickel, 1996). Vitamins are classified by solubility; there are nine water-soluble vitamins (vitamin C, thiamin, riboflavin, B6, niacin, biotin, pantothenic acid, B12, and folate) and four fat-soluble vitamins (vitamin A, vitamin K, vitamin E, and vitamin D) (Grand et al., 1987). The water-soluble vitamins are usually thought to function as coenzymes or apoenzymes. The fat-soluble vitamins play an important role in the function of the nervous system and in skin development. More than 18 disorders associated with vitamin intake (deficiency, toxicity, or both) have been reported with water-soluble and fat-soluble vitamins (Kleijnen and Knipschild, 1991; Nickel, 1996; Grand et al., 1987).

A recommended daily allowance (RDA) has been established for all vitamins by the U.S. Food and Drug Administration. Megadose vitamin therapy usually includes dosages of vitamins that are 20 to 600 times the RDA. The use of such megadoses is of concern because of potential side effects related to vitamin overdosage, particularly for the fat-soluble vitamins A and D and possibly the water-soluble vitamin pyridoxine (Kleijnen and Knipschild, 1991). Potential side effects include increased intracranial pressure, skin rashes, retinal changes, bone disorders, seizures, and liver disease.

Recent interest in vitamin therapy in individuals with developmental disabilities comes in part from a 1981 study examining the cognitive effects of nutritional supplements on children with mental disabilities (Harrell et al., 1981). In this study, 16 children were regularly treated with supplements containing 8 minerals and 11 vitamins. The authors reported that some of the children showed an increase in IQ after treatment (Harrell et al., 1981). Four or five of these individuals were children with Down syndrome. A 1983 double-blind case control study of 20 individuals with Down syndrome showed no significant group differences in appearance, growth, or health after vitamin supplement therapy (Bennett et al., 1983). The authors concluded that they could find no evidence to support the use of orthomolecular megadose vitamin therapy in school-age children with Down syndrome (Bennett et al., 1983). A 1989 placebo-controlled crossover study of high dose multivitamin and mineral supplements in 15 children with Down syndrome showed that the only documented benefit was parental impression of improved skin appearance in their child (Bidder et al., 1989). In one review of questionnaire responses of parents of individuals with Down syndrome in 1985 and 1986, 36 of 190, or 19%, indicated that they were using megavitamin therapy for their children (Van Dyke et al., 1990b).

There is much recent interest in administration of vitamin and mineral supplements along with the nootropic compound piracetam. The commercially available product is Nutrivene-D. It comes without piracetam ($75/unit container) and with piracetam ($140/unit container). Piracetam has been studied in a number of disorders including Alzheimer's disease, Raynaud's phenomenon, dyslexia, learning disabilities, preeclampsia, and certain seizure disorders (Wilsher et al., 1987; Wilsher, 1986; Ackerman et al., 1991; Herrmann and Stephan, 1992; Artieda and Obeso, 1993; Brown et al., 1993; Moriau et al.,1993). Piracetam is an orphan drug for the treatment of cortical myoclonus (Brown et al., 1993). The effects of the drug piracetam have not been clinically tested on young children with Down syndrome.

CELL THERAPY

Cell therapy consists of injections of freeze-dried or lyophilized cells derived from fetal animal tissue—typically rabbits and sheep (Schmid, 1983; Foreman and Ward, 1987; Van Dyke et al., 1990a; Last, 1990). Proponents of cell therapy have reported a perceived improvement in facial features, accelerated growth, and improvements in IQ, motor skills, social behavior, language, and memory (Schmid, 1983). In addition to treatment of Down syndrome, cell therapy has been used in other countries to treat a wide range of conditions including heart disease, poor circulation, infertility, cancer, and mental illness (Bardon, 1964).

A Canadian double-blind perspective trial showed no evidence that sicca cell therapy (a form of cell therapy originally described by Schmid) improved developmental outcome (Black et al., 1966). Another earlier study found no significant cognitive differences between subjects treated with sicca cell injections and controls (Bardon, 1964). Studies by Bremer (1975) and Schulte (1975) found no evidence that sicca cell therapy was effective in ameliorating the symptoms of Down syndrome. A retrospective study in 1990 in which 11% had received cell therapy with a control group matched for sex, age, socioeconomic status, and cardiac history showed no significant differences for a number of developmental and growth variables (Van Dyke et al., 1990a). Critics argue that all these studies demonstrate significant flaws in experimental design and that a large double-blind study of cell therapy efficacy has not been performed (Fackelmann, 1990). New variations on cell therapy include the use of freeze-dried human fetal tissue.

OTHER MEDICAL THERAPIES

Other alternative therapies in the treatment of Down syndrome have included pituitary extract, dehydroepiandrosterone, glutamic acid, thyroid hormone, 5-hydroxytryptophan, and DMSO; none has demonstrated benefits (DeMoragas, 1958; Aspillage et al., 1975, Koch et al., 1965; Tu and Zellweger, 1965; Coleman, 1975; Gabourie et al., 1975; Gadson, 1951; Van Dyke et al., 1990b). Areas of continued interest include mineral cofactors such as zinc and selenium, and human growth hormone (Allen et al., 1993; Van Dyke, 1995).

PHYSICAL THERAPIES

Craniosacral therapy attempts to restore the body's ability to heal itself through manipulation of the craniosacral system (Dinnar et al., 1982; McConnell et al., 1980). The therapy is based on the assumption that the fluid-filled cavities in the brain and spinal cord represent a semi-closed hydraulic system with its own intrinsic rhythm (Roberts et al., 1995). Proponents of craniosacral therapy believe that the physiology of this system has significant effects on other organ systems in the body, particularly the nervous, musculoskeletal, vascular, lymphatic, endocrine, and respiratory systems (McConnell et al., 1980; Roberts et al., 1995). Craniosacral therapy is thought to benefit dyslexia, attention-deficit hyperactivity, spastic cerebral palsy, and a number of other conditions (Roberts et al., 1995). Participation of individuals with Down syndrome in craniosacral therapy is not known.

Massage therapy is a method of providing gentle tactile stimulation to the body surface; proponents have claimed that it promotes growth, enhances immune function, and improves behavior as well as overall developmental function (Koes et al., 1991; Roberts et al., 1995). Other reported benefits include improvements in parent–infant bonding, digestion, sleep patterns, and pain tolerance, as well as decreases in stress level and colic symptoms (Roberts et al., 1995). Most studies of massage therapy have been done in infants and adults (Koes et al., 1991; Roberts et al., 1995). There have been no known studies of massage therapy in young infants or older children with Down syndrome.

COMMUNICATION AND EDUCATIONAL THERAPIES

Facilitated communication is a technique in which the facilitator provides physical support to the upper extremities to assist persons with communication disabilities in pointing to words and other symbols (Levine and Wharton, 1995; Hostler, 1996). The method originated in Australia, where it was used with individuals with cerebral palsy. Because communication and language problems are common in Down syndrome, facilitative communication has become an area of significant interest for children with this condition as well. The ultimate goal for users of facilitative communication is independent typing without physical support. Facilitative communication therapy often continues, however, even when it is obvious that this aim will not be achieved. Media interest and allegations of child physical and sexual abuse expressed through facilitated communication placed this modality in the national spotlight in the early 1990s (Jones, 1994). Recent studies have not been supportive of this technique (Hostler, 1996). Controversy continues about its effectiveness; it continues to be practiced in some settings.

NEUROPHARMACOLOGY

Neuropharmacology has been an area of active research in the pharmaceutical industry, particularly in Germany, Eastern Europe, and Russia. Over the past 30 years, investigations in this area have led to the development of compounds that may be or are hoped to be effective in treating such disorders as Alzheimer's disease, dyslexia, and learning disabilities (Debendt, 1994).

Nootropics are drugs that improve brain function and lead to physiological activation of adaptation (Nicholson, 1989). These agents have been studied in animal models and in humans with Alzheimer's disease. Animal models suggest it may be effective as a cognitive enhancer; however, studies in humans with Alzheimer's disease have not shown symptomatic benefits (Gottfries, 1990; Claus et al., 1991). Several compounds in this class of pharmaceutical agents are piracetam (2-thio-1-pyrrolidine-acetamide), levetiracetam, and other derivatives of piracetam (Gouliaev and Senning, 1994). A review of the literature from 1965 to 1992 shows more than 400 references to such compounds as piracetam, oxiracetam, pramiracetam, etiracetam, nefiracetam, aniracetam, and rolziractam.

Other neuroactive medications of interest include the cholinesterase inhibitors; specifically, the drug tacrine (Cognex). Most research on tacrine has been focused on its effect on individuals with Alzheimer disease, some of whom may also have Down syndrome (Croisile et al., 1993; Kurz et al., 1995; Boller and Orgogozo, 1995). Another neuroactive drug of potential interest for individuals with Down syndrome is fluoxetine (Prozac). Current areas of Prozac research include its effect on aggressive behaviors, mental disability, selective or elective mutism, and depression (Black and Ubde, 1994; Troisi et al., 1995; Wong et al., 1995). At present there are no double-blind controlled studies dealing with Down syndrome for any of these chemical compounds.

RESEARCH AND ALTERNATIVE AND UNCONVENTIONAL THERAPIES

Multiple alternative therapies are available to the interested individual, family, and health care provider; unfortunately, there is a paucity of information available to answer questions about safety and effectiveness. For parents, alternative or unconventional therapies fall into three groups: a few alternative therapies in which blinded, retrospective, or case-controlled studies have been performed in which no efficacy has been demonstrated; therapies in which controlled studies have shown possible to significant efficacy; and a large number of therapies in which no blinded, case-controlled, or retrospective studies have been performed.

In order for research to occur on alternative therapies four things need to occur: development of objective, statistically accurate, clinically relevant, and well organized research design; approval by internal review board of such proposals; approval, in some cases, of investigational drug use by the FDA; and appropriate funding for research. If any one of these four items falls short, good research will probably not be a reality.

QUESTIONS PARENTS NEED TO ASK

In order to help make appropriate decisions about such treatment, there are key questions that parents should ask their health care practitioner and themselves about alternative therapies (Van Dyke et al., 1995):

1. Has your physician, therapist, or other health care provider provided you with clearly written and easily understood information about research, documenting the benefits, lack of benefits, or side effects of the therapy?
2. What are the possible risks of the procedure or the therapy?
3. Do the benefits of the therapy outweigh the risks?
4. Does the individual want the therapy?
5. What kind of follow-up care is needed; how will the individual be monitored and who will do the monitoring?
6. Are there long-term results or long-term side effects? What documentation of side effects is needed?
7. What is the cost? Will insurance cover all or part?

SUMMARY

Alternative medicine is a political, financial, social, and medical reality. It is hoped that increased research of alternative and unconventional therapies, possibly with government sponsorship or support, will provide practitioners and parents with much needed objective information. At present, there is no cure or "ultimate treatment" for individuals with Down syndrome, and there is little objective information on alternative and unconventional therapies. As long as this situation exists, there will be continued interest and concern about alternative and unconventional therapies.

ACKNOWLEDGMENTS

We gratefully acknowledge the technical and editorial expertise of Marilyn Dolezal, Susan Eberly, M.A., and Dianne M. McBrien, M.D. in the writing of this manuscript.

REFERENCES

Ackerman PT, Dykman RA, Holloway C, Paal NP, Gocio MY (1991): A trial of piracetam in two subgroups of students with dyslexia enrolled in summer tutoring. J Learning Disabilities 24:9:542–549.

Allen DB, Frasier SD, Foley TP Jr., Pescovitz OH (1993): Growth hormone with Down syndrome. J Pediatr 123:5:742–743.

Artieda J, Obeso JA (1993): The pathophysiology and pharmacology of photic cortical reflex myoclonus. Ann Neurol 34:2:175–184.

Aspillage MJ, Morizon G, Vendano IA (1975): Dimethylsulfoxide therapy in severe retardation in Mongoloid children. Ann New York Acad Sci 243:421–451.

Bardon LM (1964): Sicca cell treatment in Mongolism. Lancet 2:234–235.

Barlow JF (1992): Freedom of choice in medicine—"it makes me feel better." South Dakota J Med 45:5:125.

Bennett FC. McClelland S, Kriegsmann EA, Andrus LB, Sells CJ (1983): Vitamin and mineral supplementation in Down's Syndrome. Pediatrics 72:5:707–713.

Bidder RT, Gray P, Newcombe RG, Evans BK. Hughes M (1989): The effects of multivitamins and minerals on children with Down syndrome. Devel Med Child Neurol 31:532–537.

Black B, Uhde TW (1994): Treatment of elective mutism with fluoxetine: a double-blind, placebo-controlled study. J Am Acad Child Adolesc Psychiatr 33:7:1000–1006.

Black DB, Kato JG, Walker GW (1966): A study of improvement in mentally retarded children accruing from sicca cell therapy. Am J Ment Defic 70:4:499–508.

Blumbalo TS (1964): Negative results: treatment of Down syndrome with the "U" series. J Am Med Assoc 361:1987.

Boller F, Orgogozo JM (1995): Tacrine, Alzheimer's disease, and the cholinergic theory. A critical review and results of a new therapy. Review. Neurologia 10:5:194–199.

Bremer HJ (1975): Comment on cell therapy in children with special reference to pediatric-metabolic issues. Mschr Kinderheik 123:9:674–675.

Brown GW (1979): Learning Disabilities: Fads, Fallacies, and Fictions. "Learning Disabilities: An Audio Journal for Continuing Education." New York: Grune & Stratton.

Brown P, Steiger MJ, Thompson PD, et al. (1993): Effectiveness of piracetam in cortical myoclonus. Movement Disorders 8:1:63–68.

Claus JJ, Ludwig C, Mohr E, Gluffra M, Blin J, Chase TN (1991): Nootropic drugs in Alzheimer's disease: Symptomatic treatment with piracetam. Neurology 21:4:570–574.

Coleman M (1975): "Serotonin in Down's syndrome." New York: Elsevier Publishers.

Croisile B, Trillet M, Fondarai J, Laurent B, Mauguiere F, Billardon M (1993): Long-term and high-dose piracetam treatment of Alzheimer's disease. Neurology 43:2:301–305.

Debendt W. Interaction between psychological and pharmacological treatment in cognitive impairment (1994): Life Sci 55:25–26; 2057–2066.

DeMoragas J.(1958): Treatment of mongolism with dehydroepiandrosterone. Rev Span Pediatr 14:545.

Dinnar U, Beal MC, Goodridge JP, et al. (1982): Description of fifty diagnostic tests used with osteopathic manipulation. J Am Osteopath Assoc 81:5:314–321.

Eisenberg DM, Kessler RC, Poster C, Norlock FE, Calkins DR, Delbanco TL (1993): Unconventional medicine in the United States. Prevalence, costs and patterns of use. N Engl J Med 328:4:246–252.

Fackelmann K (1990): New Hope or False Promise? Sci News 137:168–170.

Feurstein R (1985): Down syndrome surgery: A part of an active modification approach. Symposium on the future of seriously impaired: Where do professionals and society stand? Annual meeting of the American Orthopsychiatric Association, Boston.

Foreman PJ, Ward J (1986): A survey of paediatric management practices in Down's syndrome. Austral Paediatr J 22:3:171–176.

Foreman PJ, Ward J (1987): An evaluation of cell therapy in Down syndrome. Austral Paediatr J 23:3:151–156.

Gabourie J, Becker JW, Paterman B (1975): Oral dimethylsulfoxide in mental retardation. Part I: Preliminary behavioral and psychometric data. In Jacobs SW, Herschler R (eds.): Biological actions of dimethylsulfoxide. Ann New York Acad Sci 243:1–508.

Gadson EJ (1951): Glutamic acid and mental deficiency. Am J Ment Defic 55:521–528.

Golden GS (1984a): Controversial therapies. Pediatr Clin North Am 31:459–469.

Golden GS (1984b): Controversies in therapy for children with Down syndrome. Pediatr Rev 6:4:116–120.

Golden GS (1987): A hard look at fad therapies for developmental disorders. Contemp Pediatr 4:47–60.

Golden GS (1992): What's new in controversial therapies? Update. An abstract presented at the 12th Annual Conference on Developmental-Behavioral Disorders.

Gottfries CG (1990): Pharmacological treatment strategies in Alzheimer type dementia. Eur Neuropsychopharmacol 1:1:1–5.

Gouliaev AH, Senning A (1994): Piracetam and other structurally related nootropics, Review. Brain Res Brain Res Rev 19:2:180–222.

Grand, R.J., Sutphen JL, Dietz Jr., WH. (eds.) (1987). "Pediatric Nutrition: Theory and Practice." Boston: Butterworths, pp. 51–111.

Harrell RF, Capp RH, Davis DR. Peerless J, Ravitz LR (1981): Can nutritional supplements help mentally retarded children? An exploratory study. Proc Natl Acad Sci 78:1:574–578.

Harris SR (1981): Effects of neurodevelopmental therapy on motor performance of infants with Down syndrome. Devel Med Child Neurol 23:477–483.

Herrmann WM, Stephan K (1992): Moving from the question of efficacy to the question of therapeutic relevance, an exploratory reanalysis of a controlled clinical study of 130 inpatients with dementia syndrome taking piracetam Intern Psychogeriatr 4:1:25–44.

Hohler H (1977): Changes in facial expression as a results of plastic surgery in Mongoloid children. Aesthetic Plastic Surg 1:225.

Hostler SL (1996): Facilitated Communication. Pediatrics 87:4:584–586.

Jones D (1994): Autism, Facilitated Communication and Allegations of Child Abuse and Neglect. Child Abuse Neglect 18:6:495–503.

Karp IF (1983): New hope for the retarded. Am J Med Gen 16:1–5.

Kleijnen J, Knipschild P (1991): Niacin and vitamin B6 in mental functioning: A review of controlled trials in humans. Biol Psychiatr 29:9:932–941.

Koch R, Share J, Graliker BV (1965): The effects of cytomel on young children with Down's Syndrome (Mongolism): A double-blind longitudinal study. J Pediatr 66:776.

Koes BW, Bouter LM, Knipshild PG, et al. (1991): The effectiveness of manual therapy, physiotherapy and continued treatment by the general practitioner for chronic nonspecific back and neck complaints: Design of a randomized clinical trial. J Manip Physiol Therap 14:9:498–502.

Kunzi M (1994): Complementary medicine and health policy regulations. Schweizerische Medizinische Wochenschrift-Supplementum 62:7–12.

Kurz A, Marquard R, Mosch D (1995): Tacrine: Progress in treatment of Alzheimer's disease? Review. Zeitschr Gerontol Geriatr 28:3:163–168.

Last PM (1990): Cell therapy: A cruel and dangerous deception. A drama in three acts. J Paediatr Child Health 26:4:197–199.

Lefebvine A (1987): Should retarded people have surgery? The psychological aspects of craniofacial problems. Surgery is not enough. The International Craniofacial Institute Conference, Dallas, Texas.

Lemperle G, Radu D (1980): Facial plastic surgery in children with Down's syndrome. Plastic Reconstruct Surg 66:3:337–342.

Levine K, Wharton R (1995): Facilitated communication, What parents should know. Exceptional Parent 40–53.

McConnell DG, Beal MC, Dinnar U, et al. (1980): Low agreement of findings in neuromusculoskeletal examination by a group of osteopathic physicians using their own procedures. J Am Osteopath Assoc 79:7:441–450.

Moriau M, Lavenne-Pardonge E, Crasborn L, von Frenchkell R. Col-Debeys C (1993): Treatment of the Raynaud's phenomenon with piracetam. Arzheim Forsch 43:5:526–535.

Nickel RE (1996): Controversial therapies for young children with developmental disabilities. Infant Young Children 8:4:29–40.

Nicholson CD (1989): Nootropics and metabolically active compounds in Alzheimer's disease. Biochem Soc Trans 17:1:83–85.

Office of Alternative Medicine (OAM) (1995): Department of Health & Human Services, National Institutes of Health, Bethesda, Maryland, June 1995.

Pruess JB, Fewell RR, Bennett FC. (1989): Vitamin therapy and children with Down syndrome: A review of research. Exceptional Children 55:4:336–341.

Rimland B, Edelson SM (1994): The effect of auditory integration training on autism. Am J Speech Lang Pathol 3:16–24.

Rimland B, Edelson SM. (1995): Brief report: a pilot study of auditory integration training in autism. J Autism Devel Disorders 25:1:61–70.

Roberts DC, Johnson CP, Kratz L (1995): Alternative therapies: a critical review and parent's view point. American Academy of Cerebral Palsy and Developmental Medicine. 27–30 September 1995, Philadelphia, Pennsylvania.

Rozner L (1983): Facial plastic surgery for Down's syndrome. Lancet 11:1:8337:1320–1323.

Rudman D, Williams, PJ (1985): Megadose vitamins: use and misuse. N Engl J Med 309:8:488–490.

Schmid F (1983): "Cell Therapy: A New Dimension of Medicine." Thun, Switzerland: Ott Publishers.

Schulte FJ (1975): Comments on therapy of Down syndrome on cell therapy from a neurophysiologic-neuropediatric point of view. Mschr Kinderheik 123:9:683–685.

Sparrow S, Zigler E. (1978): Evaluation of a patterning treatment for retarded children. Pediatrics 62:2:137–150.

Spigelbaltt L, Laine-Ammara G., Pless IB, Guyver A (1994): The use of alternative medicine by children. Pediatrics 94(6 pt 1):811–814.

Starrett AL (1996): Nonstandard therapies in developmental disabilities. In Capute AJ, Accardo PJ (eds.): "Developmental Disabilities in Infancy and Childhood," 2nd ed. New York: Paul H. Brookes, pp. 593–608.

Troisi A, Vicario E, Nuccetelli F, Ciani N, Pasini A (1995): Effects of fluoxetine on aggressive behavior of adult inpatients with mental retardation and epilepsy. Pharmacopsychiatry 28:3:73–76.

Tu JB, Zellweger H (1965): Blood serotonin deficiency in Down's syndrome. Lancet 2:425:715–716.

Turkel H (1975): Medical amelioration of Down syndrome incorporating the orthomolecular approach. J Orthomolec Psychiatr 41:2:102–115.

Van Dyke DC, Lang DJ, van Duyne S, Heide F, Chang H (1990a): Cell therapy in children with Down syndrome: a retrospective study. Pediatrics 85:1:79–84.

Van Dyke DC, van Duyne S, Lowe O, Heide F (1990b): Alternative and controversial therapies. In Van Dyke DC, Lang DJ, Heide F, van Duyne S, Soucek MJ (eds.): "Clinical Perspectives in the Management of Down Syndrome." New York: Springer-Verlag, pp. 208–216.

Van Dyke DC (1995): Alternative and unconventional therapies in children with Down syndrome. In "Medical and Surgical Care for Children with Down Syndrome: A Parents Guide." Bethesda, MD: Woodbine House, pp. 288–302.

Wilsher CR (1986): Effects of piracetam on developmental dyslexia. Review. Intern J Psychophysiol 4:1:29–39.

Wilsher CR, Bennett D, Chase CH, et al. (1987): Piracetam and dyslexia: Effects on reading tests. J Clin Psychopharmacol 7:4:230–237.

Wong DT, Bymaster FP, Engleman EA (1995): Prozac (fluoxetine, Lilly 110130), the first selective serotonin uptake inhibitor and an antidepressant drug: Twenty years since its first publication. Review. Life Sci 57(5):411–441.

V. Psychosocial Issues

Finding the Reason for Problem Behavior and Planning Effective Interventions: A Guide for Parents

Jane I. Carlson and Christopher E. Smith

WHY PROBLEM BEHAVIOR OCCURS

Problem behavior in a child with a developmental disability can be one of the most difficult challenges that a parent may face. When confronted with a child who is hurting himself or others, a parent may experience a range of emotions including fear, anger, and confusion. The situation may seem hopeless and the parent may be at a loss as to how to proceed. This chapter provides a framework for determining why a child is engaging in problem behavior as well as providing ideas for intervention planning. By gaining a thorough understanding of the purpose of a child's problem behavior, a parent can turn an enormous challenge into a problem that can be effectively managed.

Historically, behavior problems such as aggression, self-injury, tantrums, and property destruction have been viewed as being manifestations of a psychotic disorder or random outbursts of uncontrolled behavior resulting from the child's disability. Interventions for these behaviors were often focused on eliminating the offending behavior at all costs. Treatments included punishment (including the use of aversives), medication (including antipsychotic drugs), and both physical and mechanical restraint (Matson and DiLorenzo, 1984).

Research from the areas of developmental and behavioral psychology has helped us to look at these severe behavior problems in a different way. Developmental psychology shows us that many behaviors displayed by children with developmental disabilities are also present in typically developing children. Crying, tantrums, and aggression in very young children serve a number of purposes. These behaviors can help a child gain access to desired items in the environment, summon assistance, or end frustrating situations (Bayley, 1932; Bell and Ainsworth, 1972). In addition, self-

Down Syndrome: A Promising Future, Together, Edited by Terry J. Hassold and David Patterson
ISBN 0-471-29686-4   Copyright © 1998 by Wiley-Liss, Inc.

injury is often seen in children experiencing discomfort (deLissovoy, 1963) such as pain related to middle ear infections. These behaviors are equally effective in influencing the behavior of adults in the child's environment and in influencing the behavior of their peers (Brownlee and Bakeman, 1981). For example, a child may scream and cry in the supermarket, which results in a parent buying a desired item for the child. On the playground, the same child may hit a peer, which results in the peer surrendering a favorite toy. Importantly, research also demonstrates that these "problem" behaviors often occur with less frequency as language develops. In other words, as a child begins to use language to influence people, they no longer need to cry or hit to communicate wants and needs. This change typically occurs between the ages of two and three (Brownlee and Bakeman,1981) when language is developing at an extremely rapid rate.

Children with developmental disabilities often experience delays in language development. Children with such delays typically are described as having more behavior problems than children with age appropriate language skills (Caulfield, Fischel, DeBaryshe, and Whitehurst, 1989; Stevenson and Richman, 1978). Thus there appears to be an inverse relationship between behavior problems and communication skills. In other words, as communication skills increase, behavior problems tend to decrease. The study of this relationship has led several researchers to develop the "communication hypothesis" of problem behavior (Carr and Durand, 1985; Donnellan et al., 1984). This hypothesis states that behavior problems are a form of communication used by individuals who do not yet have a more advanced form of communication to use in order to influence the environment.

Three main communicative functions of problem behavior have been identified in the research literature: escape, attention-seeking, and tangible-seeking. Escape-motivated behavior (Weeks and Gaylord-Ross, 1981) is seen when an individual wants to avoid an unpleasant or frustrating situation. Examples of this include escape from task demands (Carr et al., 1980), parent requests, and unpleasant social situations (Taylor and Carr, 1992b). Attention-seeking behavior is seen when an individual desires the company of an adult or a peer (Taylor and Carr, 1992a). Examples of this include wanting the teacher to spend some time with him or her, wanting a parent to end a telephone conversation, or wanting another child to interact with him or her on the playground. Tangible-seeking behavior helps the individual gain access to desired items or activities (Day et al., 1988). Examples of this include wanting candy while waiting in the supermarket check-out line, wanting to play on the swing set at the park, or wanting a Barney toy advertised on TV.

A given problem behavior can serve any one or any combination of these communicative functions for an individual (Carr and Carlson, 1993; Smith et al., 1993). For example, a child may bite her hand when asked to pick up her toys (escape from demands). She may also bite her hand when her mother is busy talking to another adult (attention seeking). In addition, she may bite her hand when she is unable to have seconds on dessert (tangible seeking). In this case, the same form or type of problem behavior (self-injury) serves many different functions.

ASSESSMENT: FINDING THE PURPOSE OF PROBLEM BEHAVIOR

In order to plan an intervention to reduce the frequency of and prevent the reoccurrence of problem behavior, it is important to do a thorough assessment of the conditions surrounding the occurrence of the behavior. In the research literature, a functional analysis (Iwata et al., 1982), defined by researchers as an experimental manipulation of consequent variables, is often performed. This type of analysis is often too complex and time consuming for a parent or teacher to perform in the home or in the classroom. Parents and teachers do, however, need to collect and analyze some data in order to assess for the factors that are motivating and maintaining the problem behavior (Repp et al., 1988).

A relatively easy way to collect a large amount of information is to keep some form of written record of the circumstances surrounding each episode of problem behavior. This can be done by keeping a log or diary, or by using standard A-B-C data sheets. Regardless of the data collection format, it is important to write down the events that occurred immediately before the behavior (the *A*ntecedent), the behavior itself (the *B*ehavior), and the events that immediately followed the behavior (the *C*onsequence). These data can then be reviewed on a regular basis to determine motivating factors and to aid in intervention planning.

A typical log entry might look like this:

9/11/96

At 8:45 AM, Jamie was watching cartoons and I told him it was time to get dressed for school. He didn't respond so I turned off the TV and told him to go get dressed. He started to scream and then he threw his toy at me. He continued to tantrum for about 10 minutes. I finally said, "Okay, you can have 10 more minutes of TV time but then you have to get dressed." He stopped crying and turned the TV back on.

In order to analyze the conditions motivating and maintaining the problem behavior, it is important to identify the antecedents, behavior, and consequences for each log entry. In this example, the antecedent (the conditions that triggered the problem behavior) was the parent turning off the TV and placing a demand on the child, in this case, asking the child to get dressed. The behaviors that followed included screaming, throwing, and having a tantrum. The consequence (the condition that immediately followed the problem behavior) was that the parent withdrew the demand and allowed the child to watch some more TV.

In this case, the problem behavior could have served one of two functions for the child. He could have been trying to escape from the demand of getting dressed or he could have been seeking the tangible activity of watching TV. Analysis of subsequent log entries will most likely reveal a pattern of behavior that will help the parent to pinpoint potential motivating factors. For example, if the child responds in a similar fashion when other preferred activities are terminated, this would suggest that the behavior is predominantly tangible seeking. If the child responds similarly whenever the parent asks him or her to perform a task, this would suggest that the behavior is predominantly escape motivated.

When using A-B-C sheets to collect data, the analysis is the same but the data is collected in a different format. Two examples of data collected on an A-B-C sheet appear in Figure 1.

The first A-B-C entry in Figure 1 is the same as the sample log entry and could be an example of either escape-motivated or attention-seeking behavior. The second A-B-C entry is an example of possible attention-seeking behavior. Jamie was fine until his mother began to interact with the neighbor. He then displayed problem behavior resulting in his mother paying attention to him and sending the neighbor home. Analysis of subsequent A-B-C entries may reveal a pattern of this type of behavior indicating that attention may be highly motivating to this child.

Parents and teachers frequently wonder how much data collection is necessary for a thorough assessment of a problem behavior. Although there is no set rule for determining length of assessment, we recommend collecting data at least until a clear pattern or set of patterns has emerged. In addition, we recommend continuing to collect data while the intervention is being implemented in order to track progress and pinpoint any additional motivating conditions that may develop.

It is important to note that sometimes the same antecedent conditions may result in very different behavior. For example, on Monday when Jamie is asked to get dressed, he immediately complies and laughs and jokes with his parent while dress-

Date	Time	Antecedent	Behavior	Consequence
9/11	8:45 AM	Jamie was watching TV and I turned it off and asked him to get dressed.	He screamed and threw a toy, then had a tantrum for 10 minutes.	I told him that he could watch TV for 10 more minutes but then he had to get dressed.
9/14	3:20 PM	The next-door neighbor came over for coffee and we were sitting in the kitchen talking. Jamie came in and kept trying to climb into my lap. I told him I was busy and would play with him later.	Jamie started screaming and threw himself to the floor and banged his head about five times.	I told the neighbor I was sorry but we'd have to postpone our talk until another time. I then picked up Jamie and told him he could hurt himself if he banged his head on the floor.

Fig 1. An example of an A-B-C (antecedent-behavior-consequence) sheet for data collection.

ing. On Tuesday when Jamie is asked to get dressed, he screams and has a 20-minute tantrum. The reason for this difference probably lies outside the typical antecedent–behavior–consequence unit of analysis. Often, conditions that exist prior to the immediate situation are influencing the way the child is reacting. These conditions are called setting events (Bijou and Baer, 1961; Bailey and Pyles, 1989). A setting event is something that influences how a person responds to an antecedent when it is presented. Examples of setting events that may lead to problem behavior include medical conditions (Carr and Smith, 1995) (for example, allergies, colds, or ear infections), temporary physical states (Carr and Smith, 1995) (for example, fatigue, hunger), or environmental events (Bailey and Pyles, 1989) (for example, losing a favorite toy, a noisy bus ride to school). In the example above, Jamie may have had a tantrum on Tuesday morning because he did not get a good night's sleep the night before. Lack of sleep may be a setting event that explains the inconsistency in his behavior from one day to the next, even though the same demands are presented to him on both days. If your review of the data indicates mixed or unclear motivations, you may need to look more closely at possible setting events that may account for this discrepancy.

PLANNING AN INTERVENTION: STRATEGIES TO PRODUCE CHANGE

When assessment has been completed, intervention planning can begin. A comprehensive intervention plan should include both strategies to reduce the probability that the problem behavior will occur (short-term intervention) and to teach the child the skills that are necessary to meet his or her needs when similar situations occur in the future (long-term intervention). Combining these approaches often helps to reduce the problem behavior immediately while building skills to ensure that a child is better able to deal with the challenges of daily living.

Short-term interventions usually address the setting events and antecedent events that have been shown to result in problem behavior. Examples of effective short-term interventions include changing the setting event and changing the antecedent (Carr et al., 1998). Changing the setting event can include providing treatment for a medical condition or changing some aspect of the environment that has been identified as mediating problem behavior. A child with an ear infection may need a pain reliever in addition to antibiotic treatment to minimize or eliminate the setting event. A child who has a bad day at school after a noisy bus ride may need to ride to school in a less crowded bus. Changing the antecedent may include removing the immediate trigger to the problem behavior or modifying the trigger in some way. A child who displays a lot of escape-motivated behavior related to school work may initially require fewer demands during the school day or may need extra time to transition into the school day (for example, a child could be given fewer tasks to complete during the first hour of school).

Long-term interventions usually address the need for additional skills either to get needs met successfully or to alleviate successfully the stressors involved in being in an unpleasant situation. Examples of long-term interventions include teaching a functionally equivalent communicative response (Carr et al., 1994) and teaching a coping skill (e.g., Schroeder et al., 1977). Teaching a functionally equivalent communicative response can include teaching a skill to access directly the desired outcome or teaching a child to ask for assistance in meeting a need. A child who displays aggression when confronted with a frustrating task can be taught to ask for a break or to summon an adult to provide additional instruction in completing the task. Teaching a coping skill may include teaching a child to avoid an unpleasant situation or teaching a child to employ a strategy to make the unpleasant situation more tolerable. A child who responds aggressively when other children are teasing him or her can be taught to walk away or tell a teacher. A child who has a tantrum when a desired activity is unavailable can be taught to select another activity from a list of preferred choices or to keep busy when he or she has to wait before a preferred activity can begin.

CASE EXAMPLES: PUTTING IT ALL TOGETHER

The following case descriptions provide real-life examples of using assessment information to design multicomponent interventions. Each case description describes the motivation for the problem behavior and provides examples of both long- and short-term intervention strategies that are likely to result in a positive outcome.

Case Example 1: Escape

Description of the Problem Situation. Sarah has frequent tantrums in the morning when getting ready for school. Her typical morning routine consists of getting up, eating breakfast, washing up, brushing teeth, and working with her mother on dressing independently. Sarah typically wakes up in a good mood but usually becomes irritable as the morning progresses. When she is asked to begin dressing herself (a hard task), she will throw herself to the floor, scream, cry, and sometimes bang her head. If her mother tries to prompt her to continue dressing, she may hit or bite her mother. When her mother leaves the room (to ignore the tantrum behavior), Sarah will stop the behavior and begin to play with her toys. On mornings when Sarah has not gotten enough sleep, the problem is much worse. She will often have trouble with even the initial steps of the morning routine. Only eating breakfast goes smoothly on these days. She will cry and tantrum until her mother completes all of the tasks for her.

An example of a log entry made by Sarah's mother appears below:

3/15/97 7:45AM

Sarah got up late this morning and we were really in a hurry. She had just finished brushing her teeth and I told her it was time to get dressed. I had laid out her clothes and was starting to prompt her to put on her socks. She started screaming and pulling her arms away from me. I kept trying to get her to put on her socks but she threw herself to the floor and screamed and thrashed around. I told her she had to calm down before she got dressed and I left the room.

Points of Intervention. Sarah's mother and father made log entries each day for three weeks and then reviewed the data to determine the variables influencing the behavior and to plan an intervention. In order to reduce the probability that the behavior will occur now (short-term intervention), Sarah's mother plans an intervention to address the setting events and the antecedents. The most obvious setting event is lack of sleep (Sarah has much more difficulty when she is tired). Sarah's parents make an effort to make sure that she is in bed at a reasonable hour each night so that she is likely to get a good night's sleep. To address the antecedents or immediate triggers for the problem behavior, Sarah's parents will do a couple of things. First, if Sarah is tired and has not gotten a good night's sleep, her mother will automatically help her through her morning routine. By not placing demands on Sarah at these times, the probability that she will display problem behavior is greatly reduced. On average mornings when Sarah wakes up in a good mood, Sarah's mother will have Sarah get dressed as the first task in her morning routine. Placing this task first will capitalize on Sarah's natural willingness to cooperate when she first wakes up.

Long-term intervention will include teaching a functionally equivalent skill so that Sarah is able to end an unpleasant task without having to exhibit problem behavior. Sarah's mother begins by prompting Sarah to ask for a break during difficult parts of her morning routine. This prompting takes place before Sarah displays problem behavior so that she learns a new way to meet her needs. To teach Sarah to cope with similar situations in the future (situations in which a lot of demands are placed in a short period of time), Sarah's mother capitalizes on Sarah's love of music. Having a favorite radio station playing during the morning routine helps Sarah to focus on singing along with the songs and minimizes the unpleasant nature of the routine. In addition, Sarah's mother makes up a song that they both sing during dressing (the most problematic part of the routine). By teaching Sarah to pair something fun (music) with something unpleasant (dressing), Sarah learns a valuable strategy for getting through difficult tasks.

Case Example 2: Attention-seeking

Description of the Problem Situation. Kristen has frequent episodes of self-injurious face slapping. These episodes often occur when Kristen is left alone or when her parents are busy. When her parents are playing with her or helping her with a task, Kristen is usually very happy. Kristen has a history of frequent ear infections. When she has an infection, she is usually in a bad mood and does not want to interact with anyone except her mother and father. She will cling to them and will not let them leave her sight without displaying severe problem behavior. Her parents know that she is coming down with an infection because Kristen will have a large increase in the number of episodes of face slapping. In addition, Kristen will have many episodes of hitting her ears. These episodes occur only when Kristen has an ear infection.

Kristen's parents document episodes of self-injury on A-B-C data sheets. The data entry in Figure 2 is an example of that theme.

Points of Intervention. Several short-term interventions could be implemented immediately in the home to reduce the probability that problem behavior will occur. To address the setting event (ear infections), Kristen's parents could use the data reflecting an increase in face slapping, along with the occurrence of hitting her ears, as indicators that Kristen may have an infection. They could then immediately take Kris-

Date	Time	Antecedent	Behavior	Consequence
9/20/97	1:15 PM	I (Mom) was on the phone in the kitchen with the babysitter. Kristen was sitting in the next room looking at me.	Kristen began screaming and started throwing her toys. When I did not respond, she came into the kitchen and started slapping her face while looking directly at me.	I told the babysitter that I had to get off the phone. I started talking to Kristen and asked her if she wanted to play with her blocks. She immediately stopped hitting herself and started to play with me.

Fig. 2. An example from Kristen's A-B-C sheets showing attention-seeking behavior.

ten to the doctor and begin the necessary medical intervention as early as possible. To address the more common antecedent factor for Kristen's behavior, being left alone, Kristen could be given more access to preferred toys that she could play with when an adult was not immediately available to interact with her. When in a situation that would involve removing attention from Kristen for more than a few minutes (such as talking on the phone), her parents could intermittently stop their activity and give Kristen attention on a frequent basis. For example, if Kristen's mother were on the phone, she could interrupt her conversation approximately every minute so that she could call to Kristen and praise her for playing quietly.

Eventually, Kristen could be taught to spend more time by herself. Therefore the long-term interventions planned would address this issue. First, Kristen's mother could further increase the amount of time between interruptions in a phone conversation to give Kristen attention. Kristen could also be taught how to tap an adult on the shoulder if she wanted an adult's attention. Initially, Kristen would be physically prompted to tap an adult. The adult who was tapped would respond by giving Kristen a big reaction (e.g., "Wow, Kristen! You did a great job tapping me! Don't you look pretty today!"). The adult would then spend a few moments interacting with Kristen before turning away. Kristen could then be prompted to tap the adult again, and the adult would respond in the same way. Once Kristen is able to independently tap a parent to get their attention, her parents could then delay Kristen's access to attention. For example, if Kristen tapped her mother while she was on the phone, her mother could respond by saying "Good job tapping me, Kristen. I'll be with you in one minute." In addition, Kristen could be taught additional play skills so that she could better occupy herself when not interacting with adults.

Case Example 3: Tangible-seeking

Description of the Problem Situation. Ben's favorite activity in his classroom at school is the computer. He loves every program that the teacher has for the computer and becomes extremely upset when another child is taking a turn. When working on a group activity, Ben will often poke at the children sitting around him. This often escalates into hitting and hair pulling until the teacher finally has to separate him from the group and give him some independent work to do. This independent work is often a lesson on the computer. When Ben is working one-on-one with the teacher or classroom aide, he is often able to finish his work very quickly and is then able to work on the computer. When Ben is working by himself on the computer, he is very quiet and does not disturb or try to hurt the other students. When the classroom is very noisy, the teacher notices Ben is more likely to engage in problem behavior such as aggression. Two times of day are particularly problematic, right after playground time and the end of the day when the students are getting ready to board their busses for home. During these times, Ben often runs around the room and hits or kicks any child who is in his path.

Ben's teacher kept a log of his problem behavior and a typical log entry appears below.

9/12/97 10:20AM

All of the students were sitting down for circle time. Ben was at the computer and I had to ask him repeatedly to join the group. I finally turned off the computer and prompted him to sit down with the other children. Ben immediately started to fidget and push the boy next to him. I asked him to stop but he kept pushing the boy and pinched his arm. I then told Ben that if he couldn't participate in the group, he would have to work by himself. I sat him at the computer and put on the math quiz program. He worked quietly while we finished the group lesson.

Points of Intervention. Short-term intervention is needed to reduce the amount of aggression that Ben is currently directing toward his classmates. Because noise and a chaotic environment seem to be major setting events, the teacher may reduce the probability of aggression by allowing Ben free access to the computer during the times that have been identified as most problematic. As soon as he comes in from the playground, the teacher directs him to sit at the computer and work on one of his favorite programs. This is repeated at the end of the day when the other students are preparing for the bus. A direct antecedent to aggression seems to be working in a group environment. For a short period of time (a week or two), it may be helpful for the teacher to allow Ben to work in a one-to-one setting with frequent breaks to work on the computer. The teacher may need to enlist the help of additional school personnel in order to implement this part of the plan.

While Ben is working with a one-to-one instructor, he needs to learn two very important skills in order to gain access to his favorite activity and to work better with his classmates. He needs to learn to ask appropriately to work on the computer (a functionally equivalent skill) and he needs to learn how to wait either when he must complete another task or when another child is working on the computer. First, his teacher prompts him to ask for the computer when he is working in the one-to-one setting. When he is able to ask successfully in this setting, the teacher then allows him to work in the group, where she again prompts him to ask appropriately to leave the group and work on the computer. When he is first learning this communicative skill, the teacher allows him to use the computer for a short time each time he asks. She will then teach him to tolerate gradually longer and longer delays between the time that he asks and the time that he gets to go to the computer. She will do this by acknowledging his request ("Sure, you can work on the computer . . .") and requiring a small amount of work before she allows him to go (". . . but first, let's do one more math problem"). When another student is working on the computer, the teacher will prompt Ben to find another fun activity to engage in until the other student is finished. Gradually, over time, Ben will learn to wait for long periods of time before his request is honored and will be better able to work within the regular routines of the classroom.

CONCLUSION

This chapter has presented the three most common social motivations for problem behavior in people with developmental disabilities. Assessment and intervention of severe problem behavior can seem like a daunting task to many parents. It is important to remember that, for any given problem behavior, there are a number of intervention approaches that will likely be effective in reducing the probability that the behavior will occur. The key to selecting an intervention is a thorough assessment of the conditions motivating and maintaining the problem behavior. We have presented several examples of assessment and intervention in this chapter that may assist the reader in a greater understanding of these processes. Parents are advised to work in cooperation with professionals in behavior analysis to plan and implement effective interventions. In closing, remember that, although problem behavior can seem difficult to deal with, it is possible to make significant changes by employing a systematic approach.

REFERENCES

Bailey JS, Pyles DAM (1989): Behavioral diagnostics. In E Cipani (ed.): "The Treatment of Severe Behavior Disorders." Monographs of the American Association on Mental Retardation, Vol. 12, pp. 85–107.

Bayley N (1932): A study of the crying of infants during mental and physical tests. J Genet Psychol 40:306–329.

Bell SM, Ainsworth MDS (1972): Infant crying and maternal responsiveness. Child Devel 43:1171–1190.

Bijou SW, Baer DM (1961): "Child Development I: A Systematic and Empirical Theory." Englewood Cliffs, NJ: Prentice-Hall.

Brownlee JR, Bakeman R (1981): Hitting in toddler-peer interaction. Child Develop 52:1076–1079.

Carr EG, Carlson JI (1993): Reduction of severe behavior problems in the community using a multicomponent treatment approach. J Appl Behav Anal 26:157–172.

Carr EG, Carlson JI, Langdon NA, Magito McLaughlin D, Yarbrough SC (1998): Two perspectives on antecedent control: Molecular and molar. In Luiselli JK, Cameron MJ (eds.): "Antecedent Control Procedures for the Behavioral Support of Persons with Developmental Disabilities." Baltimore, MD: Paul H. Brookes.

Carr EG, Durand VM (1985): Reducing behavior problems through functional communication training. J Appl Behav Anal 18:111–126.

Carr EG, Levin L, McConnachie G, Carlson JI, Kemp DC, Smith CE (1994): "Communication-based Intervention for Problem Behavior: A User's Guide for Producing Positive Change." Baltimore, MD: Paul H. Brookes.

Carr EG, Newsom CD, Binkoff JA (1980): Escape as factor in the aggressive behavior of two retarded children. J Appl Behav Anal 13:101–117.

Carr EG, Smith CE (1995): Biological setting events for self-injury. Ment Retard Devel Disabilities Res Rev 1:94–98.

Caulfield MB, Fischel J, DeBaryshe BD, Whitehurst GJ (1989): Behavioral correlates of developmental expressive language disorder. J Abnormal Child Psychol 17:187–201.

Day RM, Rea JA, Schussler NG, Larsen SE, Johnson WL (1988): A functionally based approach to the treatment of self-injurious behavior. Behav Modific 12:565–589.

deLissovoy V (1963): Head banging in early childhood: A suggested cause. J Genet Psychol 102:109–114.

Donnellan AM, Mirenda PL, Mesaros RA, Fassbender LL (1984): Analyzing the communicative functions of aberrant behavior. J Assoc Persons Severe Handicaps 9:201–212.

Iwata BA, Dorsey MF, Slifer KJ, Bauman KE, Richman GS (1982): Toward a functional analysis of self-injury. Analy Intervent Devel Disabilities 2:3–21.

Matson JL, DiLorenzo TM (1984): "Punishment and Its Alternatives: A New Perspective for Behavior Modification." New York: Springer.

Repp AC, Felce D, Barton LE (1988): Basing the treatment of stereotypic and self-injurious behaviors on hypotheses of their causes. J Appl Behav Anal 21:281–289.

Schroeder SR, Peterson CR, Solomon LJ, Artley JJ (1977): EMG feedback and the contingent restraint of self-injurious behavior among the severely retarded. Behav Therapy 8:738–741.

Smith RG, Iwata BA, Vollmer TR, Zarcone JR (1993): Experimental analysis and treatment of multiply controlled self-injury. J Appl Behav Anal 26:183–196.

Stevenson J, Richman N (1978): Behavior, language, and development in three-year-old children. J Autism Childhood Schizophrenia 8:299–313.

Taylor JC, Carr EG (1992a): Severe problem behavior related to social interaction. II: A systems analysis. Behav Modific 16:336–371.

Taylor JC, Carr EG (1992b): Severe problem behavior related to social interaction. I: Attention seeking and social avoidance. Behav Modific 6:305–335.

Weeks M, Gaylord-Ross R (1981): Task difficulty and aberrant behavior in severely handicapped students. J Appl Behav Anal 14:449–463.

Positive Behavior Support:
Analyzing, Preventing, and Replacing Problem Behaviors

Daniel B. Crimmins

Problem behaviors, such as tantrums, aggression, noncompliance, and inappropriate social interactions, are commonly encountered among persons with developmental disabilities, including Down syndrome. This leads to three questions. First, are behaviors caused by disability? No, behavior problems, in one form or another, are estimated to occur in as many as 20% of all children, and not all children with disabilities have them. Second, are behavior problems more likely in children with disabilities? Yes, events that are common in the lives of many people with disabilities, among them difficulties in communication and learning, rejection, reduced expectations, and limited opportunities can all increase the likelihood of problem behaviors occurring. And, third, are specific behavior problems associated with Down syndrome? No, people with Down syndrome seem to show the same range of behaviors as individuals with other disabilities and those without disabilities.

Problem behaviors are a significant concern for parents and teachers of children with Down syndrome. In addition to their emotional impact on the individual and family members, these behaviors present significant obstacles to developing social relationships and participating in the community (Meyer and Evans, 1989). They are often the primary reason that individuals are referred to more restrictive educational or vocational settings. Historically, these behaviors were seen as needing "management" with some procedures extending to the use of painful or highly restrictive consequences (Repp and Singh, 1990). During the 1980s, there was a strong reaction against this position by many in the field on ethical and legal grounds (Guess et al., 1987), as well as by the demonstration of a range of alternative strategies (Helmstetter and Durand, 1991). Thus, over the past 20 years, interventions for difficult behaviors have evolved from largely reactive, systems-centered strategies to more

Down Syndrome: A Promising Future, Together, Edited by Terry J. Hassold and David Patterson
ISBN 0-471-29686-4 Copyright © 1998 by Wiley-Liss, Inc.

preventive, person-centered approaches. The latter approach, generally referred to as positive behavior support (PBS), has emerged and is supported by an increasingly well-established knowledge base demonstrating its effectiveness for individuals exhibiting challenging behaviors in all life settings (Koegel et al., 1996; Lehr and Brown, 1996).

Because problem behaviors are not specific to Down syndrome, this chapter reviews three important components of PBS that have been demonstrated across a range of people and settings. The first of these is the importance of understanding why a behavior continues to occur. This is a process that can take some time, but is critically important for success. The second component involves preventing the behavior through changing one or more aspects of the environment. The third is developing long-term replacements for the problems behaviors—specifically, teaching the child to do something else in the same situations that the behavior now occurs. Note that these approaches can be carried out without the use of punishment. A fourth section of the chapter discusses the need for coordinating the efforts of parents and teachers in providing PBS.

Successful solutions *are* possible for behavior problems. The concepts in this chapter will be familiar to parents and teachers; they are often described as making "common sense." But, like many things we know we *should* do because it's the right thing, we often stop somewhere short of completion. It is important to remember that behavior problems developed over time, and will also take time to resolve.

UNDERSTAND WHY THE BEHAVIOR PERSISTS

There are many reasons that behaviors occur, but the first step in addressing behavior problems is to understand why it "makes sense" that a child engages in them. You need to ask a series of questions to understand how your child might be responding to the environment. Is the behavior triggered by specific events? Is it a form of communication? What causes the behavior to persist? What does he or she get out of it? The answers to these questions generally come from an organized approach to information-gathering called functional assessment. The functional assessment identifies specific situations that influence whether the behavior occurs or not, and helps to determine the function that the behavior serves for the child. A number of books are available that discuss strategies for conducting functional assessments (e.g., Durand, 1990; Durand and Crimmins, 1992; O'Neill et al., 1990); the following sections outline the kinds of questions that are asked and information being sought as part of this process.

Setting Events and Antecedents

One of the first steps in understanding a behavior is to look at the times, places, people, and activities associated with both the behavior occurring *and* not occurring. This helps to identify two concepts, setting events and antecedents, that are critical in the assessment process.

Setting events can be thought of as situations that make a behavior more likely to occur for a given child. Antecedents are events that immediately precede a behavior.

For example, what might we expect of a child in the morning who had a poor night's sleep due to an ear infection? Most people can immediately bring to mind a child who is fussy or perhaps clinging, and might have difficulty separating from a parent. These behaviors by themselves would be easily understood and accepted. But under these particular circumstances, many children's behaviors escalate to more problematic levels. To continue the example, the child, who normally dresses independently and happily, has a tantrum when asked to get dressed. In this example, illness and disrupted sleep are potential setting events; the request is an antecedent for the behavior. Table 1 provides a number of examples that can logically be seen to have a potential effect on a behavior. For some children, behaviors are far more likely to occur when one or more of these settings events occurs; the setting events, however, are usually not sufficient by themselves.

Table 1. Examples of Setting Events

Disrupted routine (e.g., new teacher, different order of activities)
Negative interaction (e.g., a fight, being "made" to do something)
Specific time of day or day of the week
Disrupted sleep
Physical discomfort, illness, or pain (e.g., headache, seizures, allergies)
Mood (e.g., agitated, depressed)

Antecedents may be thought of as triggers, events that make it quite likely that a behavior will occur. Determining antecedents occurs through direct observation, structured interviews, or questionnaires. Table 2 contains some examples of antecedent conditions that have been associated with behavior problems for a number of children.

Table 2. Examples of Antecedents

Left alone for a long time
Asked to do a difficult task (e.g., corrected during
    the task, frustrated in completing an assignment)
End of an interaction
Told "no" after asking for something
Interrupted during a pleasant event
Teased or called a name

Functions

Identifying setting events and antecedents assists in determining the function that a behavior might serve. We have found, for example, that behaviors often serve as a way of communicating, "Pay attention to me!" Typical antecedents for this function of a behavior would include being left alone, being left out of a conversation, or ending an interaction. Other communicative functions that are frequently observed include "I don't want to do this," "I want my way," and "Doing this is fun." The child may, however, be unable or unwilling to tell you what he wants or needs. In attempting to determine the function of a behavior, we consider a number of questions (see Table 3) that help in pinpointing the behavioral concerns, and why a behavior may persist. The answers to these questions lead directly to planning a solution to a behavior problem.

Table 3. Functional Assessment Considerations

What precisely does the individual do?
What function(s) does the behavior serve?
Is the behavior a form of communication?
Is the behavior a habit or source of pleasure?
Is the behavior a means of exerting control?
Is the behavior something to do during free time?
How effective is the behavior at getting a child what he or she might want?
Does the behavior warrant intervention?
Do several behaviors occur together or in a sequence?

MAKE THINGS BETTER FOR EVERYONE; PREVENT THE BEHAVIOR BY CHANGING THE ENVIRONMENT

Once you better understand why the behavior is occurring, you can begin to figure out ways to prevent it from occurring. What would happen if you changed certain patterns of interaction? What if you reduced demands? Do you need to avoid certain situations? What would happen if the child could do something really enjoyable more often? Understand that these questions lead to the identification of short-term rather

Table 4. Setting Event Strategies

Make accommodations for unpleasant events or difficult times
Provide social support (e.g., counseling, "cool down" time)
Set up distraction routines (e.g., exercise)
Clarify rules and expectations
Treat sleep disorder
Ensure treatment for physical conditions
Provide relaxation routine
Present with calming music

Table 5. Antecedent Strategies

Structure "down" time (e.g., increase supervision, give reminders for expected behavior)
Provide extra assistance
Change tasks to match student skills
Alternate easy with difficult tasks
Change interaction style or staffing
Signal transitions (e.g., give "2-minute warnings")
Increase access to preferred activities (noncontingent reinforcement)
Redirect at first sign of behavioral sequence
Avoid problem activity or location

than long-term solutions, but this is an important intermediate step. We find that preventing or reducing the frequency of problem behaviors gives everyone a break. Many times people are concerned that preventing the behavior through changing the environment is somehow "giving in" to the child and that this will make the problem worse. We generally find that this is not the case, rather that this approach makes things more predictable for all who are involved. Tables 4 and 5 present strategies that, when matched to the assessment information, are often dramatically effective in reducing the frequency or intensity of problem behaviors. In many ways, we are removing the need to use behaviors to control the environment.

REPLACEMENT IS THE BEST LONG-TERM ANSWER

In the long run, behaviors rarely "go away" without being replaced by something else. It is important to identify what it is you want your child to do *instead* of what he or she is doing now. What skill would serve as a replacement? Some possibilities are listed as alternative behaviors in Table 6. Teaching these skills, however, requires a plan for the child that can be carried out at home and in school. Table 6 identifies a number of considerations for these plans, which are described in detail elsewhere (e.g., Carr et al., 1994; Durand, 1990; Meyer and Evans, 1989).

In brief, the best replacement behaviors serve the same function as the problem behavior. Thus, if a behavior gets the child attention, the replacement behavior must be some means of gaining the attention of others. This could be through raising a hand in a classroom or gently tapping someone on the shoulder; it also suggests the need for teaching the child a means of maintaining the attention of others (e.g., conversation). With this type of instruction, children tend to learn better by doing rather than by being told what to do. Instruction must include the steps of showing what it is that we'd like done, making sure there is a good chance of success, and then giving the child a chance to practice. Once instruction begins in a specific skill, the plan must provide time for practice in situations that become more and more realistic with the

Table 6. Plan for Teaching Replacement Behavior

Make sure that alternative behavior serves the same function
Teach alternative behavior
  Functional communication training
  Use of leisure time
  Stress management and relaxation
  Social skills
  Anger control
  Coping
  Self-management
  Organization
Provide time for practice
Prompt use of skill in "trigger" situations
Fade supports to achieve spontaneity
Evaluate progress by skills learned, not just a reduction in
  behavior problems

ultimate goal of the child spontaneously using the alternative behavior. The final aspect of the plan is evaluating its effectiveness in terms of demonstrating the impact of this approach on the child's life—using the replacement skill, going to new places, getting along better with siblings, and learning new skills, as well as by an improvement in the problem behavior.

WORK TOGETHER

Most children do not need formal behavioral plans. But when one is needed because of a child's persistent behavior problems, it should be based on understanding of *why* the behavior is occurring (functional assessment) and a recognition of what he or she needs to learn to do instead. Too many plans only describe what should happen in response to the behavior occurring. Although this is necessary, the plan should also identify what will be done in the short term to prevent incidents of the behavior and how the replacement skills will be taught.

Providing PBS requires the coordinated efforts of parents, family members, teachers, assistants, speech therapists, guidance counselors, psychologists, principals, and potentially many others. This occurs best through a small team of the people who know the child well, with the support of someone well-versed in PBS, and when there is a shared vision for the child. These circumstances can be elusive, but are necessary for having long-term impact.

REFERENCES

Carr EG, Levin L, McConnachie G, Carlson JI, Kemp DC, Smith CE (1994): "Communication-based Intervention for Problem Behavior: A User's Guide for Producing Positive Change." Baltimore: Paul H. Brookes.

Durand VM (1990): "Severe Behavior Problems: A Functional Communication Training Approach." New York: Guilford Press.

Durand VM, Crimmins DB (1992): "The Motivation Assessment Scale (MAS) Administration Guide." Topeka, KS: Monaco & Associates.

Guess D, Helmstetter E, Turnbull HR, III, Knowlton S (1987): Use of aversive procedures with persons who are disabled (TASH Monograph Series, No. 2). Seattle: The Association for Persons with Severe Handicaps.

Helmstetter E, Durand VM (1991): Nonaversive intervention for severe behavior problems. In Meyer LH, Peck CA, Brown L (eds.): "Critical Issues in the Lives of People with Severe Disabilities." Baltimore: Paul H. Brookes, pp. 559–600.

Koegel LK, Koegel RL, Dunlap G (1996): "Positive Behavioral Support: Including People with Difficult Behavior in the Community." Baltimore: Paul H. Brookes.

Lehr DH, Brown F (1996): "People with Disabilities who Challenge the System." Baltimore: Paul H. Brookes.

Meyer LH, Evans IM (1989): "Nonaversive Intervention for Behavior Problems." Baltimore: Paul H. Brookes.

O'Neill RE, Horner RH, Albin RW, Storey K, Sprague JR (1990): "Functional Analysis: A Practical Assessment Guide." Pacific Grove, CA: Brooks/Cole.

Repp AC, Singh NN (1990): "Perspectives on the Use of Nonaversive and Aversive Interventions for Persons with Developmental Disabilities." Sycamore, IL: Sycamore Publishing Co.

The 3 Rs of Sexuality Education:
Rights, Responsibilities, and Realities

Mary Ann Carmody

The question is not *if* parents and educators should offer sex education to persons with Down syndrome. The questions are *when* and *how* they should begin. Passage of the Americans with Disabilities Act has opened the doors to housing, education, and employment for all persons. Deinstitutionalization has emptied large state-run facilities so that adults with developmental disabilities have become more visible than ever in community residences and in competitive employment. For school-age children, inclusion is occurring at a rapid pace and is reportedly successful. In all walks of life, persons with Down syndrome and other disabilities are taking more control of their lives as their social opportunities and interactions increase.

However, the same doors that are opening by legal mandate are not opening as quickly for friendship building and social dating. Myths abound about the social and sexual behaviors of persons with disabilities. Although there are many instances of inappropriate behavior, due to lack of information and social opportunity, as well as immutable patterns of acting out and/or coping, it is a fact that there is a high risk of sexual abuse to this vulnerable population. In the past, persons with developmental disabilities have not had as many opportunities to learn about and to practice safe, appropriate, and rewarding behaviors. Now, preparation for full inclusion *must* offer information about human sexuality.

As the National Down Syndrome Society's poster for Down Syndrome Awareness Month theme so poignantly states: *"None of us are the same on the outside. All of us are the same on the inside."* Within the context of sexuality education, this theme means that *all* persons need information about how their bodies work and how to take care of them, how to identify and adaptively express a wide range of feelings, and how to build and enjoy social or intimate relationships. Nationally and internationally there is a heightened awareness of the need for sexuality education for persons with developmental disabilities. Sexuality has taken on a new importance as we head to-

Down Syndrome: A Promising Future, Together, Edited by Terry J. Hassold and David Patterson
ISBN 0-471-29686-4   Copyright © 1998 by Wiley-Liss, Inc.

ward the 21st century. Persons with disabilities need neither more nor less information than their nonlabeled peers.

Throughout the life-span, information must be given to children, adolescents and adults that is relevant to their life situations. Using the 3 Rs as a frame of reference is beneficial to students and parents alike. The 3 Rs within this context are defined as follows:

1. *Rights:* Matters to which one has just claim. For example, the rights to privacy and education are guaranteed by law for every citizen. With reference to sexuality, all persons expect to be free from exploitation, to be able to engage in rewarding social activities, and to be able to express themselves as sexual beings, if they so choose.
2. *Responsibilities:* Events for which one is accountable. In the area of sexuality, these include the respect due the rights of others; the awareness of home, agency, and community standards; and the need to act as appropriately as possible based on education and life experiences.
3. *Realities:* Considerations that have impact and that are based on fact. The realities in this context include the cognitive and/or physical limitations resulting from the developmental disability; natural, human feelings and needs; restricted access to persons of same or opposite sex with whom to build relationships; negative labels; low expectations; life experiences to date; social isolation; and the list goes on.

These three components are shared by individuals and their parents or educators in an overlapping fashion. When the expression of one person's *right* begins, so does that person's *responsibility* for that action; because of his or her *reality,* another person, perhaps a parent or professional also with rights and responsibilities, enters the picture. This intertwining of the 3 Rs of students, parents, and educators, must be appreciated if sexuality education is to be relevant and successful.

EDUCATION FOR CHILDREN

The home is a natural setting in which to begin the process of sexuality education. Who better to begin this education than parents and caring relatives. Rather than leave sexuality information for others to impart to their children, parents can begin early in childhood to build the foundation of honesty and openness that will enhance their child's decision-making throughout life. Children can benefit by learning early on about their gender from parental role modeling, from being presented with choices for gender-appropriate clothing, and from hearing positive comments about the specialness of their male- or femaleness. Experience has demonstrated the importance of discussing disability issues at home to enhance self-esteem and decrease vulnerability.

Even young children have the *right* to privacy and the *responsibility* to be mindful of the privacy of others. For example, 3- to 5-year-old children typically exhibit curiosity about their own and others' bodies. They have the *right* to know correct names for their private body parts, to know who can touch them, and to begin to practice saying Rule #1: "My body belongs to me" Agency for Instructional Technology (AIT).

They have the *responsibility* not to touch the private parts of parents' or playmates' bodies, not to listen in on private conversations, and to be unclothed only in appropriate private places. Given the *reality* of their special needs, they will require that the information be repeated often over the years and presented in clear and concrete terms.

Parental *responsibilities* come into play at this age as parents decide what meaningful sexuality information they must give their children and where they can first educate themselves. They are often in a quandary because of their own discomfort and because the process does not begin naturally. Parents are reminded that two skills are to be utilized: *observation* and *anticipation*. The term "SOAP" is helpful as a buzzword for parents. It is described as follows:

- S: What $\underline{S}$eems to be happening from the parent's observations; what does the child seem to be doing or needing.
- O: What is $\underline{O}$bjectively happening based on verbal or nonverbal feedback.
- A: What does the parent $\underline{A}$nticipate happening from literature on developmental tasks, workshops, talking with other parents, etc.
- P: What $\underline{P}$lan of action or education is needed. Refer to a curriculum such as "Changes in You" to begin the process early.

Resource Suggestions

AIT video, "The Five Rules of Sex Abuse Prevention"
"Changes in You" curriculum

EDUCATION FOR ADOLESCENTS

Because of deinstitutionalization, funding cutbacks, individual choice, and other considerations, children are staying in their family homes longer. Parents know more about the sexual behaviors of their children with Down syndrome, such as masturbation, than perhaps they know of their other children's. Sometimes this behavior, which is a *right* and a normal developmental task of all children, has overstepped certain boundaries and has become public or excessive. In other words, it is not being addressed *responsibly*. The adolescent's *reality* (inability to foresee the consequences of such activity) may have caused him or her to masturbate in public.

Parents who are ready for this task will consult the SOAP model and find the following tips:

- S: Their 16-year-old son *seems to be* spending a rather long time in the bathroom and he frequently leaves the bathroom door open.
- O: When questioned, the teen says that the boys in gym class talk about masturbation and that he is trying it out.
- A: The parents have been prepared for this topic because they and their son are familiar with the "Changes in You" curriculum that discusses pubertal changes. They are able to explain clearly and calmly to their son that this is an adult behavior that must be done privately in order to be *responsible*.
- P: They plan to review the curriculum again with their son because they know the value of frequent repetition: one of his *realities*.

Another developmental task in adolescence is experimentation as teens shape their own identity to fit into the larger world as they perceive it. Teens have *rights* to information on a variety of subjects: pubertal changes that they are experiencing, personal safety, same and opposite sex intimacy, privacy, birth control, HIV, and social skills to count a few. They need this information to take on the challenges of a world that is overwhelmed by sexual innuendo. They need to know the meaning of words, to learn to mean what they say and to say what they mean, to learn to recognize bribes, and to learn how to attract positive attention.

In other words, teens with developmental disabilities need the same information as other teens; it is the "how" it is taught that is different. One helpful vehicle is peer group work as demonstrated in the video, "Roots and Wings." The video's title comes from the delicate balance that parents are trying to achieve: the gift to their children of strong family roots and values in order that they might fly with wings as independently as possible. Successful sexuality education programs for high-school-age children are partnerships between parents and teachers. This ensures a carryover of the information from school to home and gives the parents opportunities to present their value system to their teenagers.

Finally, another example of shared rights and responsibilities is the onset of menstruation. A 13-year-old girl approaching menarche has the *right* to education about menstruation and menstrual hygiene. She has the *responsibility,* within her particular capabilities, to act as appropriately as possible, for example, change her pads successfully and discuss her periods only with certain appropriate persons. But the *educational responsibility* belongs to her family and to support persons. The school-based nurse might use teachable moments to reinforce the one or two people to talk to about her periods. The nurse would then share the effective teaching techniques with the youngster's family and support network.

Resource Suggestions

Choices, Inc. video, "Roots and Wings"
"Masturbation Instruction for Men Who Have Developmental Disabilities"

EDUCATION FOR ADULTS

Adult women and men have the *right* to date if they so choose, but they often have no understanding of how to meet appropriate persons. Family or care-giving staff will have anticipated this human need for companionship, and they will know that some of the *responsibility* for broadening the social opportunities is theirs. Before facilitating more social opportunities, however, family and staff must offer assistance in exploring feelings about dating and related subjects. The mutual rights and responsibilities of sexual expression must be addressed as a framework for all healthy relationships. Then, eventually, caregivers can facilitate healthy and fulfilling social opportunities for persons with disabilities. This can mean anything from being a chauffeur to outlining the steps in relationship building to finding a therapist who will help an individual overcome paralyzing fears of social contact.

No matter how serious the cognitive disability, men and women alike need the skills with which to communicate what they want, need, and feel: a basic *right*. They need to be informed of safe and appropriate touch at any level of relationship, whether by kissing or hugging or sexual intimacy, and that there are ways to express feelings that are safe and refreshing. The *reality* of their disability means that time also has to be spent on how they learn and retain new information so that a new skill will be a lasting and valuable one.

Resource Suggestions

Choices, Inc. video, "Making Connections"

SUMMARY

Sexuality education for persons with developmental disabilities is an awesome responsibility for parents and professionals. If they keep in mind the balance of mutual *rights* and *responsibilities,* tempered with pertinent *realities,* they will be successful in leading their children and students to a better sense of themselves as valuable and competent individuals. Parents and professionals working together will gain *comfort* with the topic of human sexuality and *competence* as sexuality educators for their children and students. They will enjoy *improved communication* with adolescents and adults as they share with them the knowledge and skills needed to ensure safe and satisfying relationships throughout the life span.

RESOURCE INFORMATION*

Changes in You, Peggy C. Siegel, MS, 1990. Family Life Education Associates, 804/262-0531. Complete curriculum sold by James Stanfield Co. Inc., 800/421-6534. (Books and curriculum for children and adolescents with special needs.)

AIT Presents: Five Rules of Sex Abuse Prevention. 800/457-4509. (Video and training manual; excellent resource.)

Person to Person, produced by Mary Ann Carmody and American Film & Video, 1991. Choices, Inc., 202/364-5303, $79. (Sensitive approach to sex education for parents and caregivers. VHS format, 52 minutes, discussion guide included.)

Roots and Wings, produced by Mary Ann Carmody and American Film & Video, 1995. Choices, Inc., 202/364-5303, $79. (Educational video about the social-sexual development of adolescents with cognitive disabilities. Great for parents, caregivers, teachers, therapists, and other professionals. VHS format, 35 minutes, Discussion Guide included.)

Making Connections, produced by Mary Ann Carmody and American Film & Video, 1995. Choices, Inc., 202/364-5303, $79. (An engaging look at dating for persons with disabilities of all kinds. It is enjoyable and educational viewing for parents, professionals, and young adults with or without cognitive disabilities. The cast is made up primarily of persons with disabilities. VHS format, 31 minutes, discussion guide included.)

Masturbation Instruction for Men Who Have Developmental Disabilities, Jason R. Dura, Ph.D., Clinical Psychologist and Heidi Nunemaker, L.S.W., Human Awareness Instructor,

---

*More complete list available upon request.

and Behavior Specialist. Practical Programming Group, 230 West Evers, Bowling Green, OH 43402. (A manual intended for use as an instruction guide for teaching privacy and masturbation skills.)

A Life-Span Approach to Nursing Care for Individuals With Developmental Disabilities, Shirley P. Roth and Joyce S. Morse, 1994. Brookes Publishing Co., 800/638-3775.

Living Your Life, Ann Craft, 1991. Living and Learning, Seattle, WA, 800/521-3218. (Excellent and comprehensive curriculum.)

Group Teaching Strategies for Persons with Severe and Profound Mental Retardation. Video from the Young Adult Institute, 212/563-7474.

Circles and *Circles Stop Abuse.* James Stanfield Co., PO Box 1995E, Santa Monica, CA 90406.

STARS: Skills Training for Assertiveness, Relationship-Building, and Sexual Awareness. Wisconsin Council on Disabilities, 608/266-7826, $5. (A wonderful curriculum.)

Wings to Fly, Sally D. Bailey, R.D.T., 1993. SD Bailey, Woodbine House, Rockville, MD. "Bringing Theatre Arts to Students with Special Needs." (Comprehensive handbook for special education and drama teachers at elementary through high school levels; describes concrete, proven techniques and lesson plans to teach drama to students with a wide array of special needs in academic and theatre settings.)

Learn About Life: Sexuality and Social Skills (6 booklets covering a wide range of sexual and social concepts) and *What People Wear: Body Awareness and Dressing Skills.* Attainment Co., Inc., 800/327-4269.

Behavior Disorders in Children and Adolescents with Down Syndrome

William I. Cohen

Children with developmental disabilities often present challenging behaviors to the primary care physician: biting, throwing toys, hitting other children, temper tantrums, and unruly behavior in the community. The usual recommendations that we make for typically developing children are often found to be futile, leading to increased parental frustration.

The Down Syndrome Center of Western Pennsylvania (DSC) at Children's Hospital of Pittsburgh has developed a model for assessment and treatment of these common but nevertheless troublesome complaints. Using a team consisting of the director (a developmental-behavioral pediatrician with further expertise in family therapy) and a behavioral psychologist, children whose parents and/or caregivers identified behavioral concerns were offered referral to the clinicians for diagnostic evaluation. Selected cases were offered treatment by the same team except in those cases where the severity of the disorder required intensive intervention.

In the first 3 years of operation of the center (1990–1993), 37 patients were found to have behavioral concerns noted at the time of the initial appointment, which consisted of a review of the child's health, development, and social adaptation, using the "Preventive Medical Checklist for Down Syndrome" (Cohen, 1992): 17 of the 37 were younger than 20 years of age: 7 were children less than 12 years old, and 10 were adolescents (between 12 and 20 years of age).

CHIEF CONCERNS AND DIAGNOSES
Children

Six of the children were described as having unmanageable behavior and two of these six were aggressive toward siblings. The seventh child was described as having poor social skills.

Down Syndrome: A Promising Future, Together, Edited by Terry J. Hassold and David Patterson
ISBN 0-471-29686-4   Copyright © 1998 by Wiley-Liss, Inc.

The preliminary diagnostic formulations included one child with attention deficit hyperactivity disorder (ADHD) and oppositional-defiant disorder (ODD) and the other six children with Rule/Out ODD.

Adolescents

The chief concerns of the 10 adolescent patients were as follows: five were described as aggressive; one was suicidal; one was stealing food; one was hiding from the family and crying; one was refusing to go to school; and one was defiant.

The preliminary diagnostic formulations included four with ODD; two with major depression, single episode; two with adjustment disorder; one with post-traumatic stress disorder; and one with eating disorder, not otherwise specified.

EVALUATION AND TREATMENT

The team began eliciting a detailed history of the presenting problem. This was followed by a behavioral analysis, and the development of a program designed to modify the target behavior. The structure and belief systems of the family were utilized in presenting the behavior plan. The failure of the plan to be implemented was reevaluated from both the behavioral and family (contextual) perspectives: that is, was there a flaw in the program itself, or were there factors within the family (including grandparents) that had not been accounted for, or both.

Children

The child with ADHD and ODD was referred to a specialty psychiatric program for children with multiple disabilities. The parents of the other six children were all offered services by the in-house team of behavioral pediatrician/family therapist and behavioral psychologist. Five of these children elected to begin treatment at the DSC; one child was seen for one session, after which his mother transferred care to another program. Four children underwent treatment at the DSC.

In three of these four cases, treatment led to a change in diagnosis to *parent–child problem*. The course of treatment lasted from one to three sessions, at which time the treatment was terminated because the problems were resolved.

In the fourth case, further evaluation during treatment led to a change in diagnosis to *autistic disorder,* with a subsequent shift in the focus of treatment.

Adolescents

The four adolescents with oppositional defiant disorder (ODD) were offered services by the in-house team. The parents of one of the four elected treatment at the DSC, and three chose referral to a community agency. Both adolescents with depression were referred directly for psychiatric evaluation and required hospitalization as part of their treatment. The individual with post-traumatic stress disorder was referred to a private therapist who specializes in this condition. This patient also received a psychiatric evaluation for depression. The individual with the eating disorder was referred to a community mental health agency. One of the two adolescents with adjustment disorder was offered services at the DSC , but the family did not pursue treatment; the other was referred to a community mental health agency.

SUMMARY

Children with behavior problems such as aggression and unmanageability were successfully treated in one to three sessions by a team of behavioral pediatrician/family therapist and behavioral psychologist. These cases were often examples of *parent–child problems*. They appeared to reflect the difficulty some parents have in responding appropriately to the developmental stage of their child: the parents often expected the children to behave like a child of the same chronological age, rather than the same developmental age. When this belief was an honest error, treatment proceeded rapidly and effectively. However, when the behavioral difficulties did not respond to straightforward behavioral programming, we often found that the complaint about the problem represented a struggle within the family (not necessarily of both parents) to deal with the underlying problem of having a child with a disability.

Behavior problems in adolescents were more likely to require further psychiatric evaluation and treatment, although some problems were able to be managed by the team. The team's experience in the years following the study period has been essentially similar, in terms of the nature of the cases referred, and the results obtained.

REFERENCES

Cohen WI, Ohio/Western PA Down Syndrome Network (1992): Down Syndrome Preventive Medical Check List. Down Syndrome Papers and Abstracts for Professionals, 15(3):1–7.

Cohen W, Murray NJ, Pary RJ, Handen BL (1993): Behavioral and Psychiatric Problems in Individuals with Down syndrome. Presented at American Association on Mental Retardation 117th Annual Meeting, Washington DC.

VI. Communication, Language, and Literacy

Comprehensive Speech and Language Treatment for Infants, Toddlers, and Children with Down Syndrome

Libby Kumin

This chapter discusses a comprehensive approach to speech and language treatment from infancy through elementary school, which considers the communication strengths and challenges for children with Down syndrome, as well as the specific needs of the individual child with Down syndrome.

Speech and language are complex and present many challenges to the child with Down syndrome that need to be addressed through a comprehensive approach to speech and language treatment. There have been major historical, legislative, and financial influences on speech and language services and service delivery for children with Down syndrome; these are summarized below.

LEGISLATIVE BACKGROUND

The Education for All Handicapped Children Act (Public Law 94-142) was passed in 1975 and resulted in special education services in separate classrooms as the model for helping children with disabilities. The Individualized Education Plan (IEP) became the blueprint for each child's educational program for the school year. The law has been amended and renewed to the present day. The most recent legislation is the Individuals with Disabilities Education Act Amendments of 1997 (IDEA 97).

The important ramifications of IDEA for communication in school-age children are that *speech-language pathology is a related service and is based on a remediation model.* Related services are developmental, corrective, and other supportive services, as may be required to assist a child with a disability to benefit from special education, and includes the early identification and assessment of disabling conditions in children. A remediation model means that the child receives services only when there is a documented problem based on test results, in order to address that problem. With in-

Down Syndrome: A Promising Future, Together, Edited by Terry J. Hassold and David Patterson
ISBN 0-471-29686-4   Copyright © 1998 by Wiley-Liss, Inc.

clusion becoming more common and the regular education initiative, the child's needs for speech-language pathology services may be greater, and the goals may be higher.

Public Law 99-457 provided funding to extend services to children ages 3 to 5 years using the IEP as the child's service plan, and provided for early intervention services to children ages birth to 2 years who are experiencing developmental delays or who have a diagnosed condition that will place them at risk for developmental delay, using the Individualized Family Service Plan (IFSP) as the family's service plan. Children with Down syndrome would qualify for evaluation for services from the time of diagnosis, based on the guidelines in PL 99-457. Important ramifications of PL99-457 for speech and language treatment are that *speech-language pathology services are based on a prevention model* and that *the family is included as central to the treatment process.* When the child is 3 years of age, the educational plan changes from the IFSP to the IEP, and this represents a shift from a *prevention model* to a *remediation model,* and a shift in service delivery.

IDEA 97 has continued the funding for early intervention services for children under age 3, which was first mandated under PL 99-457. The sections related to early intervention are under Part C in IDEA 97. Whereas speech-language pathology is defined as a related service for children age 3 and older, it is defined as an early intervention service for infants and toddlers younger than 3 years. Early intervention services "are designed to meet the developmental needs of an infant or toddler with a disability in any one or more of the following areas: physical development, cognitive development, communication development, social or emotional development, or adaptive development" [Section 632(C)].

Under IDEA 97, it appears that children under age 3 with Down syndrome would be eligible for early speech-language evaluation and treatment services, audiological evaluations including hearing testing, feeding therapy, assistive communication devices, and transportation and related costs.

IDEA 97 considers several issues that have a direct impact on where services should be delivered. Part A deals with elementary through secondary school. For elementary-school-age children through high-school age, services are most likely to be delivered on site within the school. According to the statutes of IDEA 97, services should be provided in the natural environment, and the interpretation appears to be that "the natural environment" means within the classroom. There is a recognition within the legislation that inclusion within regular classrooms is increasing, and that classroom teachers in regular education settings and specialists (such as speech-language pathologists) in special education roles are working together more frequently. For example, the legislation mandates that the regular education teacher in a child's classroom be part of the IEP team for that child and provides funding for regular educators, classroom assistants, and special education and related services personnel to receive training regarding children with disabilities.

FINANCIAL BACKGROUND

Funding issues often drive service delivery in schools and community settings. Most available funding is through health insurance or through federal and state legislation that provides funding for educational budgets. Many health insurance plans do not fund long-term speech and language treatment for children with developmental disabilities. School systems are mandated to provide services based on specific criteria that they have developed to ensure compliance with federal funding. It is essential to become familiar with the entrance and exit criteria, eligibility for services through the local schools, and the criteria and guidelines through the health insurance agency.

GENERAL CONSIDERATIONS FOR SPEECH AND LANGUAGE TREATMENT

Although every child is a unique individual and therapy must be designed for the individual child, there are some general considerations that form the foundation for a speech and language treatment program.

Communication skills are important and contribute to inclusion and integration. Communication includes not only speech, but also facial expressions, smiles, gestures, pointing, high five signs, and alternative systems such as sign language and computer-based systems. Children and adults are more likely to interact when they can understand and be understood. At home, in school, and in the community, a functional understandable communication system facilitates relationships.

Although there are common speech and language problems, there is no single pattern of speech and language common to all children with Down syndrome. There are, however, speech and language challenges for most children with Down syndrome. Many children with Down syndrome have more difficulty with expressive language than they do with understanding speech and language, that is, receptive language skills are usually more advanced than expressive language skills. Certain linguistic areas, such as vocabulary, are usually easier for children with Down syndrome than other areas, such as grammar. Sequencing of sounds and of words may be difficult for many children. Many children have difficulties with intelligibility of speech and articulation. Some children have fluency problems. Some children use short phrases, while others have long conversations. All of the speech and language problems that children with Down syndrome demonstrate are faced by other children as well. There are no speech and language problems unique to children with Down syndrome. This means that there is a great deal of knowledge and experience that can be applied to helping a child with Down syndrome with his/her specific areas of challenge.

The speech and language treatment program should be individually designed based on a careful evaluation of each child's communications patterns and needs. It is especially important to include the family as part of the treatment team. The child, family (including siblings and extended family), teacher, friends, and community members can all contribute to the child's communication success. The speech-language pathologist can guide, inform, and help facilitate and enhance the process of learning to communicate effectively. But language is part of daily living and must be practiced and reinforced as part of daily life.

During the school years, speech and language treatment must relate to the child's educational setting and the communication needs of the classroom and the curriculum. Speech and language treatment should also consider the child's needs in relation to community activities such as religious groups and scouting. Communication goes on outside of therapy sessions, as well as inside the sessions. Inclusion and community involvement promote interactive communication and provide models and communication partners.

On the path from infancy to adulthood, the child may need speech-language treatment at various points, and the family may need ongoing information, resources, and guidance to work with the child at home. At different developmental stages, the child may need periods of treatment and/or a home program.

What is a *comprehensive* speech and language treatment program? It is an individually designed program that meets all of the communication needs for a specific child. Let's examine some of the areas that could be targeted in a comprehensive program at different speech and language learning stages.

During the birth to one-word period, the most important intervention occurs at home. Families need to be the focus of the treatment program. In the program at Loyola College, families observe the therapy sessions 100% of the time, and discuss all of the activities with a clinical supervisor. For each session, they are provided with home activities so that speech and language experiences will continue in the home environment (Kumin et al., 1991). For infants, one focus of the treatment program will be sensory stimulation: providing activities and experiences to help the infant develop auditory, visual, and tactile skills, including sensory exploration and sensory feedback and memory. The child will experience what a bell sounds like, or the different sensations while touching velvet or sandpaper. It is essential to monitor hearing status for every infant with Down syndrome, since they are at high risk for otitis media with effusion (Roberts and Medley, 1995). The most recent literature (Gravel and Wallace, 1995) is finding strong relationships between OME (otitis media with effusion, or fluid in the middle ear without signs or symptoms of ear infection), language development, and academic achievement in typically developing children. Some of the delays in language that we see in children with Down syndrome may be related to the presence of OME. The pediatrician or otolaryngologist and the audiologist will be able to monitor hearing status and treat fluid accumulation in the ear.

Speech is an overlaid function in the human body. Feeding and respiration involve many of the structures and muscles used in speech. Therefore, feeding therapy, sensory integration therapy, and other complementary therapies may have a poistive impact on speech function.

Many infants and toddlers whom we see are very sensitive to touch. They do not want to be touched, don't want their teeth brushed, or do not like certain textures of foods or perhaps mixed food textures. The term "tactilely defensive" is sometimes used. We have found that by using oral massage, direct muscle stimulation, and an oral normalization program (using the NUK massager), infants and toddlers are able increasingly to tolerate touch in the lip and tongue area. The massage program begins with the arms and legs and gradually moves toward the face and intra oral area. A detailed description of the program is included in an article by Kumin and Chapman (1996). We find that babbling and sound making increase after the oral normalization activity. Once the child can tolerate touch and can freely move the articulators, an oral motor skills program is introduced. This might include blowing whistles, blowing bubbles, making funny faces, and sound imitation activities. Generally, the clinician will imitate the child rather than providing a model to imitate.

The basis for communication is social interaction, and certain conversational skills such as turn taking can be developed at a very young age through play (MacDonald, 1989). Peek-a-boo games and handing a toy or musical instrument back and forth are ways of developing turn taking. There are many pre-language skills that can be addressed in treatment before the child is able to talk, so therapy should begin early, before the child speaks the first word (Kumin et al., 1991).

Infants with Down syndrome, by 8 months to 1 year, have a great deal to communicate with the people around them. If they do not have some way of communicating their messages, young children become frustrated by their inability to be understood. A transitional communication system is very important until the child is neurophysiologically able to speak (Gibbs and Carswell, 1991). Although speech is the most difficult communication system for children with Down syndrome, more than 95% of children with Down syndrome will use speech as their primary communication system. Total communication (use of sign language plus speech), communication boards or computer communication systems may be used as communication systems until the child is ready to transition to speech. (Kumin, 1994; Kumin et al., 1991; Meyers, 1994). Research has shown that children with Down syndrome will discontinue using the sign when they can say the word so that it is understandable to those around them.

ONE-WORD TO THREE-WORD PERIOD

Once the young child begins to use single words (in sign or speech), treatment will target horizontal as well as vertical growth in language. Treatment may address single word vocabulary (semantic skills) in many thematic and whole language activities, such as cooking, crafts, play, and trips (Kumin et al., 1996). So there may be a great deal of horizontal vocabulary growth. Treatment will also target increasing the length of phrases, the combinations of words that the child can use; this is known as increasing the mean length of utterance (Manolson, 1992). There are many meaningful relations that the child learns in two word phrases (e.g., agent-action, possession, negation), and then further expands into three word phrases.

We have found that the pacing board provides a visual and motoric cuing system that capitalizes on the strengths of children with Down syndrome, and helps children to expand the length of their utterances (Kumin et al., 1995). The pacing board is usually a rectangular piece of tag board with separate circles that represent the number of words in the desired utterance (e.g., "throw ball" would have two circles). The pacing system concept can also be implemented by putting a dot under each word in a book.

Pragmatics skills such as making requests and greetings, as well as conversational skills would be taught during this period.

Vocabulary, pragmatics, and other language activities would generally be approached through play activities. Play would also be used to increase auditory attending and on task attention skills (Schwartz and Miller, 1996). Language skills would be supported through the use of appropriate computer activities, such as First Words or First Verbs by Laureate or Living Books or Bailey's Book House by Edmark (Kumin et al., 1996).

The basis for developing speech during this period is sensory integration (translating auditory to verbal messages) and oral motor abilities. Most children with Down syndrome understand messages, and are able to produce language (through signs) well before they are able to use speech. So sensory integration and oral motor skills therapy are used to strengthen the readiness for speech during this period.

PRESCHOOL THROUGH KINDERGARTEN

The young child is usually far more advanced in receptive language skills than in expressive language skills, but both areas are targeted in therapy. During this stage, receptive language work may focus on auditory memory and on following directions, which are important skills for the early school years. It will also focus on concept development such as colors, shapes, directions (top and bottom), prepositions through practice, and play experiences. Expressive language therapy will include semantics, expanding the mean length of utterance, and will begin to include grammatical structures (word order) and word endings (such as plural or possessive). Pragmatics skills such as asking for help, appropriate use of greetings, requests for information or answering requests, as well as role playing different activities of daily living may be addressed. Again, play activities such as dressing and undressing a doll, crafts activities such as making a card, or cooking activities such as making cupcakes may be used. The same activity may target semantic, syntactic, and pragmatics skills, for example, how many cupcakes should we make, what color frosting should we use, and following the directions to make the cupcakes. Many children with Down syndrome learn to read effectively, and this can help in learning language concepts (Buckley, 1993).

During this stage, sounds and specific sound production would be targeted; articulation therapy could begin. But the therapy would also include oral motor exercises and activities on an ongoing basis to strengthen the muscles and improve the coordination of muscles. Intelligibility is the goal of the speech component of therapy.

ELEMENTARY SCHOOL YEARS

During the years in elementary school, there is a great deal of growth in language and in speech. Speech-language pathology may involve collaboration with the teacher and may be based in the classroom. Often, the curriculum becomes the material used for therapy, both proactively, to prepare the child for the subject and reactively, to help if problems occur. This makes sense, because school is the child's workplace, and success in school greatly affects self esteem.

Receptive language work becomes more detailed and advanced (Miller, 1988), including following directions with multiple parts, similar to the instructions given in school. Receptive language might include comprehension exercises, reading and experiential activities, and specific comprehension of vocabulary, morphology (word parts such as plurals), and syntax (grammatical rules).

Expressive language therapy would also focus on more advanced topics in vocabulary, similarities and differences, morphology, and syntax. Expressive language work might also include work on increasing the length of speech utterances. The pacing board, rehearsal, scaffolds, and scripts have been found helpful in facilitating longer speech utterances.

Pragmatics becomes very important during this stage; using communication skills in real life in school, at home, and in the community is the goal. Therapy might address social interactive skills with teachers and peers, conversational skills (discourse), how to make requests, how to ask for help when the child doesn't understand material in school, how to clarify statements that people do not understand, and so forth. As the child matures, the communicative activities of daily living will change. Treatment and/or home practice must keep pace with the child's communication needs at every stage.

Speech skills with emphasis on articulation and intelligibility would be targeted in therapy during this period (Swift and Rosin, 1990). An individual analysis of oral motor strengths and challenges is important to determine what specific skills need to be addressed, for example, does the child have low muscle tone or muscle weakness in the oral facial area? difficulty with motor coordination? difficulty with motor planning? Are other speech areas such as voice and fluency affecting intelligibility? Each of these areas can be worked on if they are affecting communication ability for an individual child.

There are many different approaches to speech and language treatment that can be used, and some may be used simultaneously as part of a comprehensive individually designed program.

Therapy may be programmed based on linguistic skills, that is, there may be individual goals for semantics, morphology and syntax, pragmatics, and phonology. Therapy may also focus on different channels. So the goals for therapy may target auditory skills or speech and oral motor skills, or encoding a language message or producing a language message. One channel, such as reading, may be used to assist another channel such as expressive language or written language. Therapy may also be approached through the needs of the curriculum. In this approach, vocabulary would be taught based on the vocabulary that the child needs for success in science or social studies. The therapy may be proactive, teaching in advance the language skills that the child will need for the official curriculum, formal and informal classroom interactions, following directions in class and learning the rules and routines, and skills for interacting with peers. Curriculum-based therapy may also be reactive, targeting areas of difficulty as they occur and providing assistance with study skills and strategies to meet classroom expectations or to overcome difficulties when they occur. The speech-language pathologist can also suggest adaptive and compensatory strategies such as seating in front of the room, using a peer tutor, and visual cue sheets.

Whole language is a current approach in which reading, understanding, writing, and expressive language are taught as a whole. This often is based on children's literature and thematic activities accompanying the books; for example, a book about weather might also involve weather reporting, building a weather station, or drawing pictures or taking photographs of different weather conditions. Whole language does not teach in discrete linguistic units, such as focusing on plurals or verb tenses.

Rather, it teaches in larger themes using meaningful multisensory experiences to teach concepts.

Communication in context is a pragmatics approach often used in classroom-based collaborative programs. It considers the entire communication situation including the participants (child, teacher, other children, school staff), the various settings in which the child communicates, and the differences between settings. This approach is very real-world oriented. Therapy might work on scripts and may provide assistance through scaffolds (e.g., fill-in sentences) to help the child learn to communicate more effectively with specific people or in specific settings based on a variety of objectives.

Speech and language treatment is complex and can include different approaches, a variety of goals, and many different activities. The goal is to find treatment approaches and methods which will enable each child to reach his communication potential.

RESOURCES

Communicating Together
PO Box 6395
Columbia, MD 21045-6395
Telephone: 888-816-8501, or 410-995-0722
FAX: 410-997-8735

Communicating Together provides workshops for parents and professionals and a subscription newsletter devoted to speech and language issues in infants, toddlers, children, and adolescents with Down syndrome. Workshops are held in different parts of the country throughout the year. Local workshops can be arranged. The newsletter is published six times per year. Written and edited by Dr. Libby Kumin, each issue includes a major topic article (e.g., IEPs/IFSPs, oral motor skills, intelligibility), questions and answers, home activities and reviews of current research articles. Call Dr. Martin Lazar for more information.

REFERENCES

Buckley S (1993): Language development in children with Down's syndrome: Reasons for optimism. "Down's Syndrome: Research and Practice." 1:3–9.

Gibbs ED, Carswell L (1991): Using total communication with young children with Down syndrome: A literature review and case study. Early Childhood Devel 2:306–320.

Gravel J, Wallace I (1995): Early otitis media, auditory abilities, and educational risk. Am J Speech-Language Pathol 4:89–94.

Kumin L (1994): "Communication Skills in Children with Down Syndrome: A Guide for Parents." Bethesda, MD: Woodbine House.

Kumin L, Chapman D (1996): Oral motor skills in children with Down syndrome. Communicating Together 13:1–4.

Kumin L, Councill C, Goodman M (1995): The pacing board: A technique to assist the transition from single word to multi-word utterances. Infant-Toddler Intervention 5:293–303.

Kumin L, Goodman M, Councill C (1996): Comprehensive communication assessment and intervention for school-aged children with Down syndrome. Down Syndrome Quart 1:1-8.

Kumin L, Goodman M, Councill C (1991): Comprehensive communication intervention for infants and toddlers with Down syndrome. Infant-Toddler Intervention 1:275–296.

MacDonald JD (1989): "Becoming Partners with Children—From Play to Conversation." San Antonio: Special Press.

Manolson A (1992): "It Takes Two to Talk," (2nd ed.). Idylewild, CA: Imaginart.

Meyers L (1994): Access and meaning: the keys to effective computer use by children with language disabilities. J Special Educ Technol 12:257–275.

Miller JF (1988): Facilitating advanced speech and language development. In C Tingey (ed.): "Down Syndrome: A Resource Handbook." Boston, MA: College-Hill Press, pp.119–133.

Roberts JE, Medley L (1995): Otitis media and speech-language sequelae in young children: Current issues in management. Am J Speech-Language Pathol 4:15–24.

Schwartz S, Miller J (1996): "The New Language of Toys: Teaching Communication Skills to Special Needs Children." Bethesda, MD: Woodbine House.

Swift E, Rosin P (1990): "A remediation sequence to improve speech intelligibility for students with Down syndrome." Language, Speech Hearing Services Schools 21:140–146.

Individualizing Reading for Each Child's Ability and Needs

Patricia L. Oelwein

Contrary to previous beliefs that children with Down syndrome were generally unable to learn to read, and if they did, their comprehension was so poor that reading was a useless skill, today most children with Down syndrome are expected to learn to read *and* to use reading as a valuable tool to enable them to function with greater competence and confidence in all areas of life, throughout their lives.

Although there has been a general change in attitude among educators, and reading skills appear on most Individualized Education Plans (IEPs) of elementary-school-age children with Down syndrome, many of these children make very little progress in reading and, based on their lack of progress and response to the instruction, reading is dropped. Even if they are given additional opportunities to learn to read, they frequently fail again or make little progress. Fowler et al. (1995) state that it is estimated that 40% of adolescents with Down syndrome acquire at least *some* reading skills. This suggests that 60%, more than half, have *no* reading skills. This is unacceptable. I believe that at least 90% of adolescents with Down syndrome should have at least some reading skills.

My theory as to why so many young people with Down syndrome do not learn to read, even in this day and age, is that those responsible for teaching reading to them lack understanding of the learning differences *individuals* with Down syndrome have, and, in addition, they do not have the tools to individualize and adapt materials, methods, and techniques to fit these differences. Not only is there confusion about how to teach reading to these students, there is also considerable confusion about *what* to teach them to read and *how* to measure student progress in reading.

MEASURING READING SUCCESS FOR CHILDREN WITH DOWN SYNDROME

The goal for educating children with Down syndrome is not to "cure" or "fix" the learning differences and disabilities. The diagnosis has been made, and we need to ac-

Down Syndrome: A Promising Future, Together, Edited by Terry J. Hassold and David Patterson
ISBN 0-471-29686-4   Copyright © 1998 by Wiley-Liss, Inc.

knowledge it. We must respect the person and treat him or her with dignity. The goal should be to teach the child the skills that will facilitate his or her ability to function with the highest degree of independence feasible *with* these differences, just as the child who is blind will be taught the skills that will facilitate his or her ability to function to the highest degree of independence feasible, *with* his or her blindness. In both cases, the instruction will have to be individualized, and often specialized, to meet the needs of individual learning differences and disabilities. In addition, the degree of independence *feasible,* the degree of independence *reached,* and the *measurement* of "success" will vary with the *individual.*

Being able to read certainly facilitates one's ability to function independently. We live in a world in which the written word provides us with information that assist us in just about everything we do. We cannot do the laundry, plant seeds, or shop in the supermarket with *competence* and *independence* without the ability to read. We need to read clothing labels to choose the proper washing and drying cycles, laundry product labels to know which products to use and how much, and the washing machine and dryer controls to turn on the chosen cycles. Directions on the seed package tell us where (sunny, shady, well drained) to plant the seeds, what time of the year to plant them, the amount and kind of fertilizer to use, and how close together and how deep to plant them. Labels on the food containers help us to buy the products we want and provide instruction as to how to prepare and serve them.

Reading these things is often referred to as *functional* reading. However, it is *functional* only if the person to whom it is being taught has a *use* for it. Reading that is functional for one person may not be functional for another. The above-mentioned skills are functional only to the person who does the laundry, plants the seeds, and shops in the supermarket; they are *not* functional for a person who does not do these things *currently.* Learning to read these things would be of little value for most elementary-age children, although in the future they may be useful. Wait until there is a use for them and teach them in the context of actually *doing* these things. An elementary-age child should be taught the words that are *functional* for him *currently,* such as words that he or she could use to write in his journals and words used in classroom curriculum.

Lack of understanding of this concept has led to misuse of the term "functional" in special education. As one parent told me, "*Functional* is a dirty word in Texas." I have had experiences (not in Texas—it happens everywhere) that enabled me to understand just what the parent meant by that statement. When I have been shown the "functional" reading programs for some children with Down syndrome, I have been appalled. One 13-year-old girl was being taught the sight words NO TRESPASSING, PRIVATE, and EMPLOYEES ONLY. A 9-year-old boy was taught NO CYCLING, DEER CROSSING, and NO LOITERING. Their teachers had ordered kits of functional words (often referred to as "survival" words) and were teaching children these words and calling it "functional" reading. I can think of no other words that could have been farther from functional for these children. The 13-year-old girl had no opportunities to respond to those signs and most likely did not understand what they meant. Indeed, the aide that was teaching her had trouble explaining them. The 9-year-old boy lived in a group home, never went out alone, and did not ride a bicycle, and there were no such signs in the community in which he lived. (I asked the teacher, and she admitted it!) Not only were the words the wrong words, but the teaching method was deplorable. It was not teaching—it was *testing*. The teacher held up signs and said, "What does this say?" The student guessed or did not say anything at all. The program—curriculum and methods used—were totally off-base. When I refer to *functional reading,* I am referring to reading that the *individual* has an *immediate* and *ongoing* use for. And, furthermore, it is not limited to reading single words taught by sight. It includes maps, directions, sentences, paragraphs, chapters, books, and manuals, such as the driver's manual used in drivers' education, and students can be taught to use the phonological skills they have to read new words—to apply them to whatever they read. In addition, they can continue to learn new phonological skills. It is *functional* use that all meaningful reading leads to. The difference for these children is the way that we teach it. Rather than following a "developmental" program by progressing from the pre-primer to the sixth-grade reader, children in a "functional" program will be learning to apply their reading skills to other subject matter and activities throughout the day. This will take considerable time and effort on the part of the teacher, because materials will have to be adapted or developed for each student in the functional program. This is also referred to as *applied academics.* There are no kits available that will be appropriate to meet the special needs of individual students. Individualizing to meet special needs is what is so *special* about it, and it is *education*—very *special education,* which is a *service* these children deserve. It is not a placement.

Reading is a valuable skill to teach children with Down syndrome, and it is a *feasible* skill for most of them, although there is a wide range in the levels of reading achievement. Some will do very well with functional reading; others will do well in a basal reader. Both groups can develop reading skills to the degree that reading is their primary form of obtaining information and both groups can read for recreation as well. Intelligence or general ability as measured by standardized instruments does not predict or determine the level of "success" in reading children with Down syndrome acquire as determined by reading measures. In fact, the reading scores are higher than the general ability and intelligence scores. This further confirms my conviction that for many children with Down syndrome, reading is a relative *strength*. And this *strength* can be used to compensate for other areas in which many children show relative weaknesses—such as short-term verbal memory—and to facilitate learning in all areas. The written word can remain for as long as one needs it, and it can be recovered, because it is permanent until someone destroys it; the spoken word vanishes, never to be recovered. Can you imagine having a poor short-term verbal memory and not being able to take notes, write down lists, and look up needed information? (Can you imagine having a *good* short-term verbal memory and not being able to do these things?) Can you imagine going to school and never having a textbook? Can you imagine what is like to be known as a person who is illiterate? Well, that is what happens to about 60% of the children with Down syndrome, *if* an estimate by Fowler et al. (1995) is accurate. Another very important aspect of reading for children with Down syndrome is that being able to read enhances verbal language in many children. Buckley (1985, 1995) agrees.

What we are looking for are *matches:* a good *match* of the *student's needs* with *goals* and *objectives* (often referred to as appropriate goals and objectives); a *match* of a *curriculum, learning activities,* and *instruction* with the *goals* and *objectives;* a *match* of the *evaluation* (the measurement of the effectiveness of the program) with the *goals* and *objectives.*

Measurements used to evaluate the reading success of students with Down syndrome should be selected to *match* the reading goals for the individual. For example, if a student is in the basal reading program with her classmates, and her reading goal is that she will increase her reading skills to reach a specific reading grade level, then it is appropriate to obtain reading scores for this student by using the same measurements that were used for the other students in obtaining reading grade levels. This is often appropriate for the more talented readers.

There may, however, come a point when the student shows little or no progress in reading using these measures (she is "stuck" on a level); interventions with adaptations, additional individualized instruction, and additional practice have been tried, and still the grade-level measure shows no progress in reading. The *evaluation* (reading grade-level measure) has done its job. It has informed us that the *program* is not effective in reaching the student's goals; it has not increased the reading grade level. The goal is not a good match with the student's needs. The student may be having problems understanding and applying the phonological skills presented at the higher level; the vocabulary in the reading material may be too difficult (she may be able to sound out the words, but not know what they mean); perhaps the stories in the readers are uninteresting and meaningless to the student, causing the student to lose interest and motivation. Teachers and parents are often in a dilemma over this. If they insist on measuring her progress by grade level, they may never see any real measurable progress, and the child will stay stuck there forever (And, I am told, she plateaued at the third-grade level.). Whose goal is it anyway? Is the student's goal to read on the fourth-grade level, or is it the parent's goal? Whom will this benefit?

If, however, the reading goal is changed to meet the student's needs—to help her *use* her reading to succeed in other subjects and activities, and the measurement is changed to match the goals, then considerable progress can been measured. The student can succeed at going "horizontal"—appplying reading to more and more activities and subjects rather than "vertical"—to a higher reading level.

The change in the goals should reflect practical *use* of the student's reading skills, *applying* and *embedding* reading in activities throughout the day (a *real* functional program). Her reading goals will, of course, depend on the curriculum and activities in the student's program. An example of a good reading goal for a student in an inclusive classroom, who is "stuck" on the third-grade level might be as follows: The student will increase her reading vocabulary to include words used in science, geography, social studies, and health in areas that are important and useful to her; she will receive 20 minutes of individualized instruction during the reading period daily in applying word attack skills to new words; she will practice new words by playing games with peers and working on projects during cooperative learning periods; and she will use these words throughout the day and practice reading by reading adapted subject-matter material, completing adapted work sheets, and by keeping a word bank by category, and using the word bank as a reference. Reading vocabulary will be measured by daily probes and comprehension by completing adapted work sheets and following written directions. A recreational reading goal may be added: She will read at least one book, of her own choice, per month, for pleasure. (These can be the low-vocabulary, high-interest books such as *The Riddle Street Mystery Series* by Elaine Pageler.)

Having a goal of increasing grade level is, in my opinion, futile. It is teaching her for the sake of the score—the score is the goal, rather than what will best benefit the child. Teach her to *use* the reading skills she has to *function well* in that classroom. And she will learn to read words that will help her to understand her world better, select a good diet, and someday vote for the candidate of her choice.

A distraught mother sent me an audio tape of an Individualized Education Plan (IEP) conference for her 16-year-old son who has Down syndrome. At the meeting, she asked that reading goals be included in his IEP. The school psychologist became upset with this request, and reacted quiet emotionally with comments that were offensive to his mother (and to me as well—but I was not face to face with him). He said, "You want *reading goals* for him when he is *16 years old* and has an *IQ of 36,* and can read only on the *first-grade level? Forget it!* He qualifies only for a *vocational training program!*"

Before commenting on this anecdote, I first would like to look more closely at the Fowler, et al. study cited previously. The researchers had requested "adult readers with Down syndrome" for their study; therefore, those referring these young adults (ages 17 to 25 years) to the research project classified them as literate. These young adults obviously used reading in their everyday lives and had demonstrated this to those referring them. When they were placed in reading groups, 22 of the 33 (67%) were placed in the novice and emerging reading groups (mean age-equivalent scores for these two groups were: word attack, 6.2 years; word identification, 7.4 years; comprehension, 6.4 years, general ability test, 5.7 years—the remaining 33%, placed in the developing and skilled groups, mean age-equivalent scores were: word attack skills, 12 years; word identification, 11 years; comprehension, 8 years; general ability test, 6.7 years). When their "success" in reading was measured by the researchers using tests, the novice and emerging groups' scores did not classify them as successful readers. "Success" was measured differently by friends and family referring them. And this is as it should be. Reading success for children with Down syndrome should be measured by how *useful* reading is to the individual-how it *benefits* them. Keeping in mind the discrepancy between their mental ages or general-ability ages and their age-equivalent reading scores, one could judge them as "successful" readers because they were reading above their mental ages. Typical children whose "discrepancy" is the other way—reading level significantly lower than their mental age or general-ability level—are classified as having a "learning disability" and therefore qualify for special education services. Typical children who are reading at their chronological age (they should have a mental age to match) are considered successful readers (they are at grade level). However, when their reading level significantly exceeds their grade level (chronological age), they are considered gifted readers, and are usually referred to be tested for the "gifted" program. These tests will identify them as "gifted" if their mental or general ability age is significantly higher than their chronological age. If it is not, but they are reading sidnificantly above their mental-age or general-ability score, they are generally referred to as "overachievers." Refer to the summary of the data above, and you will observe that all of the mean reading scores are higher than the general-ability scores—for all "levels" of readers (67%, novice and emerging readers, 1.7 years; 33%, developing and skilled readers, 4.3 years).These mean scores suggest to me that most individuals with Down syndrome, *who have been taught to read*, are "overachievers" in reading, based on the discrepancy between their mental age or general-ability age and reading age. In addition, when examining all data that I have seen, where both reading and mental ages are reported, the reading age always exceeds the mental age. I find this an intriguing and refreshing perspective.

Now, back to the school psychologist: If his testing was accurate (and if it means anything at all), and the student at 16 demonstrated an IQ of 36, and read on the first-grade level, then this student was reading at or above his mental age (5.8) (exact reading age not given, but if it was first grade, it would be somewhere between 6 and 7 years). Given this information, it is not at all unreasonable (or stupid, as he had implied) for the mother to request reading goals for her son. This does not mean that he should be placed in a first-grade reader (a developmental program), and that his reading success should be measured by reading-grade level. His reading program should be designed to help him to use—to *apply*—his existing reading skills to learn to read the words that will help him to *function* more independently in the vocational training program, in the community, and at home. His reading success will not be measured by reading-grade level, nor will his success in the vocational program be measured by his IQ; his success will be measured by his competence and independence on the job, in the community, and at home. Having the ability and *opportunity* to read bus schedules, street signs, the name of the building and department where he works, his job title, his job trainer's name, his employer's name, work routines and sequences, menus, directions, notes, weather reports, greeting cards, television schedules, and the name of his bank will certainly play a major part in enabling him to reach a higher degree of competence and independence. Reading and vocational training are not mutually exclusive.

BUILDING A FOUNDATION FOR READING

One of the most frequently asked questions about teaching reading to children with Down syndrome is, "When do you start?" Buckley and I agree that "prerequisite" or "readiness" tests are not generally useful to determine when to start reading using the basic method we both use. This reading program has the "readiness" skills embedded in activities. In reality, it *is* a "readiness" program. The program we advocate starts from the "top down," a whole language approach that is meaning- and context-based, starting with the whole word and then to phonological skills (to the degree that each individual is successful), rather than the "bottom up" approach which starts with phonological awareness. Watkins and Bunce (1996) describe these approaches and stress the importance of providing early literacy experiences in preschool intervention programs for children with special needs. Therefore, this being a readiness program, I recommend starting during the preschool years. The only difference in the activities that Watkins and Bunce recommend and those that I recommend is that I am recommending *adaptations* in teaching techniques and materials that present the words, letters, and letter sounds in a systematic way that allows the child with Down syndrome to *succeed* in learning them. If the child is *succeeding* without adaptations, he is "getting it" the regular way, no adaptations are necessary. However, I do believe that even the more verbal and talented children with Down syndrome, who can "get it" the regular way, benefit from this program. It gives them a real boost, taps into their potential early, and allows them to move beyond the preschool or kindergarten curriculum. Some of these children who have this "head start" are able to succeed in regular basal reading programs and are included in the same instruction as their same-age typical peers. More typical children with Down syndrome may need to continue in this "readiness" program before moving into a basal reader or other reading programs, and some will make the most progress by staying in this individualized program, progressing at their own rate beyond the readiness stage.

The typical preschool and kindergarten "readiness" and "phonological awareness" activities provide the children with "exposure" to the printed word and phonological awareness. These activities are not generally adapted for individual impairments, and children with Down syndrome often fail to grasp the concepts presented. Wang (1996) reports data that reinforce previous data that show that children with Down syndrome generally show a weakness in verbal short-term memory skills and a relative strength in visual-motor skills. He states, "Effective educational intervention must take such impairments (verbal short-term memory) into account during the development of individualized educational plans" (page 102). That is just what I recommend. *Use* the research and *apply* methods that compensate for deficits and take advantage of strengths. *Assure* student progress by implementing systematic instruction: (1) state specific objectives—what the child is *to do* that lets you know that she is learning—how she will respond; (2) plan and implement appropriate learning activities to meet objectives, and give her opportunities for fun and meaningful practice at her success level; and (3) take data to determine if, indeed, she is successful and making progress, and make program decisions—to continue, change, or stop the program—based on these data.

"When do you start?" You can start any time during the preschool and kindergarten years. The more "talented" children generally respond well in their third year, but most children with Down syndrome are more responsive during their fourth or fifth year. Some will not respond well until later during the elementary years, and you can "start" at any age after that. Adolescents and adults have responded well to reading programs that are individualized, systematic, and designed for their success and generally make rapid progress once they experience the joy of such an awesome accomplishment.

A more important question for parents and teachers of preschoolers is, "When do you stop?" You can *start* at almost any age and it will do no harm, but if you *continue* when the child is *not successful,* you can do considerable harm. You can "turn him off" to reading, and he will run the other way when he sees the written word. If you start and the child does not respond well, *put it away* and try again later. You can "take a sampling" from time to time and see if he is receptive. Use family photos to catch his interest—few children turn away when the photos are brought out. Motivation is always of most importance. Remember, you are using systematic instruction as described above, and this method is designed to assure child success. If you continue when the child is not successful, you are not using the systematic method. This program that I recommend, that was developed in the Down syndrome program at the University of Washington in 1972, is a *fun* program in which the child experiences the joy of learning; it builds a foundation for future reading. It is most important that the child has *positive* and *successful* experiences with the printed word. This program is based on "errorless" learning—if he is making a lot of errors and/or is not cooperative, his foundation is crumbling.

Perhaps the single greatest reason so many children with Down syndrome aren't taught to read is because the educators are following the traditional rules and waiting for them to acquire the "prerequisite" skills—skills necessary to pass the "readiness" test, or to reach the proper mental age before *starting* reading instruction. Many children with Down syndrome are never able to pass these tests; they are not able to learn these skills that don't make sense to them, and lacking these skills, they are never given the opportunity to learn to read. Parents say, "He never learned to read because he never learned the alphabet." On the other hand, there are a few children with Down syndrome (two in my acquaintance) who were able to learn the "readiness skills," from the "bottom up," and master a "phonological awareness" program. They could "sound out" every letter, but were unable to blend those sounds into words when presented with the printed word. Instead, these children insisted on saying each letter sound. They were unable to transfer their phononetic skills into actually reading a word. They were unable to *read*.

The individualized, systematic method that I recommend is a "top-down" approach. It gives each child an opportunity to learn to read at his or her own rate and to continue to grow in reading skills throughout his or her lifetime. If the child is able to learn phonological skills—and most are able—he or she is taught those which are feasible for him or her to learn. In the individualized, systematic method, we do not continue where there is failure, but we do *continue* where there is success. Two interesting findings from the Fowler at el. study were that productive decoders had less phoneme awareness than expected and that a little phoneme awareness goes a long way. They can generally make good use of the skills they have. If the child is unable to learn phonetic skills, he or she will continue learn by sight; he or she will have the opportunity to continue to grow as a reader.

I describe this method in detail in *Teaching Reading to Children with Down Syndrome* (Oelwein, 1995). The child learns to read words that are meaningful and useful to him (usually starting with his/her own name, mommy, daddy, and in the classroom, classmate names and classroom words) by sight, using an almost errorless method of *matching* words first, then *selecting* words on verbal cue, and finally *naming* (reading/saying or signing words). This gives the child immediate success and comfort with reading words. These words are embedded in games and activities for practical use (place cards on the table at home, names on chairs and on lockers or coat hooks at school) and practice (lotto games, matching words with pictures, sorting words by first letter, and simple books). When the child is successfully using the words he/she can read, then letters and letter sounds are introduced, starting with the first letter of the child's name and gradually adding the initial letter of all the words he/she can read. Again, opportunities for practical use and practice are embedded in activities throughout the day. The words and letters are systematically taught, and new words and letters are introduced based on the child's data (proficiency with the words and letters that have been introduced must be met before new words and letters are introduced). Individualizing for each child and making decisions based on each individual's data are of greatest importance. This method taps into the potential of children with Down syndrome, what ever it may be, and each child is allowed to succeed at his or her own rate. One size does not fit all, and we have a lot of sizes among children with Down syndrome.

SUMMARY

As we approach the end of the twentieth century, children with Down syndrome are expected to learn to read, and they should be given an opportunity to meet this expectation. The research demonstrates that reading is a relative strength for readers who have Down syndrome. There is a general discrepancy between cognitive ability and reading skills, with reading skills of those who have been taught to read higher than their cognitive ability. There is a wide range in reading ability among individuals with Down syndrome, with some becoming skilled readers, some with good functional reading skills, some with minimal reading skills, and some who have no reading skills. It is my belief that most of these nonreaders have the potential to read, but that this potential has not been tapped owing to the lack of understanding of the needs of the students and their learning differences and to the lack of the use of effective methods and techniques for teaching this population. Measurement for success in reading should be measured by how effectively the student is able to use his or her reading skills to function in everyday life, rather than by grade-level scores. Educators should learn about learning differences in children with Down syndrome and develop truly individualized education plans for them, applying systematic instruction and methods that have been effective in teaching these children. A foundation for learning to read should start for most children with Down syndrome during the preschool years, and the "top-down" approach is recommended. Reading is a valuable and necessary tool for developing independence and competency and for compensating for a poor verbal short-term memory. It is a feasible skill for most children with Down syndrome to obtain.

REFERENCES

Buckley S (1985): Attaining basic educational skills: Reading, writing and number. In Lane D, Stratford B (eds.): "Current Approaches to Down's Syndrome." New York: Praeger.

Buckley S (1995): Teaching children with Down syndrome to read and write. In Nadel L, Rosenthal D (eds.): "Down Syndrome: Living and Learning in the Community." New York: Wiley-Liss.

Fowler AE, Doherty BJ, Boynton L (1995): The basis of reading skills in young adults with Down syndrome. In Nadel L, Rosenthal D (eds.): "Down Syndrome: Living and Learning in the Community." New York: Wiley-Liss.

Oelwein PL (1995): "Teaching Reading to Children with Down Syndrome: A Guide for Parents and Teachers." Bethesda, MD: Woodbine House.

Wang PP (1996): A Neuropsychological profile of Down syndrome: cognitive skills and brain morphology. Ment Retard Devel Disabilities Res Rev 2:102–108.

Watkins RV, Bunce BH (1996): Natural literacy: Theory and practice for preschool intervention programs. Topics Early Childhood Special Educ 16:2, 191–212.

The Challenge of Linguistic Mastery in Down Syndrome

Anne E. Fowler

In this chapter I will speak to a number of questions about language learning in persons with Down syndrome (DS), informed by recent research. I first consider whether language merits particular concern in DS; despite well-documented success stories, research suggests that persons with DS are at high risk for language difficulty. I then ask whether the linguistic challenges faced by persons with DS can be attributed to across-the-board learning difficulties; this does not seem to be the case, in light of evidence from other neurodevelopmental disorders in which language is not as severely and consistently affected, but where general cognitive function is as impaired as, or more impaired than, it is in DS. The third question concerns specific areas of weaknesses within language; research suggests that persons with DS are especially vulnerable to difficulties with grammatical function (morphology and syntax), with relative sparing of semantic knowledge (i.e., vocabulary), and with communication skills that extend beyond language per se.

On these issues, researchers are in agreement, by and large. The question for which we continue to seek answers is *why* persons with DS are at such risk for language failure. And why do some, but not other, persons with DS succeed in achieving full linguistic mastery? My goal is to review and motivate informed hypotheses presently under consideration, acknowledging that existing data are consistent with several different hypotheses. In this paper, I choose to place particular emphasis on the link between grammatical difficulties and more fundamental phonological weaknesses (including articulation, speech perception, naming, and verbal memory capacity). In exploring how these phonological weaknesses may contribute to linguistic function more generally, I draw parallels with a growing body of research implicating phonological difficulties in normally intelligent children and adults with specific reading and/or language impairment.

Down Syndrome: A Promising Future, Together, Edited by Terry J. Hassold and David Patterson
ISBN 0-471-29686-4   Copyright © 1998 by Wiley-Liss, Inc.

Although research to date offers no definitive answer as to why persons with DS have particular language difficulties, I wish to draw attention to the potential role that fundamental phonological processes may play in achieving full linguistic function. My hope is that more intensive intervention efforts will be made toward improving phonological function in persons with DS at all ages. Ultimately, research is necessary to determine whether improving phonological function (articulation, perception, naming, and memory) leads to demonstrable gains in grammatical function. However, even if such a link is not supported, and we must explore other means to improve grammatical function, I would argue that we already have ample evidence to suggest that improving phonological function is a worthwhile end in its own right.

IS LANGUAGE AN AREA OF PARTICULAR CONCERN IN DS?

Despite improved educational opportunities and heightened expectations, full mastery of the linguistic system remains a major challenge for many persons with Down syndrome (DS). Notable exceptions notwithstanding, many schoolchildren, adolescents, and adults with DS continue to experience frustration in making themselves understood and in mastering the intricacies of grammar* so readily achieved by most young children without DS. And yet, recent research suggests that these linguistic difficulties cannot be dismissed as a reflection of general cognitive function. Nor is it the case that all persons with DS are equally affected.

Evidence of the linguistic difficulties faced by persons with DS derives from a variety of sources. Particularly compelling are parent reports suggesting that language difficulty can be a major barrier to fulfilling their children's potential. In one recent survey involving 937 families, 58% of the parents reported that their children with DS "frequently" had difficulty being understood, whereas only 5% reported that their children "rarely or never" experienced difficulty (Kumin, 1994). In contrast, Kumin notes that children without disabilities typically achieve 100% intelligibility by 4 years of age. Intelligibility problems were similarly prevalent in a group of British adolescents studied by Buckley and Sacks (1987). Although between 78 and 88% of their parents reported being "usually" able to understand what their adolescents were trying to communicate, they acknowledged that between 32% (girls over 14 years) and 67% (boys between 11 and 14 years) had "frequent" difficulty being understood

---

*Morphosyntax—or grammar—refers to knowledge and use of rules governing word formation and sentence structure. Examples of word formation (morphology) include use of inflectional morphemes to modify nouns (e.g., plurals and possessives), verbs (e.g., progressive or past tense markers), and auxiliaries (e.g., to indicate subject–verb agreement for tense and number). Examples of syntactic knowledge include canonical word order in English and how this must be permuted for passive voice sentences, wh-questions, or relative clause constructions. Such grammatical knowledge of language structure can, in principle, be distinguished from knowledge of individual word meanings (semantic, vocabulary, or lexical knowledge), from pronunciation of those words (phonology, articulation), and from appropriate usage in a social context (pragmatics, communicative function). In practice, of course, it is often difficult to distinguish between a grammatical (failure to mark plural endings) and a phonological weakness (failure to pronounce a final "s") or even a semantic one (failure to distinguish single from multiple forms). In order to improve overall communicative function, our challenge is to see if we can tease apart— and remediate—more specific risk factors that may jeopardize communication in general.

by strangers. Although these difficulties surely reflect significant phonological problems, only about half of the parents also reported that their adolescents "speak in full sentences," with approximately 20% stating that their children speak in sentences of three words or fewer.

Research studies involving direct assessment of language skill confirm these parental impressions and indicate that linguistic problems are greater than would be expected solely on the basis of overall cognitive function. For example, when compared to typically developing youngsters of equivalent mental age, older children with DS typically produce shorter, less complex sentences with only limited use of grammatical devices (for reviews and some representative studies see Miller, 1987; Fowler, 1990; Scarborough et al., 1991). Although general verbal comprehension appears to be less impaired than speech production in older children with DS (e.g., Chapman, 1991; Marcell et al., 1990), studies targeting comprehension of particular grammatical constructions have revealed some striking difficulties with grammatically complex structures (e.g., Naigles et al., 1995; Fowler, 1984; Marcell et al., 1994; see Fowler, 1997, for a review).

Comparisons across a variety of neurodevelopmental syndromes provide further evidence that DS puts persons at particular risk for language difficulties. As a group, persons with DS typically display more severe language impairments than comparison groups matched in age and overall level of cognitive function. This is almost always the case when the comparison group is of "unspecified" or "mixed" etiology. That it is not necessarily the case is evident from research on individuals with fragile (X), who may be even more severely affected in language and communication than persons with DS (e.g., Dykens et al., 1992). Intriguingly, though still open to much interpretation, persons with autism can sometimes master complex grammatical function, far more advanced than typically seen in DS, but at the same time be far less sophisticated than persons with DS in their use of verbs and pronouns that depend on social inferencing skills (e.g., Tager-Flusberg, 1994).*

Perhaps the most dramatic evidence of a dissociation between grammar and cognition derives from recent research on Williams syndrome (WS), a rare disorder leading to moderate to severe retardation and uneven cognitive profiles. Whereas very young children with WS, like those with DS, begin with markedly delayed syntactic development, the children with WS, *unlike* most with DS, typically move ahead to acquire full syntactic complexity by middle to late childhood. By adolescence, the WS language advantage is pronounced. When IQ- and age-matched adolescents have been compared, those with DS produced only short, simple, and grammatically inaccurate constructions, whereas those with WS displayed extensive and spontaneous usage of passives, questions, embedded clauses, conditionals, and multiple embeddings, with nearly accurate grammatical morphology (Bellugi et al., 1990). When

---

*The case of autism is particularly problematic owing to well-appreciated difficulties in diagnosis and the wide range of cognitive levels associated with the condition. What can be learned, however, from comparing the linguistic effects of DS to those of other established neurodevelopmental conditions is the demonstration of distinctive cognitive profiles. Linguistic difficulties do not extend equally across all areas of communication, nor can they be dismissed as an inevitable outcome of general cognitive weaknesses.

presented with models to imitate, the group with DS could reproduce very few constructions; the group with WS could imitate sentences of almost any verbal complexity. When asked to tell the story depicted by a wordless picture book, adolescents with DS provided minimal descriptions using ill-formed sentences, while those with WS produced three times as many utterances speaking in complex well-formed sentences three or four times as long as the DS utterances (Reilly et al., 1991),

What is especially interesting about these comparisons is that the linguistic deficits in DS do not indicate more severe cognitive deficits across the board. Rather the linguistic weaknesses in DS are offset by some striking visual-spatial deficits in WS. Adolescents with DS can reproduce simple shapes, draw figures from memory in a recognizable fashion, and navigate in space sufficiently well that they often achieve considerable self-sufficiency in adulthood, riding buses, participating in a variety of sports, and living in independent apartments. In contrast, the impressive linguistic skills in WS coexist with severe impairments in reconstructing even the simplest shape or figure from memory; extreme spatial limitations create huge obstacles to independent living.

These comparisons across syndromes make it clear that language difficulties are not a direct reflection of general cognitive ability, but require intervention specific to an individual child's cognitive–linguistic profile. Bellugi and her colleagues make much of the fact that language has somehow been "spared" in the effects of WS; I would argue that equal attention should be paid to the fact that language has somehow been "impaired" in DS. It is intriguing that receptive vocabulary level exceeds general cognitive level in adolescents with WS; it is distressing that grammatical function in DS tends to lag even further behind their already weak receptive vocabulary scores (e.g., Chapman, 1993; Fowler, 1990; Miller and Chapman, 1984).

Although the typical person with DS has more difficulties with language than would be predicted on the basis of overall cognitive function, absolute levels of final attainment vary dramatically. For example, it is clear that the adolescents with DS selected by Bellugi et al. (1990) for comparison with the WS group do not adequately represent what *can* be achieved by persons with DS; they may not even be representative of what is typically achieved. For example, Rondal (1994a, 1994b) presents the case of a mildly retarded young woman named Francoise whose spontaneous productions are both long and complex (with utterance averaging 12 morphemes in length), whose grammatical morphology (and comprehension) is consistently accurate, and whose phonological skills include absolutely normal articulation, fluency, and intonation patterns. Although Francoise's case is unusual in the extent to which it has been studied, numerous articulate young people with DS, including a trilingual young woman from Spain, have begun speaking and writing in their own voices (see Levitz and Kingsley, 1995; Nadel and Rosenthal, 1995; Seagoe, 1964).

Longitudinal research has documented significant variation in the rate at which language is acquired and in the achievements that are ultimately attained in persons with DS. For example, Miller et al. (1995) measured the rate at which preschoolers with DS acquired their early language milestones (first words, size of spoken vocabulary, and two-word combinations); resulting growth curves suggest two quite distinct trajectories differentiated by progress or no progress. Working with somewhat older children, Fowler (1988) tracked language development over a period of several years in 11 children with DS. Three youngsters made steady improvements in sentence length and complexity between 6 and 9 years of age; during these very same years, another four children attending the same classes in the same school remained stalled at limited language levels, speaking in simple two- to four-word phrases. Four older children whose linguistic development was followed from when they were 10 or 11 years old began with the limited skills evident in the "slower" trajectory at the early ages and made upward progress only late in adolescence after years of nongrowth. Two of their adolescent peers had already acquired complex syntax by 10 or 11 years and maintained a sizable advantage throughout the teenage years.

Apparently, some children with DS are far more restricted in language development than others; the limited data available suggest this difference may be evident early on and persist over time. To document and understand better the incidence and context of linguistic proficiency in DS within a larger sample, my students and I (Fowler, 1995; Fowler et al., 1995) interviewed 33 young adults, aged 17 to 21 years, who were referred through word-of-mouth as representing what might be achieved in terms of language when provided with adequate medical care, dedicated commitment of parents, and informed educational practices. Despite having skewed our sample toward high achieving, hard-working, and self-assured young adults, we found that the only verbal measure to exceed general cognitive levels was receptive vocabulary, as assessed on the Peabody Picture Vocabulary Test (Dunn and Dunn, 1981). Where comparative data on verbal and non verbal tasks from a single test (Kaufman and Kaufman, 1983) could be submitted to statistical analysis, verbal scores were consistently and significantly below nonverbal scores. A statistically significant nonverbal advantage was evident in the individual profiles of more than half of our sample; a statistically significant verbal advantage was observed exactly once. Even in this high-functioning sample, verbal skills were identified as a significant weakness relative to overall cognitive profile in more than half the sample (Doherty, 1993; for similar findings, see Pueschel, 1988).

Among this group, we were fortunate in interviewing a group of five impressively articulate—and literate—young adults, with reading and language levels not unlike those reported by Rondal (1994a, b) for Françoise. These young people had acquired the receptive vocabulary of a typical 11 year old, the arithmetic skills of a 9 year old, and listening and reading comprehension skills near an 8-year-old level. Reading skills in word recognition and decoding exceeded 12-year-old levels. In terms of spoken language, these adults could imitate sentences with complex verbal auxiliaries. And yet, in terms of their cognitive profiles, these most proficient adults were quite similar to the larger group as a whole, and to persons with DS generally. Three of the five displayed a significant "strength" on a nonverbal measure, and only one a strength on a verbal measure.

Such well-documented cases of linguistic proficiency make it clear that DS does not categorically preclude linguistic mastery. A "ceiling" on linguistic success in DS has not been established, and is not likely to exist. At the same time, however, linguistically proficient individuals seem to be have cognitive profiles that are quite similar to persons with DS generally. What this seems to suggest is that despite also being "at risk" for language impairment, these young adults have somehow managed to gain spoken and written proficiency in English. The strategy in the second half of this chapter is to consider risk factors for linguistic failure. To this end, I shall introduce characteristics that distinguish DS from other developmental disorders less associated with difficulties in learning language. I shall make the case that these same factors also appear to distinguish *among* persons with DS who differ in linguistic proficiency, as well as among normally intelligent children and adults with and without specific difficulties in language and literacy.

POSSIBLE FACTORS CONTRIBUTING TO LANGUAGE DIFFICULTIES
Language Learning Strategies

To account for specific difficulties in acquiring grammatical structure, it is conceivable that children with DS posit different kinds of rules or entertain hypotheses not observed in the normal process of language learning. However, as has been reviewed extensively, quests for "deviant" processes have proven futile to date: both the structures acquired by children with DS and the errors made in the process are indistinguishable from those observed in much younger nondisabled children matched on language level (see Fowler, 1990; Fowler et al., 1994; Miller, 1987; Naigles et al., 1995). Importantly, studies of other subgroups characterized as language-delayed have also yielded little support for deviant language processes within the area of morphosyntax, suggesting that development in both production and comprehension largely parallels that observed in typically developing children, even if stopping short of full mastery. As but one example, in a study refuting prior suggestions that children with mental retardation apply "abnormal" strategies to understand passive voice sentences, Bridges and Smith (1984) demonstrated that the erroneous strategies observed constituted a normal language "stage" also seen in younger children, rather than a "deviant" strategy. (For a review of the extensive literature reporting "delay without deviance" in a variety of populations, see Fowler, 1997; Johnston, 1988; Rosenberg and Abbeduto, 1993).

Critical Period Hypothesis

In an alternative explanation for limited language learning in DS, Lenneberg (1967) suggested that the capacity for language learning slows dramatically in adolescence after a biologically imposed shutdown of the critical period for language acquisition. Recent estimates, looking at effects of age on first and second language learning (including sign language), place the end of this hypothesized critical period at approximately 7 or 8 years age (Newport, 1990), emphasizing that the shutdown is not absolute. The limited longitudinal data currently available for children with mental retardation suggest relatively rapid growth in the preschool years, followed by more limited growth in the school-age years and beyond (Dykens et al., 1994; Fowler, 1988; Fowler et al., 1994; Miller; 1988, Tager-Flusberg et al., 1990). Consistent with a slowdown rather than shutdown, Fowler (1988) observed a modest increase in syntactic comprehension and production during late adolescence among persons with DS observed (see also Chapman, 1993; Marcell et al., 1994).

As was illustrated in the earlier discussion of children with WS, general cognitive delay apparently exerts a strong and consistent effect at the very earliest stages of language learning across a variety of syndromes. Where children with DS seem to stand apart more dramatically is during the school years. For example, Smith and Stoel-Gammon (1983) report that children with DS display a slower rate of improvement in phonological skill over time, lagging further and further behind the language-matched controls on which they were initially matched. We noted a similar pattern in longitudinal research: children with DS made their most rapid gains between 4 and 8 years of age, making only brief and inconsistent gains beyond that point (Fowler, 1988; Fowler et al., 1994).

Newport (1990) raises the possibility that these critical period phenomena may stem from changes in overall cognitive function: whereas young children are forced to analyze utterances to accommodate their cognitive limitations, older children are more likely to store unanalyzed utterances. Such an explanation cannot, however, account for the slowdown in children with MR, who by those standards should be open to language learning for many more years. In a somewhat different approach to critical period phenomena, Locke (1994) has argued that impoverished language results when the child is deprived of a full data base (from either environmental or cognitive factors), during what he refers to as a "critical period for activation of species-typical linguistic mechanisms" (page 37). Beyond that time, the child can continue to acquire "utterances," which Locke describes as a right brain function, but these will not undergo the kind of analysis that characterizes early language learning.

Clearly, more definitive data are needed to evaluate these hypotheses better, both within and beyond the relatively well-studied case of DS. The growing disparity between mental age and language level even in children without DS is of interest (e.g., Abbeduto et al., 1989), but it would be especially worthwhile to learn just when highly verbal children with DS (or WS or autism) achieve their impressive skills. It would also be of great interest to examine susceptibility to language therapy as a function of chronological age and language status.

Specific Linguistic Deficit

As one alternative to deviant learning strategies, it is been suggested that focuses on certain linguistic relationships are not—and potentially cannot be—appreciated in individuals with language difficulties. That is, what *is* acquired is acquired normally. More interesting perhaps is what is *not* acquired. In the most explicit account of such a hypothesis, Gopnik (1990a, b) speculated that some particularly pronounced cases of specific language impairment (SLI) may stem from a (genetically transmitted) insensitivity to grammatical features (plural, gender, tense). As evidence, she cited data from an extended family of affected individuals, none of whom produced morphological overgeneralizations. Although the hypothesis is appealing in its simplicity, in SLI, as in DS, the evidence for such an isolated deficit is not well substantiated. Investigators familiar with the family studied by Gopnik report both that some grammatical morphemes *are* acquired and that the ostensibly isolated deficit extends well beyond grammatical morphemes to affect other aspects of syntax, semantic naming, phonological memory, and receptive vocabulary (Fletcher, 1990; Vargha-Khadem and Passingham, 1990). Although a frequent failure to acquire the complexities of verbal auxiliary system suggest that this may qualify as an area of weakness (e.g., Fowler et al., 1995) the fact that some persons do and others do not move beyond this apparent linguistic ceiling makes it highly implausible that there is a "missing piece" in the language learning apparatus of persons with DS.

Although it is unlikely we will find evidence for a syndrome-wide gene that categorically precludes mastery of some linguistic feature, it remains possible that certain prerequisites to complex syntax are specifically affected in language-impaired groups. For example, describing specific syntactic deficits associated with SLI, Clahsen and colleagues (Clahsen, 1989; Clahsen et al., 1992) point to particular problems in establishing agreement relations in grammar. If that is an accurate account of the pattern observed, plurals (which are a semantic marker not dependent on agreement within the sentence) should not be problematic for language-impaired children, despite their status as a syntactic–semantic feature and despite their low acoustic salience. In contrast, the theory would anticipate difficulty with verbal auxiliary markers, gender agreement within noun phrases, and subject–verb agreement. Clahsen reports just such a pattern in German-speaking children with SLI, suggesting they do not have a general morphological deficit, but one specific to agreement relations (see also Rice and Oetting 1993).

Although Clahsen's data have not been specifically tested in DS, his account is consistent with the facts on face value. Children with DS do acquire plurals with relative ease, and have tremendous difficulty with agreement relations. If this is in fact an apt characterization of their deficits, however, one is left to ask *why* agreement relations are so difficult. This is one of several reasons to look to the processing deficits that may underlie the difficulties with grammatical relations.

Verbal Memory Limitations

Quite apart from current work on morphosyntactic weaknesses in DS, researchers have long identified specific and dramatic weaknesses in verbal memory* as a hallmark of the cognitive profile associated with DS (e.g., Bilovsky and Share, 1965; Graham, 1974; Hulme and MacKenzie, 1992). Unfortunately, however, given the complexity of the memory system, and the diversity of ways to assess morphosyntax, we have little understanding as yet as to how verbal memory bears on morphosyntactic development. We can only note intriguing parallels.

---

*Verbal memory has, over time, been referred to as verbal short-term memory, immediate-span, working memory, and, most recently, phonological memory. I refer here to the ability to encode information (presented verbally or visually) into a verbal store, to maintain that information in memory for a brief period, and to reproduce it (orally or otherwise) as it was initially presented (e.g., Baddeley, 1986).

The cognitive profile of persons with DS is characterized not only by weaknesses in morphosyntactic function, but by a memory span well below what is ordinarily achieved. When presented with a random sequence of digits (1 through 9) at a rate of one per second, English speaking adults display an average "digit span" of 7, plus or minus 2, recalling the initial and final digits with greatest accuracy. Persons with DS, presented with the same task, show the same pattern, but recall far fewer digits. Most recall no more than two or three, and very few achieve a span greater than four digits. For example, only 25% of the 16-year olds studied by Hulme and MacKenzie (1992) and 33% of the young adults studied by Fowler (1995) could recall four digits in order; exactly one adult across these two studies reliably reproduced five digits in the correct order. The linguistically proficient young woman studied by Rondal (1995a, b) also had a span of four digits. The consistently limited span observed in persons with DS can be contrasted with the variability observed in IQ-matched adolescents of "mixed etiology," also studied by Hulme and MacKenzie (1992): in that sample, half recalled four, some recalled six, and virtually none recalled fewer than three digits.

Providing further evidence for a specific linguistic weakness, the verbal memory limitations in DS contrast with relatively intact skills in visual or motor sequencing (e.g., Doherty, 1993; Marcell and Weeks, 1988; Marcell and Armstrong, 1982; Pueschel, 1988). Most people find it easier to remember the serial order of items, such as letters or familiar shapes that can be named, than of items, such as nonsense doodles, that cannot be easily labeled. However, this standard verbal advantage is not usually found in persons with DS. For example, when adults with DS were compared to typically developing youngsters with comparable digit spans, the standard advantage was evident only in the non-DS group (Racette, 1993). Wang and Bellugi (1994) also failed to find the usual verbal advantage in adolescents with DS, but did observe it in an IQ- and age-matched group with WS. Importantly, the verbal memory limitations in DS cannot be contributed to simple auditory or articulatory difficulties; weaknesses in remembering namable stimuli remain evident whether or not the presentation is visual or oral (e.g., Varnhagen et al., 1987), and whether the response requires speaking or pointing (Marcell and Weeks, 1988).

Like grammatical function, verbal memory in DS is relatively independent of progress and variation in general cognitive factors. For example, despite a relatively high correlation between memory and cognition in typically developing 4 to 8 year olds, MacKenzie and Hulme (1987) report a substantially weaker correlation among schoolchildren (with and without DS) with moderate levels of impairment. In a further parallel with grammatical function, growth in memory span seems to slow with in creasing age in persons with DS. In adolescents studied by MacKenzie and Hulme, digit span was below mental-age-level expectations at age 10 and fell further and further behind, with mean span increasing only from 3.1 to 3.6 over the next 6 years. This contrasted with an average of 16 months' growth in general cognitive development over the same period.

Although somewhat independent of general cognition, verbal memory appears to be more closely allied with production and comprehension of grammatically complex structures in persons with DS and other disabilities (e.g., Graham, 1974). For example, adolescents and adults with DS studied by Marcell et al. (1990) achieved overall language comprehension scores equivalent to those of an IQ- and age-matched comparison group, but performed considerably less well on measures of verbal memory, sentence production, and comprehension of complex structures, all of which were strongly correlated with each other in both groups. An association between sentence production and memory was also observed in the sample of young adults studied by Fowler (1995); those participants with a memory span of less than four digits were uniformly unable to reproduce complex verbal auxiliaries modeled for them. An association between memory and syntax is also evident across populations. Whereas verbal memory is consistently an area of weakness in DS, it is an area of relative strength in cases where morphosyntax is spared despite generally low cognitive function, such as in people with WS (e.g., Crisco et al., 1988; Wang and Bellugi, 1994), and some highly functioning persons with autism (Tager-Flusberg et al., 1990).

If, in fact, limited phonological memory is an obstacle to acquiring complex syntax, there may be a minimum threshold for full linguistic mastery. Such a threshold would be not only consistent with the results from Fowler (1995), but also in keeping with the findings of Rondal (1994a, b) and Cromer (1994). Both these authors express surprise that the complex syntax they observed could coexist with a span of only four digits. This should not be surprising, however, in light of the fact that highly complex syntax is *typically* acquired in the first four or five years of life, apparently before memory span exceeds four digits (see Racette, 1993, for relevant data). Although verbal memory may not be relevant to degree of syntactic skill in language learners who meet the minimum threshold, a more limited memory capacity may constitute an important obstacle to linguistic success.

UNDERLYING PROCESSING DEFICITS THAT MAY CONTRIBUTE TO DEFICITS IN MEMORY AND MORPHOSYNTAX

Although verbal memory deficits in DS are undeniable, and parallels with grammatical function merit further investigation, the specific relevance of memory for morphosyntactic development is not clear in any group of language learners. On the one hand, measures of morphosyntactic function surely vary in their dependence on memory, depending upon whether they involve production, comprehension, and imitation, and whether additional demands are made by syntactic or phonological complexity or by lexical unfamiliarity. On the other hand, limitations on memory span may derive from poor initial encoding, weak or absent rehearsal, and delayed access to long-term memory, which itself may be impoverished. Competing demands for attention, weak formulation skills, and output difficulties also contribute to failure on the digit span task (e.g., Brady, 1997; Dempster, 1981). Indeed, these various factors may contribute to variability within a given child across tasks, across content areas, and across days (Lahey and Bloom, 1994).

As a result of this complexity, combined with the possibility of a threshold effect of memory on language learning, a failure to obtain a correlation between any two measures of syntax and memory does not categorically rule out an important role for memory in language function. We must, for instance, consider carefully how to interpret two studies that have tested for and failed to find any correlation between syntactic comprehension and digit span in non-DS adolescents with developmental disabilities (e.g., Dewart, 1979; Natsopoulos and Xeromeritou, 1990). At the same time, a positive association by itself tells us little about *how* verbal memory bears on language learning. In this regard, we are fortunate that a growing body of research is examining the intersection of memory and language in a number of subgroups, with potential for converging evidence across studies. I review here three recent explanations of individual and developmental differences in memory derived from various subgroups, and consider their potential relevance for explaining language difficulties in DS.

Rehearsal Strategies

One hypothesis for individual differences in memory derives from Baddeley's model of working memory, in which verbal material is temporarily stored and rehearsed in an articulatory loop (Baddeley, 1986). In typical adults, there is substantial evidence that the amount of material that can be articulated in a brief period of time is a good approximation of the amount of material that can be maintained in working memory; we can, for example, recall more monosyllabic than multisyllabic digits in working memory. Furthermore, study of developmental changes in working memory, and of individual differences among normally intelligent adults, suggests that variation in speed of articulation may set a limit on the amount of information that can be stored and rehearsed within an articulatory loop (Gathercole and Baddeley, 1990; Hulme et al., 1984).

Although this research is potentially relevant to explaining gains in memory observed after typically developing children reach school age, the major milestones in morphosyntactic development have already been achieved by this point in development. There is little evidence for rehearsal in very young children (e.g., Gathercole and Adams, 1993) or in persons with DS (e.g., Varnhagen et al., 1987). Hence it is unlikely that rehearsal in the articulatory loop is an important factor in basic acquisition of grammar.

Speech Perception

Yet a different account of variation in memory span refers to the initial perception (or encoding) of the verbal information to be stored and retrieved. This line of research, primarily involving poor readers with memory deficits, has documented a strong association between poor perception and poor short-term memory. Indeed it would seem that lowering the perceptual quality of stimuli limits memory in any listener (see Brady, 1997, for a recent discussion).

If poor perception limits memory, then a plausible link with morphosyntactic weaknesses can be constructed. For one thing, consistent with Gleitman and Wanner's (1982) phonological salience hypothesis, the very markers that are most often omitted in immature speech, and about which agreement relations must be inferred, are just those that are acoustically nonsalient (see the forthcoming volume by Morgan and Demuth for several papers considering the relevance of phonology to early syntactic function in typical development). An emphasis on perception also makes sense in light of the fact that perceptual deficits are highly prevalent in the language-delayed population (e.g., Leonard et al., 1992), just as language problems are highly prevalent in children first diagnosed for phonological impairments (Shriberg and Kwiatkowski, 1988). Arguing that specific language impairment (SLI) may have its roots in more basic phonological skill, Leonard et al. (1992) found that even 4- and 5-year olds with SLI who produced appropriate phonemic contrasts in spontaneous speech were less able to discriminate such contrasts as das/dash, ba/da, or dabiba/dabuba than age-mates with normal language development.

With regard to DS and other neurodevelopmental syndromes, the parallels are obvious but as yet untested. Persons with DS are well-known to have perceptual weaknesses (e.g., Marcell, 1992), just as they are to have weaknesses in morphosyntactic development. Conversely, unexpected strengths in syntax often co-occur with well-developed phonology, as is true in persons with WS and other cases of exceptional language recently discussed in the literature (e.g., Curtiss, 1988a, 1988b; Cromer, 1994; Rondal, 1994a, b). It remains to be determined whether variation in perception accuracy among persons with DS or WS—or in typically developing language learners—is causally linked to variation in grammatical skill.

Lexical Retrieval

A still different account of verbal memory deficits attributes individual differences to variation in speed of lexical retrieval from a long term store (Gathercole and Adams, 1993; Hulme et al., 1991). For instance, Gathercole and Adams (1993) found that slower access to the names of individual digits is associated with shorter spans in very young children.

Varnhagen et al. (1987) observed severe deficits in speed of lexical retrieval from a long-term store in persons with DS; in that group there was a significant correlation between retrieval speed and memory span not found in other children (see also Marcell et al., 1990). In contrast to the slow word retrieval skills observed in DS, IQ- and age-matched adolescents with WS displayed rapid lexical access when asked to generate names of animals. The group with WS produced twice as many items over trials, including such unlikely choices as *unicorn, Brontosaurus, yak, ibex,* in contrast to more typical responses from the adolescents with DS (Bellugi et al., 1990).

SUMMARY AND CONCLUSIONS

In this chapter, I have considered a number of possible explanations for the challenges faced by many persons with DS in attaining full linguistic mastery. Despite generalizations that can be drawn about morphosyntactic and phonological difficulties in many people with DS, we are much encouraged by the fact that variation exists among persons with DS, and that some individuals do succeed. This variability suggests that the obstacles that do exist may be overcome and lends greater urgency to the need to identify factors relevant to linguistic success.

I have placed particular emphasis in this chapter on the parallels that exist between verbal memory capacity and grammatical proficiency in DS, in part because these domains have been studied separately until very recently. Despite the plausibility of such an account, further research is required to establish definitively that it is phonological factors that limit morphosyntactic development; such research must involve language learners with and without DS. Observations worth pursuing in a more systematic fashion include parallels between the weak gains in verbal memory and the weak gains in morphosyntax among older disabled children, and the association between memory and grammatical skill within and across linguistically diverse samples.

It is important to acknowledge that many investigators are skeptical about the association between phonology and syntax. As noted earlier, some are struck by the low memory levels observed in linguistically proficient adults studied. Others are pessimistic about constructing meaningful and appropriate tools for assessing verbal memory capacity, morphosyntax, and even phonology. Clearly, we must continue to develop cleaner measures of morphosyntax (separate from semantics) and of phonology (separate from articulation) than are currently available. It will be essential to consider production separately from comprehension, and within comprehension to better identify the grammatical devices in question. Crucially, if a threshold is important, we should focus on potentially relevant stages of language and memory development.

In seeking the source of grammatical deficits, an important goal for future research will be to assess more accurately any syntactic competence that may be masked by processing difficulties, guided by recent methodological advances with very young language learners. One possible approach is to examine implicit knowledge of whether a given utterance is grammatical or not, a skill that turns out to be intact in agrammatic aphasics who show extreme impairment in production and comprehension of grammatically complex constructions (e.g., Linebarger et al., 1983). Although use of standard grammaticality judgment tasks has previously been restricted to normally intelligent schoolchildren and high-functioning persons with mental retardation (e.g., Bellugi et al., 1994; Cromer, 1994), the serendipitous results of a recent study suggest that it may be possible to assess sensitivity to different grammatical structures in more typical persons with mental retardation. In that study, we noticed over the course of testing that children, with or without DS, took significantly longer to begin acting out those sentences that violated constraints on verb argument structure (e.g., *the lion fall the giraffe*) than to initiate enactment of sentences that were grammatically sensible. Both groups displayed this apparent sensitivity to grammatical structure even when their comments and enactments did not reveal the same degree of understanding (Naigles et al., 1994). Relying on these and other manipulations that reduce processing demands, it may be possible to reveal intact grammatical capacities that have been masked in the more traditional measures relied on to date. It is possible that limited memory capacity does not prevent acquisition of grammatical knowledge as much it precludes demonstration and use of this knowledge in production and comprehension tasks.

Because verbal memory capacity is itself a multi-faceted skill, I also spent some time considering what factors specifically limit memory in DS, noting that some more basic weakness may affect both memory and grammatical development. In fact, it seems unlikely that we will be able to isolate just one factor that puts persons with

DS at risk for memory difficulties, given the evidence for slow word retrieval and speed of articulation, poor linguistic perception, and lack of strategic rehearsal. On the other hand, whatever the precise mechanism(s) involved, it seems clear from a wide variety of studies that individual differences in verbal memory depend importantly on one or more aspects of phonological processing. A better theoretical understanding of verbal memory may require further isolation of critical factors, but it seems already clear that intervention efforts should focus on promoting accurate and efficient production and perception of linguistic information. Whether this phonological intervention leads to improved grammatical development is an empirical question that merits investigation. Independent of that outcome, improved articulation, perception and word retrieval are important goals in their own right.

ACKNOWLEDGMENT

The writing of this chapter was supported by a grant from NICHD #HD-01994 to Haskins Laboratories.

REFERENCES

Abbeduto L, Furman L, Davies B (1989): Relation between receptive language and mental age in persons with mental retardation. Am J Ment Retard 93:535–543.

Baddeley A (1986): "Working Memory." Oxford: Oxford University Press.

Bellugi U, Bihrle A, Jernigan T, Trauner D, Doherty S (1990): Neuropsychological, neurological, and neuroanatomical profile of Williams syndrome. Am J Med Genet 6(suppl):115–125.

Bellugi U, Wang PP, Jernigan TL (1994): Williams Syndrome: an unusual neuropsychological profile. In Broman SH, Grafman J (eds.): "Atypical Cognitive Deficits in Developmental Disorders: Implications for Brain Function." Hillsdale, NJ: Lawrence Erlbaum Associates, pp. 23–56.

Bilovsky D, Share J (1965): The ITPA and Down's syndrome: an exploratory study. Am J Ment Defic 70:78–82.

Brady SA (1997): Ability to encode phonological representations: An underlying difficulty of poor readers. In Blachman B (ed.): "Foundations of Reading Acquisition and Dyslexia: Implication for Early Intervention." Mahwah, NJ: Erlbaum Associates, pp. 21–48.

Bridges A, Smith J (1984): Syntactic comprehension in Down's Syndrome children. Brit J Psychol 75:187–196.

Buckley S, Sacks B (1987): "The Adolescent with Down's Syndrome." Portsmouth, England: Portsmouth Polytechnic.

Chapman R (1993): Longitudinal change in language production of children and adolescents with Down syndrome. Presented at Sixth International Conference for the Study of Child Language, Trieste, Italy.

Chapman RS (1991): Language development in children and adolescents with down syndrome. Presented at Workshop on Deviant Language Acquisition, University of Groningen.

Clahsen H (1989): The grammatical characterization of developmental dysphasia. Linguistics 27:897–920.

Clahsen H, Rothweiler M, Woest A, Marcus A (1992): Regular and irregular inflection in the acquisition of German noun plurals. Cognition 45:225–255.

Crisco JJ, Dobbs JM, Mulhern RK (1988): Cognitive processing of children with Williams syndrome. Devel Med Child Neurol 30:650–656.

Cromer RF (1994): A case study of dissociations between language and cognition. In Tager-Flusberg H (ed.): "Constraints on Language Acquisition: Studies of Atypical Children." Hillsdale, NJ: Lawrence Erlbaum Associates, pp. 141–153.

Curtiss S (1988a): Abnormal language acquisition and the modularity of language. In Newmeyer FE (ed.): "Linguistics: The Cambridge Survey," Vol. II, "Linguistic Theory: Extensions and Implication." Cambridge, England: Cambridge University Press, pp. 96–116.

Curtiss S (1988b): The special talent of grammar acquisition. In Obler L, Obler FD (eds.): "The Exceptional Brain." New York: Guilford Press, pp. 364–386.

Dempster F (1981): Memory span: Sources of individual and developmental differences. Psychol Bull 89:63–100.

Dewart MH (1979): Language comprehension processes of mentally retarded children. Am J Ment Defic 84:177–183.

Doherty BJ (1993) Relationships between phonological processes and reading ability in young adults with Down syndrome. Master's thesis. Bryn Mawr, PA: Bryn Mawr College.

Dunn L, Dunn L (1981): "Peabody Picture Vocabulary Text—Revised." Circle Pines, MN: American Guidance Service.

Dykens EM, Hodapp RM, Evans DW (1994): Profiles and development of adaptive behavior in children with Down syndrome. Am J Ment Retard 98:580–587.

Dykens EM, Hodapp RM, Leckman JF (1992): "Profiles and Development of Adaptive Behavior in Children with Fragile X Syndrome." Thousand Oaks, CA: Sage Publications.

Fletcher P (1990): Speech and language defects. Nature 346:226.

Fowler A (1984) Language acquisition in Down's Syndrome children: Production and Comprehension. Doctoral dissertation. Philadelphia: University of Pennsylvania.

Fowler A (1988): Determinants of rate of language growth in children with Down syndrome. In Nadel L (ed.): "The Psychobiology of Down Syndrome." Cambridge: MIT Press.

Fowler A (1990): Language abilities in children with Down syndrome: evidence for a specific syntactic delay. In Cicchetti D, Beeghly M (eds.): "Children with Down Syndrome: A Developmental Perspective." New York: Cambridge University Press, pp. 302–328.

Fowler A (1995): Linguistic variability in persons with Down syndrome: research and implications. In Nadel L, Rosenthal D (eds.): "Down Syndrome: Living and Learning in the Community." New York: Wiley-Liss, pp. 121–136.

Fowler A (1997): Language in mental retardation: associations with and dissociations from general cognition. In Burack J, Hodapp R, Zigler E (eds.): "Handbook of Mental Retardation and Development." New York: Cambridge University Press, pp. 290–333.

Fowler A, Doherty B, Boynton L (1995): The basis of reading skill in young adults with Down syndrome In Nadel L, Rosenthal D (eds.): "Down Syndrome: Living and Learning in the Community." New York: Wiley-Liss, pp. 182–196.

Fowler A, Gelman R, Gleitman R (1994): The course of language learning in children with Down syndrome: longitudinal and language level comparisons with young normally developing children. In Tager-Flusberg H (ed.): "Constraints on Language Acquisition: Studies of Atypical Populations." Hillsdale, NJ: Erlbaum Associates, pp. 91–140.

Gathercole S, Adams AM (1993): Phonological working memory in very young children. Devel Pscyhol 29:770–778.

Gathercole S, Baddeley AD (1990): Phonological memory deficits in language-disordered children: Is there a causal connection? J Memory Language 81:439–454.

Gleitman L, Wanner E (1982): Language acquisition. The state of the art. In Wanner E, Gleitman L (eds.): "Language Acquisition: The State of the Art." New York: Cambridge University Press, pp. 3–48.

Gopnik M (1990): Dysphasia in an extended family. Nature 344:715.

Gopnik M (1990): Feature blindness: a case study. Language Acquisition 1:139–164.

Graham NC (1974): Response strategies in the partial comprehension of sentences. Language Speech 17:205–221.

Hulme C, MacKenzie S (1992): "Working Memory and Severe Learning Difficulties." Hillside, NJ: Lawrence Erlbaum Associates.

Hulme C, Maughan S, Brown G (1991): Memory for familiar and unfamiliar words: Evidence for a long-term memory contribution to short-term memory span. J Memory Language 30:685–701.

Hulme C, Thomson N, Muir C, Lawrence A (1984): Speech rate and the development of short-term memory span. J Exp Child Psychol 38:241–253.

Johnston J (1988): Specific language disorders in the child. In Lass N, McReynolds L, Northern J, Yoder D (eds.): "Handbook of Speech-Language Pathology and Audiology." Philadelphia: B. Decker, pp. 685–715.

Kaufman AS, Kaufman N (1983): "Kaufman Assessment Battery for Children." Circle Pines, MN: American Guidance Service.

Kumin L (1994): Intelligibility of speech in children with Down syndrome in natural settings: parents perspective. Percep Motor Skills 78:307–313.

Lahey M, Bloom L (1994): Variability and language learning disabilities. In Wallach GP, Butler KG (eds.): "Language Learning Disabilities in School-age Children and Adolescents." New York: Merrill, pp. 353–372.

Lenneberg EH (1967): "Biological Foundations of Language." New York: Wiley.

Leonard LB, McGregor KK, Allen GD (1992): Grammatical morphology and speech perception in children with specific language impairment. J Speech Hearing Res 35:1076–1085.

Levitz M, Kingsley J (1995): "Count Us In: Growing Up With Down Syndrome."

Linebarger MC, Schwartz MF, Saffran EM (1983): Sensitivity to grammatical structure in so-called agrammatic aphasics. Cognition 13:361–392.

Locke JL (1994): Gradual emergence of developmental language disorders. J Speech Hearing Res 37:608–616.

Mackenzie S, Hulme C (1987): Memory span development in Down's syndrome, severely subnormal and normal subjects. Cognitive Neuropsychol 4:303–319.

Marcell MM (1992): Hearing abilities of Down syndrome and other mentally handicapped adolescents. Res Devel Disabilities 13:533–551.

Marcell M, Armstrong V (1982): Auditory and visual sequential memory of Down syndrome and nonretarded children. Am J Ment Defic 87:86–95.

Marcell MM, Croen PS, Mansker JK, Sizemore TD (1994): Language comprehension by Down syndrome and other mentally handicapped youth. Presented at the International Down Syndrome Conference, Charleston, SC.

Marcell MM, Croen PS, Sewell DH (1990): Language comprehension in Down syndrome and other trainable mentally handicapped individuals. Presented at the Conference on Human Development, Richmond, VA.

Marcell MM, Weeks SL (1988): Short-term memory difficulties and Down's syndrome. J Ment Defic Res 32:153–162.

Miller JF (1987): Language and communication characteristics of children with Down syndrome. In Pueschel S, Tinghey C, Rynders J, Crocker A, Crutcher C (eds.): "New Perspectives on Down Syndrome." Baltimore: Brookes Publishing, pp. 233–262.

Miller J (1988): The developmental asynchrony of language development in children with Down Syndrome. In Nadel L (ed.): "The Psychobiology of Down Syndrome." Cambridge, MA: MIT Press.

Miller JF, Chapman RS (1984): Disorders of communication: investigating the development of language of mentally retarded children. Am J Ment Defic 88:536–545.

Miller JA, Leddy M, Miolo G, Sedey A (1995): The development of early language skills in children with Down syndrome. In Nadel L, Rosenthal D (eds.): "Down Syndrome: Living and Learning in the Community." New York: Wiley-Liss, pp. 115–120.

Morgan JL, Demuth K (1996): "Signal to Syntax: Bootstrapping from Speech to Grammar in Early Acquisition." Mahwah, NJ: Erlbaum.

Nadel L, Rosenthal, D (1995): "Down Syndrome: Living and Learning in the Community." New York: Wiley-Liss.

Naigles L, Fowler A, Helm A (1995): Syntactic bootstrapping from start to finish with special reference to Down syndrome. In Tomasello M, Merriman W (eds.): "Beyond Names for Things: Young Children's Acquisition of Verbs." Hillsdale, NJ: Erlbaum Associates, pp. 299–330.

Natsopoulos D, Xeromeritou A (1990): Language behavior by mildly handicapped and nonretarded children on complement clauses. Res Devel Disabilities 11:199–216.

Newport E (1990): Maturational constraints on language learning. Cognitive Sci 14:11–28.

Pueschel S (1988): Visual and auditory processing in children with Down syndrome. In Nadel L (ed.): "The Psychobiology of Down Syndrome." Cambridge: MIT Press, pp. 199–216.

Racette K (1993) Phonological bases of memory in normal preschoolers and young adults with Down syndrome. Master's thesis. Bryn Mawr, PA: Bryn Mawr College.

Reilly J, Klima ES, Bellugi U (1991): Once more with feeling: Affect and language in atypical populations. Devel Psychopathol 2:367–391.

Rice ML, Oetting JB (1993): Morphological deficits of children with SLI: evaluation of number marking and agreement. J Speech Hearing Res 36:1249–1257.

Rondal J (1994a): Exceptional cases of language development in mental retardation: the relative autonomy of language as a cognitive system. In Tager-Flusberg H (ed.): "Constraints on Language Development: Studies of Atypical Children." Hillsdale, NJ: Erlbaum Associates.

Rondal JA (1994b): Exceptional Language Development in Down Syndrome. A Case Study and Its Implications for Cognition-language and Other Language-modularity Issues." New York: Cambridge University Press.

Rosenberg S, Abbeduto L (1993): "Language and Communication in Mental Retardation." Hillsdale, NJ: Erlbaum.

Scarborough HS, Rescorla L, Tager-Flusberg H, Fowler AE, Sudhalter V (1991): The relation of utterance length to grammatical complexity in normal and language-disordered groups. Appl Psycholinguistics 12(1):23–45.

Seagoe MV (1964): Verbal development in a mongoloid. Exceptional Children 31:269–273.

Shriberg LD, Kwiatkowski J (1988): A follow-up study of children with phonological disorders of unknown origin. J Speech Hearing Disorders 53:144–155.

Smith BL, Stoel-Gammon C (1983): A longitudinal study of the development of stop consonant production in normal and Down's syndrome children. J Speech Hearing Disorders 48:114–118.

Tager-Flusberg H (1994): Dissociations in form and function in the acquisition of language by autistic children. In Tager-Flusberg H (ed.): "Constraints on Language Acquisition: Studies of Atypical Children." Hillsdale, NJ: Lawrence Erlbaum Associates, pp. 175–194.

Tager-Flusberg H, Calkins S, Nolin T, Baumberger T, Anderson M, Chadwick-Dias A (1990): A longitudinal study of language acquisition in autistic and Down syndrome children. J Autism Devel Disorders 20:1–21.

Vargha-Khadem F, Passingham R (1990): Speech and language defects. Nature 346:226.

Varnhagen CK, Das JP, Varnhagen S (1987): Auditory and visual memory span: cognitive processing by TMR individuals with Down syndrome and other etiologies. Am J Ment Defic 91(4):398–405.

Wang PP, Bellugi U (1994): Evidence from two genetic syndromes for a dissociation between verbal and visual-spatial short-term memory. J Clin Exp Neuropsychol 16:317–322.

VII. Education

Inclusion Is a Process, Not Just a Philosophy

Michael L. Remus

Much debate during the past few years has centered around the issue of including students with disabilities in the general classroom. One will hear the same debate or question being asked in every state across the nation. The question from my perspective is a "value" question and must be answered by saying that *all* children can learn and succeed—now how do we go about making sure that all students' needs are being met. We could philosophically debate this issue for the next 100 years, but we must act now if we are going to prepare students for their future.

All individuals can learn, and it is the schools' responsibility to make sure this is done. This is where inclusion becomes a process and not just a philosophy. In the next few pages I would like to take you through a process of ensuring that students with disabilities are being included in the general scheme of public education. I know this can be a reality, because students are included in their neighborhood schools and integrated into the regular school day in the districts where I worked. I was employed by Educational Service Unit #7 (ESU #7) which is an organization serving 68 school districts in a geographical area of 4500 square miles. ESU #7 serves nearly 3000 students who have been identified as needing special education services.

When making school reform or a major systems change within a school or district, one has to target and focus on specific audiences who must be involved to make the system change. In the area of inclusion it was found that there are seven audiences that must make a change in thinking and the way of providing services. These audiences comprise school board members and administrators, teachers (both general and special support staff), parents, students, higher education faculty, community leaders, and governmental officials. The inclusion process must be embraced by these audiences before inclusion can become a reality. Once these entities are brought into the process for systems change then inclusion moves from the philosophy of rhetoric to the process stage to make inclusion a reality for students.

Down Syndrome: A Promising Future, Together, Edited by Terry J. Hassold and David Patterson
ISBN 0-471-29686-4   Copyright © 1998 by Wiley-Liss, Inc.

The first stage in our process was to develop vision and mission statements with belief statements to follow. We worked with each audience named above and described below to help them believe and support the mission, vision and belief statements. Each audience was asked to be a part of a core advisory group, to report to their prospective constituency, and to gain their constituency's support. They were also to bring their concerns, ideas, barriers, and so on to the table for discussion. This was, in the beginning, to help the target audiences feel ownership of the process. Potential obstacles were identified early, and the groups were given the responsibility of overcoming these barriers. It was then the goal of ESU #7 to make sure the activities and policies of each school district were harmonious with the mission and belief statements we adopted.

BOARD MEMBERS AND ADMINISTRATORS

The first audience in the systems change process is the school officials, including board members and administrators. A primary concern of this audience is cost. They had to be convinced that inclusion is a much more productive and efficient use of district resources than segregated special education programs. As the administrator in special education, it was my job to work with this audience and show specifically how dollars can be redirected and used more effectively by the inclusion of students with disabilities in general education.

It was found five years into the process that the resources were serving more students, and money was saved. Areas focused on included transportation; if students are educated in their neighborhood schools, added transportation costs are avoided. In addition, if special education support staff is in the general classroom, then students who do not qualify for special education services are also being served alongside identified students. The "at risk" students are serving as peer models while their own needs are being met. Also, costs are saved by not contracting for core services outside of the school district, which is much more expensive. Again, to obtain the administrator "buy-in" we primarily talked of how inclusion can be cost efficient and productive in the future. By redirecting district dollars into inclusion programs, it was found that many more students could be served with the same amount of funding.

TEACHERS

The second audience is teachers (general and special support staff). Districts must provide much more in-service training regarding strategies, curriculum adaptations, and so forth, to assist teachers in including students with disabilities into the classroom. We adapted curricula to be taught in a multimodality format that enabled many students with different learning styles to benefit. For example, any concept that is taught must be presented in the visual, auditory, and kinesthetic or hands-on format. Activities using the total modality instruction will utilize all of these formats. We invited many consultants to introduce teachers to many teaching methods and techniques, and to prepare them for students with varying disabilities in their classrooms.

Among some of the consultants and areas we have brought in are Dan Hobbs of Gentle Teaching, which incorporates strategies for students with behaviors; Marsha

Forest of Circle of Friends, which teaches how to plan and uses students in planning for a student with a disability; Wayne Sailor of Comprehensive Local Schools, which provides ideas for system change within the school building incorporating inclusion; and Floyd Hudson of Class Within a Class, which teaches strategies within the general classroom. Each year several national speakers continue the in-service training with the teachers. In-service training was also provided in the classroom on a day-to-day basis, and many teachers were able to travel to other schools to observe inclusive practices. The Educational Service Unit only provided in-service training to teams of school personnel because of the need to develop the team concept with children. Each school is required to send the general classroom teacher, special education support person, parent, administrator, and a board member to each in-service. When each audience attended in-services together, they were better able to support system change.

PARENTS

The third audience is parents of both general education students and special education students. We asked parents what they felt were the top priorities for their children. Most parents of children with disabilities want the following outcomes: students should be prepared for a job, have friends, be able to live independently, and become involved in the community. These priorities are the same for parents of all children. Parents want their children to learn social skills needed to get along independently in the community. At parent meetings, I always point out that parents do not see academics as a priority, but schools are focused on teaching academics. There is something wrong with this picture.

We then ask parents how schools should be teaching these social skills, and parents ask for inclusion on a trial basis. We have always given parents the right to change their mind about having their children included, after each semester. Parents rarely choose a return to self-contained classrooms.

STUDENTS

The fourth audience is the students. We had to prepare students to accept their peers with disabilities in the classroom. We developed a disability awareness curriculum for students to develop empathy for their peers. This helped students understand why certain students may have difficulty learning, and how they can help. Peer tutoring and buddy systems were established, so everyone in the classroom felt welcome. It was set up with the idea of helping everyone develop a sense of success.

COMMUNITY LEADERS

The fifth audience is community businesses and leaders. This audience was particularly selected to become involved in the students' transitioning into the work world. The community has to be ready for an inclusive environment. We educated business leaders regarding work incentives for hiring individuals with disabilities. We stressed that they could help these students become tax paying citizens, which would, in turn, make their businesses successful. We invited business leaders into school to teach work ethics and support teachers in career curricula. This starts at the elementary level and extends into the secondary level when students graduate. The goal is to have every student go on to post secondary education or be employed within the community.

GOVERNMENT LEADERS AND EMPLOYEES

The sixth audience that must be addressed in the change process is government leaders and employees at the state and federal level. We asked our representatives in the legislature to visit our schools and to talk with parents about their expectations for their children with disabilities. We also asked the state officials to become a part of our educational team and attend our workshops and in-services. This helps them see things from our perspective, and should inspire them to make changes to support our system. We also requested waivers to enable districts to go beyond regulations creatively so they may try new approaches to inclusion. Government leaders have worked well as part of our team, and have even helped with funding and in-service training to the other audiences.

HIGHER EDUCATION

The seventh audience is higher education. Schools must work with the teacher training institutions if we are to make changes in the public schools. New teachers must be prepared to work with a diversity of learners. As we retrained our teachers in inclusive practices, we asked local universities and colleges to allow our current teachers to share what they've learned. Our teachers taught a person-centered approach to Individualized Education Plans, as well as teaching methods including thematic instruction, behavior management skills, and different scheduling patterns.

ESU #7 has been implementing this process for five years. In the first year we dissolved our four segregated facilities. In the second year, students with disabilities were transported to cluster schools that had self-contained classrooms. In the third year these classrooms were dissolved and students were placed in their neighborhood schools with brothers, sisters, and friends. In the fourth year we concentrated on integrating students into the general classroom, and in the fifth year we have focused on even more inclusion within the classrooms.

I would caution against moving too quickly through the process and placing students with disabilities in the general classroom without adequate support or preparation. School districts that have placed students with disabilities in the classroom without planning are doing what we call "main-dumping." Without proper planning and preparation, the system can set both teachers and students up for failure. This "main-dumping" is taking place in many parts of our country under the name of inclusion. This is not true inclusion, and is dangerous because it could prejudice many of our key audiences against inclusion. If you have any questions please do not hesitate to contact me at Kansas State Department of Education, 120 SE 10th Avenue, Topeka, Kansas 66612.

Curricular Adaptations to Support Elementary Age Students with Disabilities in Inclusive Settings

Marquita Grenot-Scheyer

INTRODUCTION

Carla and her classmates are engaged in building a castle with sugar cubes, glue, sequins, and other art materials as part of the class unit on classic fairy tales. Although Carla, a third-grade student with Down syndrome, does not like the sticky feeling of glue, she does enjoy working with her peers and listening to them read excerpts from the story. Together Carla's group has delegated work responsibilities for the day. Carla agreed to be responsible for distributing and collecting materials and to provide suggestions regarding the design of the castle. It was okay with Carla and her peers if she did not want to get involved in the actual construction of the castle. Later during this period, an instructional assistant helps Carla write a short entry for her journal on what life in a castle might have been like.

This vignette is presented to illustrate how a student with disabilities can be included in general education activities and curriculum. Inclusion is generally regarded as the placement of students with disabilities in neighborhood schools and general education classrooms with peers their own age. Primary placement in the general education classroom allows for membership and the development of a sense of community for all learners (Grenot-Scheyer et al., 1996). The practice of including students with disabilities into general education schools and classrooms continues to grow and is supported by legislation (see Falvey et al., 1995 for a review) and a growing body of research (Hunt and Goetz, 1997; Meyer, 1994; Staub et al., 1994). This increasing interest and practice has resulted in many resources and strategies for parents, teachers, and others to use as they include students with disabilities into general education settings.

Generally, teachers, administrators, and other school personnel are familiar with the concept and practice of inclusion, either through their professional preparation

Down Syndrome: A Promising Future, Together, Edited by Terry J. Hassold and David Patterson
ISBN 0-471-29686-4   Copyright © 1998 by Wiley-Liss, Inc.

programs, which have incorporated principles of inclusion and diversity into the curriculum, or more likely, through direct experience "on the job" (Roach et al., 1995). Although prevailing attitudes toward diversity of learners in schools is slowly changing, the curricular demands presented in contemporary classrooms challenge even the most experienced classroom teacher.

The purpose of this chapter is to present a curriculum modification process that parents, teachers, and other professionals can use when developing educational plans for students with and without disabilities in inclusive settings. An introduction to the critical values underlying inclusive education is presented first, followed by questions to guide the process of curricular modification. The chapter concludes with several examples of strategies and classroom activities to facilitate the inclusion of students with disabilities into general education settings.

INCLUSIVE SCHOOLS & CLASSROOMS: NECESSARY VALUES

In schools that include all learners, including those students with disabilities as part of the educational community, teachers and other professionals must demonstrate on a daily basis *that all students belong, can benefit from the learning community, and can have individualized needs met.* One of the goals of inclusion is to enhance the educational experience of all students. Most importantly, the education of students with disabilities is seen as *integral to school reform efforts* and not viewed as a separate agenda for special education faculty.

In inclusive schools all students are valued (Lewis et al., 1996). Through their daily interactions with a diverse student body, *teachers model caring interactions and a belief that all students can learn.* Such heterogeneous classrooms require *collaboration and shared responsibility* among professionals and parents for the benefit of all students. Students with disabilities and other diverse learners are only successful in heterogeneous classes where *interdependence is required and supported,* and where *specific structures such as cooperative grouping* (Johnson and Johnson, 1989) (Gibbs, 1995) *are in place to foster such interdependence.*

In inclusive classrooms, an important variable related to student success is *how curriculum is designed and instruction delivered. Different ways of knowing are fostered and such contributions are valued* (Armstrong, 1994). *Curriculum accommodations* are developed and *multilevel instruction* is used based upon recommendations of the *school site team* during their planning process (Thousand and Villa, 1990). The school site team is typically composed of the general education teacher, the special education support teacher, parents, related services staff, and others. This team has the responsibility to plan, implement, and monitor the educational program.

GETTING STARTED: QUESTIONS TO GUIDE THE CURRICULUM MODIFICATION PROCESS
Where Do We Start?

Teachers, parents and other members of a school site team should review the student's Individualized Educational Program (IEP) and the district's core curriculum or state framework as a starting point in the design of an educational plan. The district's core curriculum reflects both the broad content or academic skills essential to learning and the social or moral skills necessary to be an effective citizen. In addition, unlike their peers without disabilities, students with disabilities also have additional help in determining their needs because of the "blueprint" laid out in the IEP. The IEP objectives are considered by the team and infused into curricular units based upon academic skills to be developed and/or broader skills to be practiced and reinforced within given classroom activities.

How Will All the Needs of the Student Be Met?

The Inclusion Support Planning Grid (Fig. 1) may assist the school site team in determining the adaptations to the core curriculum that a student with disabilities may require. The grid provides information regarding levels of assistance and specific areas of the curriculum that will require modification. Just as the core curriculum or district framework serves as a roadmap for planning an educational year, the IEP serves as an additional tool for planning the educational program for a student with disabilities. The teacher, along with the support of the school site team, then has the responsibility to merge the classroom map and the student's map. The planning grid can help the team decide what individual needs can be met throughout the daily routine of the classroom. It allows parents and staff to "see" how the individual student goals are interwoven and part of the entire day across the curriculum.

Completion of the planning grid allows the teacher and school site team to determine the activities and time of day where *no assistance* is needed. For many students with disabilities, curricular content, classroom activities, and daily routines require no modification. The curriculum can be presented as it is usually presented to all students. For example, Carla needs no assistance or modification during the morning routine or when it is time to put materials away in preparation for recess. She has demonstrated the ability to follow the instructions that the teacher gives to the whole group.

The school site team may decide that Carla needs *physical support* to participate more fully in a lesson or activity. For example, Carla sometimes has difficulty buttoning small buttons on her pants and needs assistance to turn the faucet off completely after washing her hands. Nondisabled girlfriends are likely to be eager and willing to provide this necessary support. Carla may also need *material adaptations* to enhance her participation. For example, Carla benefits from raised glue outlines on art projects to indicate the edges of shapes, and is most successful when the number of items on a page is reduced and when enlarged print is used. Nondisabled peers are a reliable and useful resource when determining and selecting both physical means of support and material adaptations, and the school site team should rely on them for age appropriate suggestions.

Determining *additional personnel needs* is also accomplished with the planning grid. In reviewing a student's typical week, the team can decide when a student will require additional support from an instructional assistant, related service personnel (i.e., communication specialist, physical therapist), and/or nondisabled peers. For example, Carla and several of her nondisabled peers receive instruction from the communication specialist who visits once a week. She assists Carla to expand her vocabulary and to increase her volume when contributing to a small group activity.

Student: **Carla S.**

Age/Birthdate: **8/6-20-88**

Grade/Regular Education Teacher: **3/Peggy A.**

Support Teacher: **Debbie W.**

Date: **10/96**

School: **Playa Vista**

Class Schedule:

Student IEP Obj.'s	OPENING	LANG. ARTS	A.M. RECESS	MATH	LUNCH	SUST. SILENT RDG.	JOURNAL	SCIENCE SOC. STUD.	P.M. RECESS	ART/ MUSIC	DISMISSAL
Identify & use key vocabulary		D/2								D/5	
Dictate story to peer or adult							D/8				
Use estimation & prob. solving				E/3,6	E/5						
Improve writing		C/3					D/5	C/3		C/3	
Stay on topic		D/2					D/5,8	D/2,3			
Raise hand to gain attention	B/8	D/2		D/2,3	E/5					D/2,3	
Use appr. tone and volume	D/2	D/2									
Remain in seat – group time	B/8	B/8				E/5					
Check self after restroom			B/8		B/8				B/8		
Enter peer group appr.			D/5		D/5				D/5		

Key: Curriculum Adaptations:
(A) As Is (B) Physical Support (C) Material Adaptations
(D) Multilevel Goals (E) Goals Outside Content Area

Levels of Assistance:
(1) No Additional (2) DIS/Related Service (3) Support Teacher
(4) Aide (5) Staff (6) Cross-age Tutor (7) Peers (8) Parents

Fig. 1. Inclusion support planning grid (Grenot-Scheyer et al., 1992).

The communication specialist also works with the nondisabled students who present a variety of communicative needs.

Will Every Classroom Activity Have to Be Adapted Every Day?

As indicated previously, there will be many activities in which students with disabilities can participate without any modification. There will also be specific daily activities that occur regularly for which *accommodations can be predetermined and used*. For example, journal writing takes place in Carla's classroom for 15 minutes every morning. Carla's school site team has decided that she can choose between drawing a story, dictating a three-sentence story to a peer, then copying the sentences into her journal, or cutting and pasting a story with pictures from a magazine during this time. Because the team has made these predetermined choices for Carla, it is not necessary to make specific adaptations for this activity every day.

Modifications can also be developed for *typical instructional routines* present in classrooms. Many teachers use common instructional routines that vary depending upon the curricular area. For example, during lecture time when the teacher is first introducing content material, the school site team may determine that Carla is more successful if she is given an outline on which key points of the lecture are printed. She then can participate in the follow-up group discussion activity with her peers while also working on specific vocabulary development.

How Are Specific Lessons or Activities Adapted?

To meet further the student's individual needs and to ensure successful participation, some lessons will need further modification. The school site team may consider selecting *multilevel goals* and/or *goals outside the content area*. To best match the individual student objectives with the core curriculum, the school site team may need to vary the goals and objectives of particular lessons. For example, during sustained silent reading, Carla listens to a favorite story on tape with a headphone. Although she is not engaging in reading as are her nondisabled peers, she is working on a related goal of attending to a story for longer and longer periods of time. At other times, Carla concentrates on basic goals and skills outside a particular content area. For example, during prolonged discussion times in class, Carla is encouraged to monitor her tone of voice and to stay on the topic. The emphasis is on the basic skills of conversation and attending to the topic the class is engaged in.

To assist school site teams to modify individual lessons or activities, an Activity Analysis worksheet may be helpful. This process and worksheet is based upon the work of Neary and Mintun (1991). In the first column, Classroom Activity Steps, the behaviors demonstrated by any student are listed. In the second column, Student Skills, the behaviors demonstrated by the student with disabilities are listed and described. The point of this comparison is to determine where specific adaptations may be needed. In the third column, the Specific Adaptations are listed. The final column, Skills in Need of Instruction, allows the teacher and the school site team to target particular behaviors for direct instruction. A completed Activity Analysis for Carla in language arts is presented in Figure 2.

Name of Student: **Carla S.**   Date: **12/96**
Teacher: **Peggy A.**
Activity: **Language Arts: Group Report on Castles**

Classroom Activity Steps	Student Skills	Specific Adaptations	Skills in Need of Instruction
1. Teacher outlines report	Has difficulty following sequence of steps	Provide cue card with written steps.	Follow teacher outline by reading cue card.
2. Students gather in small groups.	Same as peers	—	—
3. Students decide on group responsibilities.	Has difficulty deciding on a specific role within a group.	Have a peer "coach" her; give her two choices, let her choose one.	Choice-making
4. Distribution of writing and reference materials.	Enjoys distributing materials in small group.	—	—
5. Students take notes.	Has difficulty writing from a reference source.	Pre-made note cards with key points.	Locate main points.
6. Students contribute to group report.	Tends to contribute, but "off-topic."	(same as above)	Contribute original ideas to group discussions.
7. Students share report with large group.	Enjoys sitting with group; does not want to report out.	—	—

Fig. 2. Classroom activity analysis worksheet.

WHAT CAN WE EXPECT?

The premise of this chapter and the work of many parents, teachers, and others is reflected in the belief that all students can learn, but not on the same day, and not in the same way. Students with and without disabilities need a curriculum that is accessible by all, and that allows for and supports meaningful interaction. As teachers, parents, and other professionals continue to work together to develop innovative ways of including students with diverse needs, such efforts can't help but benefit *all* students.

ACKNOWLEDGMENT

Preparation of this chapter was supported in part by Cooperative Agreement No. HO86A20003 to Syracuse University, with a subcontract to California State University, Long Beach, from the Office of Special Education Programs, U.S. Department of Education. This material does not necessarily reflect the position or policies of the U.S. Department of Education, and no official endorsement should be inferred. Portions of this chapter were presented at the National Down Syndrome Society Conference, Phoenix, Arizona, June, 1996.

REFERENCES

Armstrong T (1994): "Multiple Intelligences in the Classroom." Alexandria, VA: Association for Supervision and Curriculum Development.

Falvey MA (ed.) (1995): "Inclusive and Heterogeneous Schooling: Assessment, Curriculum, and Instruction." Baltimore, MD: Paul H. Brookes.

Falvey MA, Grenot-Scheyer M, Coots JJ, and Bishop, KD (1995). Services for students with disabilities: Past and present. In: M Falvey (ed.), Inclusive and heterogeneous schooling: Assessment, curriculum, and instruction (23–39). Baltimore, MD: Paul H Brookes

Gibbs J (1995): "Tribes: A New Way of Learning and Being Together." Sausalito, CA: Center Source Systems.

Grenot-Scheyer M, Jubala KA, Bishop KD, Coots JJ (1996): "The Inclusive Classroom." Westminister, CA: Teacher Created Materials, Inc.

Hunt P, Goetz L (1997): Research on inclusive educational programs, practices, and outcomes for students with severe disabilities. J Special Educ 31(1):3–29.

Johnson DW, Johnson RT (1989): "Cooperation and Competition: Theory and Research." Edina, MN: Interaction Books.

Lewis CC, Schaps E, Watson MS (1996): Educ Leadership 54(1):16–21.

Meyer LH (ed.) (1994): Understanding the impact of inclusion. J Assoc Persons Severe Handicaps 10(4):251–252.

Neary T, Mintun B (1991): Classroom activity analysis worksheet. Sacramento: California State Department of Education.

Roach V, Ascroft J, Stamp A, Kysilko D (eds.) (1995): "Winning Ways: Creating Inclusive Schools, Classrooms and Communities." Alexandria, VA: National Association of State Boards of Education.

Staub D, Schwartz IS, Gallucci C, Peck CA (1994): Four portraits of friendship at an inclusive school. J Assoc Persons Severe Handicaps 19(4):290–301.

Thousand J and Villa R (1990). Sharing expertise and responsibilities through teaching teams. In W Stainback & S Stainback (eds), Support networks for inclusive schooling: Integrated interdependent education. (151–166) Baltimore, MD: Paul H. Brookes.

The Meaning of Inclusion and Down Syndrome

Gloria Wolpert

Inclusive education is based on the premise that children of different abilities and backgrounds can benefit both academically and socially in a learning environment that is programmed along with typically achieving students (Banarji and Dailey, 1995). Salisbury et al. (1995) have stated that "the diverse needs of all children can be accommodated to the maximum extent possible within the general education curriculum." Children with Down syndrome have different learning styles that usually require more thought to be given to curricular choices and experiences, which previously has prompted educational programming to be more segregated in nature, involving specialized services and smaller groupings. Recently, parents of children with Down syndrome have felt that their children's education in a more specialized program was isolating, particularly when adolescence is reached. They want their children to have friends and be with peers during early childhood and the school years, in preparation for adulthood where they must get along with their peers and function in society. Some parents have gone so far as to forego academic achievement in order to maximize socialization (Salisbury et al., 1995; Stainback and Stainback, 1992). Many parents have questions on the outcomes of inclusive programming and concerns about which methods work best.

THE STUDY

The National Down Syndrome Society was asked by parent constituents to conduct a survey of parents and teachers of children with Down syndrome to determine the success or lack of success of inclusive practices, and to survey what was happening nationwide with inclusion programs and children with Down syndrome. This prompted the development and dissemination of two types of questionnaires, one designed to elicit parent case studies and opinions, and the second to examine school organization and what classroom practices teachers were using. More than 320

Down Syndrome: A Promising Future, Together, Edited by Terry J. Hassold and David Patterson
ISBN 0-471-29686-4   Copyright © 1998 by Wiley-Liss, Inc.

questionnaire pairs were mailed to affiliate parents and their children's teachers, with steps taken to match up the responses of parents and teachers. Several other school districts were also solicited.

The parent study was designed to obtain write-in responses for the following areas:

background and previous experience with the school district
basic classroom information (teaching arrangement and ratio)
the transition process/degrees of preparation
parental involvement
the child's adjustment and experiences
the evaluation of parent and professional attitudes

Parents also rated how successful they felt that inclusion was for their child in the following areas: academic, socialization, independence, language, and self-esteem.

The teacher study included questions referring to the following:

background/teacher information (experience, knowledge of special education and inclusion)
preparation for inclusion and the transition process
classroom information on curriculum, class arrangement, therapies, and support services
classroom management, instructional and behavioral strategies, and teacher attitude

Teachers then rated the inclusion experience on how much extra work it was, and how it related to their expectations. The questionnaires were disseminated in the spring of 1995, and responses were collected through the fall of 1995.

125 parent responses and 120 teacher responses were returned. Out of this population, 90 parent/teacher pairs were received. The evaluation was conducted in three parts: a parent survey, a teacher questionnaire, and parent anecdotal records. The intent of this three part approach was to examine all relevant factors of the questionnaire pairs from different perspectives and to systematically gather and evaluate evidence from various resources to arrive at conclusions regarding the effects of inclusion on education. No judgments were made on the quality of programs, the responses received complete confidentiality, and analyses were descriptive in nature to reflect what practices were currently existing.

DISCUSSION OF RESULTS OF PARENT SURVEY

Correlation analyses and multiple regression were used to determine the relationships between the variables. Teaching arrangement did not affect parent report of successful inclusion. More important than co-teaching (between special educators and regular educators) in a collaborative fashion, use of a resource room teacher, or the extra help of an aide was the teacher style with the child. This leads to the conclusion that the match of any teacher personality and skill to the student is important to successful inclusion practice. This also ties into the many teacher requests for further information on learning characteristics of children with Down syndrome and teaching methods.

It is a bit surprising that teacher preparation was not more highly correlated with parent perception of success. Teacher preparation for inclusion has been a focus of much recent research in education (Chalfant and Pysh, 1989; Fuchs, Fuchs and Bahr, 1990; Knackendoffel et al., 1992). It is possible that this relationship was not indicated because 55% of the teachers reported no preparation or inclusion training at all before the inclusion took place, which may have skewed results.

Another surprise was that administrative attitude did not seem to play a role with parent report of success. Research on organizational change and leadership in education has shown that principal and administrative attitude are important to school change and educational achievement (Owens, 1981; Stogdill, 1974). However, the unity between special education and regular education personnel was a highly predictive factor of parent perception of success, which suggests that administrative attitude may play an indirect part in the fostering of a bonding or collaborative team between the special and regular educators. There is also much anecdotal report by parents in this study on the relationships between regular educators and special education personnel. Also, when parents reported an easy, productive placement process, they found the inclusion experience successful. Those parents who had difficulty with the initial placement reported less satisfaction with the experience. It seems that first contact impressions tend to set up parent expectations for success or failure. This also indirectly indicates the need for preparation planning.

There did not seem to be any relationship between how involved the parents were in the education of their child and how satisfied they were with inclusion. This could be due to the fact that there was a small range of variability in this parameter, with almost all parents being involved with meetings, their child's Individualized Education Plan, and the daily operations. However, parents who had confidence in the professionals associated with the education of and decision-making for their child found inclusion to be more successful than parents who did not have confidence in their related professionals.

Whether or not the child was encouraged by his or her peers or was a behavior problem in class had no effect on parent perception of successful inclusion. However, parents who reported that their child had friends in class also rated the inclusion experience as successful. This supports the research and anecdotal information that it is important to parents that their children have friends in the educational environment. Parents stated that they were pleased to have their children join in socially in both formal and informal activities. The variable that showed the highest degree of relationship with report of successful inclusion was the format of the curriculum in the classroom. Teachers who were flexible with the type of student participation and who could alter their use of materials to be more concrete in nature were reported to be highly successful catalysts of achievement for students with Down syndrome. Also of importance was curricular style with visible cues, not predominant reliance on auditory language, notetaking, and workbooks.

To summarize, parent perception of successful inclusion relied on the factors of initial placement experience, teacher style with the child, the format of the curriculum, the unity between special and regular education, confidence in professionals, and whether or not their children have friends in class. This would suggest that it would be prudent to prepare teachers for skillful curricular design and learning styles of students with Down syndrome.

DISCUSSION OF RESULTS OF TEACHER SURVEY

Learning Arrangements and Materials

As can be expected from previous research, teachers found that 1:1 instruction or small group instruction worked much better than large groups or the whole class. This was one of the original reasons for the design of separate smaller special education classes in the 1950s and 1960s (Kirk and Gallagher, 1983). Materials that worked best were concrete activities, or manipulatives, and computer-assisted instruction and drill. Sometimes the same materials were used in different ways. One teacher reported that while the rest of her first-grade class used Uniflex cubes for counting and adding, the child with Down syndrome sorted the cubes by color.

Workbooks were not useful at all. This is not surprising because most workbooks either depend heavily on language comprehension (a problem area for students with Down syndrome) or have too many distractions or problems on a page, which is confusing and overwhelming for the student with Down syndrome. Doing a workbook page also requires a level of independence that may not be possible for poor learners. Teachers stated that written performance in a workbook does not adequately reflect what the student with Down syndrome knows and can do. Computer-assisted instruction is ideal for students with Down syndrome because it is interactive, nonthreatening, and self-paced, and programs usually contain small, sequenced steps with lots of repetition and drill. However, caution should be taken to ensure that computers are only a medium of instruction and do not replace instructional teacher contact. The humanistic nature of teacher–student interaction is necessary for good social development (Hasselbring and Goin, 1989). Also, a few teachers reported that their included students with Down syndrome did not have adequate fine motor coordination to use a keyboard or mouse effectively.

Grading and Behavior Management Strategies

Teachers found that considering daily physical performance or participation in class and effort of the student was a much better indicator of learning or grades for the students with Down syndrome than tests or homework. This could be tied into the fact that many parents helped their child with homework, and this did not reflect independent work of the student with Down syndrome. However, teachers did feel that homework was very important for the students with Down syndrome because it helped to bridge the gap between home and school, reinforce concepts discussed in class, and inform the parents about what the child was learning. Threat of lower grades was not an effective motivator for students with Down syndrome to work harder and try their best. Teachers stated that they usually graded the students with Down syndrome against themselves rather than norms or the other students. Praise from the teacher was by far the most widely reported best practice for inclusion of students with Down syndrome. One teacher with six years of inclusion experience said that "my children with Down syndrome soak up praise—the more they get, the more they want and the harder they will work to get it."

Punishment and ignoring did not work effectively as behavioral and instructional strategies. It is possible that the students with Down syndrome did not understand what they were being punished for and it was not adequately explained, so the unwanted behavior continued. Ignoring was not an effective method for learning and changing behavior, possibly because poor learners generally need highlighted cues and more direct instruction to link concepts of cause and effect. They may not understand the relationships between behavioral causes and consequences unless these are explained. Teachers are generally better off calmly pointing out what behavior is or is not appropriate for the consequences. Following through on rules and contingencies is most important to facilitate learning. Emotional outbursts and punishments are also ineffective because these cause bad feelings for everyone (Westling, 1986).

Teachers reported that they want more 1:1 instructional time with the student with Down syndrome, and more planning time for instruction. This is especially important if the teacher collaboration (team teaching) paradigm is used in schools. Planning time must be built in for teachers to work together in a consistent fashion. Teachers also requested more information on the learning characteristics of children with Down syndrome. Teachers did not complain about extra work or added paperwork. They also stated that they did not want more input from parents, but this statistic could be misleading because most teachers said that they had already gotten a lot of information from the parents. In many cases teachers said that although they were not prepared by the school district for inclusion, parents prepared them informally, with written material and personal information on their children. In over a third of the cases, parents also came into the classroom prior to the onset of inclusion, to prepare the prospective classmates.

The overall sense of the results of this study is that inclusion of children with Down syndrome, as it exists now, is successful according to both parents and teachers, although there is always room for improvement. Parents mainly report benefits in areas of social interaction, friendships, communication, independence, and self-esteem. Teachers find the experience challenging, rewarding, and of great value to their regular education students as well as the child with Down syndrome. It was surprising that teacher preparation by the school district had no relationship to parent perception of success. Perhaps the type of training that was given was not relevant to teacher needs or requests. It was often difficult to pinpoint direct relationships mainly because of the overlap of factors such as involvement, cooperation, preparation, personality, attitude, and parent perception of success. It is also possible that results are skewed by respondents who chose to return their surveys.

RECOMMENDATIONS

These results encourage continuing to push for inclusion of students with Down syndrome. The benefits are many to both the students who are included, and to the regular education students as well. These results also have implications for teacher training for inclusion, especially in the areas of behavioral management, instructional strategies, and learning characteristics of students with Down syndrome. School districts are also encouraged to schedule more planning time between the teachers, therapists, parents and support personnel, in order to facilitate communication among staff, ensure educational collaboration, and provide a smooth process for initial placement. It is recommended that preparations for inclusion should begin early; usually one year before placement. Initial placement in this study has been shown to be very important to parent rating of successful inclusion experiences.

REFERENCES

Banerji M, Dailey R (1995): A study of the effects of an inclusion model on students with specific learning disabilities. J Learning Disabilities 28(8):511–522.

Chalfant JC, Pysh MV (1989): Teacher assistance teams: five descriptive studies of 96 teams. Remedial Special Educ 19(6):49–58.

Fuchs D, Fuchs LS, Bahr MW (1990): Mainstream assistance teams. A scientific basis for the art of consultation. Exceptional Children 57:128–129.

Hasselbring T, Goin L (1989): Use of computers. Best practices in mental retardation. Reston, VA: Council for Exceptional Children.

Kirk S, Gallagher J (1983): "Educating Exceptional Children," 4th ed. Boston: Houghton Mifflin.

Knackendoffel EA, et. al. (1992): "Collaborative Problem Solving." Lawrence, KS: Edge Enterprises.

Owens R (1981): "Organizational Behavior in Education." Englewood Cliffs, NJ: Prentice Hall.

Salisbury CL, et al. (1995): Strategies that promote social relations among elementary students with and without severe disabilities in inclusive schools. Exceptional Children 62(2):125–137.

Stainback S, Stainback W (1992): "Curricular Considerations in Inclusive Classroom: Facilitating Learning for all Students." Baltimore: Brookes Publishing.

Stogdill RM (1974): "Handbook of Leadership: A Survey of Theory and Research." New York: The Free Press.

Westling D (1986): "Introduction to Mental Retardation." Englewood Cliffs, NJ: Prentice Hall.

VIII. Transitions To Adulthood

Life Issues of Adolescence and Adults with Down Syndrome

Dennis E. McGuire and Brian A. Chicoine

Life issues is a term that can cover a broad range of ideas. Our focus is on medical and psychosocial health issues (Chicoine and McGuire, 1996). Health is more than freedom from disease. Health is a state of physical and mental well-being and includes such issues as health promotion, exercise, diet, and activities of daily life that promote a sense of well-being. In order to understand what makes sombody ill we need to understand what keeps people healthy. This is as true for people with Down syndrome as it is in the general population. At the turn of the century, life expectancy for a person with Down syndrome was about 9 years, and now it is about 56 years (Eyman et al., 1991). People with Down sydrome are obviously living longer and fuller lives, and there is a greater need to attend to their health issues. This chapter presents findings from a multidisciplinary center serving the health and psychosocial needs of close to 500 adolescents and adults with Down syndrome (see Chicoine et al., 1994, for more details on this center). Life issues discussed include the person's adaptive living skills, health promotion, and health screening issues.

PSYCHOSOCIAL ISSUES: ADAPTIVE LIVING SKILLS

Owing to the cognitive and expressive limitations of adults with Down syndrome (DS), the psychosocial issues that caregivers and professionals often emphasize are adaptive skills. Adaptive skills can be more narrowly defined as the degree of skill and independence one has in completing the activities of daily living (ADLs). To this we would add a number of skills and beliefs that we have found to play a critical role in adaption for persons with DS including expressive language, personal beliefs and attitudes, social and interpersonal skills, and creativity and flexibility in dealing with life changes.

Down Syndrome: A Promising Future, Together, Edited by Terry J. Hassold and David Patterson
ISBN 0-471-29686-4   Copyright © 1998 by Wiley-Liss, Inc.

ACTIVITIES OF DAILY LIVING (ADLS)

We use a standard measure of daily living skills, the Developmental Disability Profile, which is quick, easy to use, and has good reliability and validity (Brown et al., 1986). We look at daily living skills to assess three things: a person's most basic skills, independence issues, and functional changes and losses that occur as a result of normal aging or of mental health or health conditions.

Assessment of Basic Skills

We have found that most individuals are capable of routine grooming, hygiene, housekeeping, and food preparation tasks. Many are also capable of more moderately difficult tasks such as use of stove or microwave, laundry, choosing clothes appropriate to weather, and crossing the street with some guidance. Other tasks that need more hands-on assistance include the use of public transportation, shopping and meal planning, free movement about the community, and money management.

Assessment of Independence

Working with more than 500 individuals with DS enabled us to determine which skills people should be able to complete independently. If a person is capable and yet not doing tasks, this may indicate a lack of challenge or overprotection by caregivers. We have identified a number of situations where caregivers were extremely overprotective, resulting in some serious problems. People have a basic drive to be independent. If this drive is stifled, the resulting frustration may lead to depression or behavior problems.

More often, however, we have found a more benign type of overprotectiveness. For example, caregivers often do such tasks as the laundry or meal preparation, which most individuals with DS are capable of doing with some initial guidance. In fairness to caregivers, there is a balance between the needs of the household and the needs of the person with DS. For example, when both parents work, some key tasks such as food preparation may need to be completed efficiently, and adults with DS are not always fast or efficient. Whenever possible, however, people with DS should be allowed to perform their own daily living tasks, particularly those tasks that require the development of new skills and trial and error approaches to task completion. The more experience people with DS have in completing new and challenging tasks, the more experience and confidence they will have in dealing with new and challenging situations in the community (such as the difficult transition from school to the world of work).

On the other hand, we have found instances where people were given too much independence, resulting in safety and health risks as well as a loss of self-esteem. For example, one older woman in an agency-run apartment was unable to manage. Her apartment was a shambles, with spoiling food, unpaid bills, and soiled laundry scattered everywhere. She was also frequenting a local tavern, which was creating an alcohol addiction and extreme safety risk. She was moved into a small group home with on-site supervision, and the problems were resolved. She was pleased to make this change because it allowed her to regain her sense of competence and self-esteem. Other individuals have had problems controlling food intake, which has resulted in significant weight gains affecting their health. Again, in these situations supervision was helpful in resolving the problem. People should be allowed challenge and independence in their lives, but not at the risk of their own health and safety.

Assessment of Skill Loss as an Indication of Normal Aging, as well as Mental Health, Sensory, and Health Conditions

For persons with DS who have expressive language limitations, a loss of daily living skills is a very telling indicator of problems, life issues or concerns. Skill losses may occur as a result of normal aging, mental health conditions, sensory problems, or medical conditions.

Many years of gathering information on daily living skills enabled us to track changes due to the normal aging process and to inform persons with DS and caregivers of these changes better. This is important because adults with DS age prematurely, approximately 10 to 20 years earlier than the general population. Thus a person with DS in his late 40s or 50s may be more like a person in the general population in his 60s or 70s. Caregivers of older adults may experience this process as a shortened middle age, or as a rapid onset of aging. Many caregivers are struck by the seemingly rapid change from a youthful and active lifestyle to the more sedentary lifestyle of an older person.

Despite this early aging, we inform caregivers that individuals who live in community settings and stay active are more likely to maintain their skills and moderate the aging process. Even when the premature aging process results in a lack of interest or retirement from formal work pursuits, a high level of social or recreational activities should be maintained. Similarly to retirees in the general population, older adults with DS who remain active are more likely to live longer and healthier lives.

Caregivers' knowledge of the premature aging process may prevent a cutoff of services from agencies that are unfamiliar with this occurrence. Uninformed staff who misinterpret slowdowns in work or other activities as symptoms of Alzheimer dementia or oppositional behavior may move to discharge the individual from their programs. These staff need to be encouraged to design new programs and services that meet the needs of "prematurely" older adults with DS.

Aside from a loss of skills due to aging, we have found that a significant loss in daily living skills may also be a symptom of a mental health disorder such as depression, or of a medical condition such as hypothyroidism or Alzheimer dementia. Skill loss may also be a symptom of a visual or hearing loss, which occurs more frequently in adults with DS than the general population (Evenhuis, 1990). Because of a tendency to association of Alzheimer disease with DS in previous research, a loss of skills may be misdiagnosed as Alzhiemer dementia (AD), which is untreatable and irreversible (Dalton and Crapper-McLauchlan, 1984; Lai and Williams, 1984; Oliver, 1986). More recent research has found that AD occurs earlier in adults with DS, possibly due to premature aging in this population, but it is not clear whether this disorder occurs at a greater rate then in the general population (Devenny et al., 1996; Wisnewski and Rabe, 1996).

In our own clinical sample of 447 people, 123 individuals (30%) showed a loss of skills. Of the 123 with skill loss only 11 individuals (9%) were diagnosed with AD.

For the age group over the age of 40 who were most at risk for AD, 11 of 53 with skill loss were diagnosed with AD, accounting for only 21% of this older age group. The remaining 42 individuals with skill loss who were over 40 showed a positive response to medical and mental health treatments or to remedial treatments for sensory impairments. For caregivers, the implications of these more recent findings are obvious: You need not assume or accept a diagnosis of AD, paticularly if a rigorous attempt to rule out other causes of the skill loss has not been made.

EXPRESSIVE LANGUAGE

Expressive language is a critical factor in adults with DS because of limitations in this area. There are three key issues related to expressive language: intelligibility, the expression of thoughts and feelings, and self-talk.

Intelligibility is the degree to which spoken language is understood by others. Although we have found a wide range of intelligibility, from nonverbal to very verbal, most adults with DS fall in the middle and have difficulty being understood by anyone other than caregivers. This lack of intelligibility often results in a dependence on caregivers who are most able to understand the person's wants and needs. Problems may develop with the absence of this interpreter. Many are lost and disoriented by these individuals' absence and may be more succeptible to depression and adjustment reactions. Some of the most difficult losses reported include the loss of a supervisor on the job, a parent due to death or impairment, a sibling who moves out of the family home, or a group home staff person. To lessen the effect of these changes, we have found that people with a wider network of family and friends have less difficulty with the loss of one member. Learning sign language or other means of communicating with a wider network of people may also be helpful to prevent too great a dependence on a small number of caregives.

The expression of thoughts and feelings is also difficult for many adults with DS, even if there is intelligible spoken language. We have found that relatively few are able to express personal thoughts and feelings verbally. Many are able to show strong emotions (disappointments, frustrations, anger, unhappiness) through face and body gestures. But it is not always possible for caregivers to interpret the source or meaning of these expressive behaviors, particularly when these issues occur in other settings such as a work site. We have found that this inability to express feelings verbally may increase the likelihood and duration of such problems as depression. To lessen the effects of this expressive limitation, caregivers may teach staff in work or residential settings how to interpret the individual's expressive face and body gestures better. The more people in various settings who are able to understand and respond to the expressed needs of the adult with DS, the more adaptive and competent this person will feel. Also, the more responsive caregivers there are, the less effect the loss of one will have on the person with DS. As an additional recommendation, involved family members should participate in work or residential staffings to ensure the most accurate interpretation of the adult with DS's expressed needs.

Self-talk is a conversation with one's self that is expressed out loud. We have found that at least 82.5% of the people seen at the center talk out loud to themselves. For example, families commonly report people talking in their rooms or bathroom about events of the day, much as we would review our daily activities through an internal conversation. As a humorous example, one parent's response to his son's particularly loud self-talk conversation in his bedroom was to knock on the door and ask, "WHO are you talking to in there?" Her son's immediate response was to yell back, "MY-SELF . . . who do you think?"

We believe that self-talk is developmentally appropriate given the cognitive level of most adults with Down syndrome. Younger children in the general population regularly talk out loud to themselves, especially when engaged in a task (Berk, 1994; Diaz and Berk, 1992). Self-talk is usually internalized between the ages of 5 and 7 in the general population. For adults with Down syndrome, self-talk continues through adulthood and serves a number of adaptive purposes. It helps one to plan and practice alternatives of action, review daily thoughts and actions, entertain oneself when alone, and vent feelings and frustrations that are not easily expressed to others.

Self-talk may also be a symptom of a more serious problem such as depression or anxiety. In these instances, caregivers report a dramatic change in the quality and quantity of the self-talk. These changes often include an increase in animation and angry content, hallucinatory-like conversations with imagined others, self-absorption, and an increase in self-talk in public places. Presented in this way, self-talk can look very odd and even "psychotic-like." Even so, we have found antidepressants to be very effective in the treatment of this and other accompanying symptoms of anxiety or depression. It has also been noted that the oddness of these behaviors may lead to a misinterpretation as psychosis (McGuire and Chicoine, 1995; Sovner, 1986). This, in turn, may increase the use of antipsychotic medications, which have a greater risk of severe side effects compared to antidepressants (Sovner and Des Noyers, 1995). If the need arises for treatment, caregivers and mental health practitioners should be informed and alerted to these issues so as to avoid the unnecessary use of antipsychotic medications.

BELIEFS

Clinical researchers have identified two key areas of beliefs that affect adaptiveness: one's view of self, or self-esteem, and one's sense of competence in dealing with the world (Bandura, 1971; Beck, 1976). Compared to the general population, adults with DS have a disadvantage in acquiring positive beliefs in these two areas. Persons with DS are minority members who are defined and treated differently by others, and this may have a profound effect on their self-esteem (Reiss et al., 1982). They also have far fewer occupational opportunities and far less independence and control in their lives, which affects their sense of competence (Weyman et al., 1988). As a result of these differences, we have identified three unique areas of beliefs for adults with DS: stigmatization, acceptance of disability, and demoralization.

Stigmatization

Owing to identifiable physical features and cognitive limitations, persons with DS are often defined and treated differently by others in society (Gibbons, 1985; Reiss et al., 1982). For younger children these differences may not be as readily apparent. A younger child with DS may play with neighborhood children and attend the same schools and even be in the same classrooms. As persons with DS reach adolescence there is often a growing awareness of the stigmatization in their lives, especially when comparing themselves to siblings who leave home to attend college or establish their own careers. For example, one young woman was cross, moody, and withdrawn for a long time after her younger sister's wedding. In time she was able to explain to her sister that she was upset because she would probably never marry, live independently, or have an "important job" like her sister. For many others, the ability to identify and discuss these issues is more limited and the resulting feelings of demoralization and frustration may result in anger or depressive resignation and withdrawal. Although some reaction to these stigmatizing realities is inevitable, we have found that individuals who have more choice and opportunity in work, social, or recreational spheres are less likely to be affected by limitations and stigma in their lives.

Acceptance of Disability

Just as in the general population, we have found that most people with DS deal with identity issues (who am I, what am I) at some point in their adulthood. We have found that many people have not had an opportunity to discuss a basic identity issue: the fact that they have Down syndrome. We believe that people are aware that they are treated differently by others. Discussing this issue at an appropriate time may minimize self-blame for the reaction of others, such as when people stare in public. More importantly, people with a better understanding and acceptance of disability are often happier and more likely to use and develop their own resources and skills, and to advocate for their own rights and needs more effectively.

A similar issue of acceptance is the attitude of the person with DS toward peers with disabilities. There are some individuals who have an aversion to socializing with persons with disabilities. This aversion is a major problem because it cuts one off from the key pool of possible friends. People tend to associate with individuals at our same cognitive level. Thus individuals who refuse to associate with other persons with disabilities are often caught between two worlds. They are not fully accepted by the general population, and they voluntarily cut themselves off from people with disabilities. For some, this aversion is relatively short-lived. For others, it is more serious. This issue seems to be more common for "higher functioning individuals," who may be more sensitive to the stigmatizing realities of their lives. Assuming that a negative view of self is at the core of this attitude, we have found that individuals who are given an opportunity to become leaders or helpers with their peers are often able to aquire a more positive view of self and others.

Demoralization in the Workplace

Studies have found a profound sense of frustration and demoralization by many persons with disabilities in the workplace (Zetlin and Turner, 1985; Weyman et al., 1988). These studies indicate that many people fall far short of meeting life goals. We have found evidence of demoralization in our clinical sample, and we have found demoralization to be a factor for many individuals who have been diagnosed with depression.

There are studies that suggest ways to decrease demoralization in the workplace (Weyman et al., 1988). Research has shown that individuals with experiences in community jobs prior to graduation from school are more likely to obtain and keep community jobs (Hasazi et al., 1985). Equally important, success and competence on the job may not depend on paid employment. Volunteer positions bring meaning and purpose to many people's lives.

Similarly, jobs need not meet family expectations to be satisfying. Many people are demoralized by jobs that are not of their own choosing. For example, family members may push for a community job whereas the person with DS may wish to be with his friends in a workshop program. Often in these situations the person with DS cannot express his or her own wishes, and may behave in ways to sabotage the job. As examples, one young man working in a grocery store tossed carts into the road; a second individual simply sat down on the job to communicate his dislike for his position. Caregivers should not impose their own wishes and needs onto the person with DS. Whenever possible, people should be given several choices among work sites. Persons with DS are less likely to be demoralized if given a choice among even a limited number of options. Adaptation to the workplace may also increase if one has had opportunities throughout their lives to complete their own daily living tasks.

SOCIAL AND INTERPERSONAL SKILLS

A large body of research exists showing the importance of social and interpersonal skills for adaptiveness and well-being (Greenspan and Grandfield, 1992). A lack of social skills is associated with maladjustment and mental health problems, and a strong association has been shown between poor social skills and depression (Reiss and Benson, 1985). A lack of social skills is also a key factor in job failure (Greenspan and Shoultz, 1981; Martin et al., 1986).

We have found relatively few instances of rude or offensive social behavior. There have been more occasions of inappropriate affection, primarily involving hugging others when it was not appropriate. For most people, this inappropriate hugging is easily corrected by some training and experience.

We have found more severe limitations in terms of social interactional skills. Relatively few individuals with DS exhibit such interactional skills as initiating and maintaining conversations, or the ability to show interest and take another person's perspective in social situations (Greenspan and Grandfield, 1992). Because of these limitations, some authors have questioned the quality of friendships for persons with cognitive disabilities (Clegg and Standen, 1991). Despite this lack of interactional skills, caregivers report that relationships with peers are generally strong, long-standing, and critically important. They say that these friendships develop over much time and familiarity, such as when people are in the same job site or school program for many years. The value of time and familiarity for peer relationships has been shown even for people who are profoundly retarded and may have been thought to have little or no relationships with others. For example, Heller (1982) looked at people who were moved when a large residential facility was closed. She found that people who transferred with those from their original units were far more likely to survive the move than people who were put with new residents.

Because time and familiarity are so important in the development of friendships, life changes that separate friends may be devastating. A move into a new home or school may eliminate friendships cultivated over many years. Starting over with new people may be overwhelming when expressive and social skills are limited. We have found these types of losses to be associated with depression and adjustment reactions. These types of friendship losses may be minimized if people have more outlets than just school or work for connecting to prospective friends. Special recreation and park district programs, church groups, and community college programs are all possible sites for meeting people, especially if they are continuous and allow contact with a regular group of participants over time.

Social skills problems may also exist at the work site. Most problems on the job result from a lack of social skill training and feedback. For example, many job coaches have little ability or interest in dealing with social skill issues, which is the most common reason for job failure (Greenspan and Shoultz, 1981). Coaches are in place to teach the job, but are often unable or unwilling to teach job etiquette skills that allow people to keep their jobs. Examples of behaviors that should be addressed by a job coach include restricting self-talk to home environments, showering and dressing appropriately, and learning when and how to address fellow employees and the supervisor.

MENTAL AND BEHAVIORAL FLEXIBILITY

For many adults with DS, life changes are difficult because of the need for a routine schedule and pattern of behavior. In the general population, this type of repetitious behavior is regarded as an obsessive–compulsive tendency. Given that this is a personality trait for many with DS, the key is to have the obsessive–compulsive tendency work for the person's benefit. Many adults with DS do well when tasks are clearly laid out and schedules are fairly routine. Problems arise when changes in schedule and routine occur, especially major changes such as leaving school, entering a group home, or unexpected changes such as an illness or death in the family. Although many will adapt if given time and preparation, some individuals have more difficulty with changes, and an obsessive–compulsive disorder results (Vitello et al., 1989). These symptoms often manifest as extremely repetitive behaviors, slowdown in behavior, or an over-reliance on a set pattern of behavior (McGuire and Chicoine, 1995). An obsessive–compulsive tendency may not be eliminated. However, the possibility that the tendency will become a disorder can be reduced by giving people opportunities to learn and gain mastery over day-to-day challenges. Under these circumstances people may be less likely to be overwhelmed by larger life changes.

SUMMARY OF PSYCHOSOCIAL LIFE ISSUES

The psychosocial life issues emphasized in this chapter include the following adaptive living skills: activities of daily living, expressive language, personal beliefs and attitudes, social and interpersonal skills, and creativity and flexibility in dealing with life changes. There are a variety of means for supporting psychosocial health and well-being. Opportunities for completing one's daily living skills and exposure to a wide variety of job tasks will promote competence, self-esteem, and flexibility in dealing with life changes and challenges. Success with job and self-care activities will also lead to a decrease in stigma and an increase in acceptance of self and one's disability. The encouragement of various verbal and nonverbal means for expressing feelings will increase adaptiveness. Exposure to a number of social and recreational settings over an extended period of time will increase opportunities for making and maintaining friendships.

The development of a wide network of caregivers as opposed to just one is recommended as a source of support. This will also minimize the effect of one caregiver's loss or absence. Caregivers should be aware that loss of skill is not necessarily a symptom of Alzhiemer dementia, even among older individuals. In most cases, skill loss is far more likely to be the result of premature aging, sensory loss of hearing or vision, medical issues such as hypothyroidism, or mental health issues such as depression.

HEALTH PROMOTION

Health promotion involves activities both inside and outside the physician's office, including nutrition and exercise.

NUTRITION

Although coronary artery disease (heart attacks) and hypertension (high blood pressure) are less common in adults with DS (Brattstrom et al., 1987), the dietary and exercise recommendations for people with DS are similar to those for the general population. These include following a diet based on the the "pyramid" program, which recommends limiting fat intake and encourages a diet high in complex carbohydrates.

Obesity is more common in persons with Down syndrome. A recent study found that children with DS have a basal metabolic rate that is lower than that seen in the general population (Luke et al., 1994). On average, those with Down syndrome burned 200–300 fewer calories per day while at rest. Reduction in calories alone led to nutritional deficiencies; therefore, it is necessary for people with DS to burn 200–300 calories more per day through physical activity to prevent weight gain. When making dietary recommendations to prevent weight gain or promote weight loss, offer low-fat snack choices such as fresh fruit, vegetables, popcorn, or pretzels rather than prohibiting desserts or snacks. Just as in the general population, better long-term success is achieved by following good general nutrition principles and regularly exercising than by dieting.

EXERCISE

Twenty to thirty minutes of aerobic exercise at least three days a week is recommended. Aerobic exercise includes such activities as walking, running, swimming, biking, and cross country skiing. Prior to starting an exercise program, a physical exam and health screening are needed. Forty to fifty percent of babies born with DS have congenital heart disease (Greenwood and Nadas, 1976). Some adults with DS have had these surgically corrected and only need antibiotics when they visit the dentist (see below). Others have not had the heart condition corrected, and many need ongoing treatment. Sylvester (1974) found that some adults with DS develop disease of their heart valves later in life. Exercise restriction may be necessary depending on the type of congenital or acquired problem. Physical examination and an echocardiogram and/or stress test (treadmill test) may be necessary to determine the safety of exercise.

Another health problem that may make modification in exercise necessary is atlantoaxial instability. This condition, in which the first vertebra (bone) in the neck slips on the second, is more common in persons with DS (Pueschel and Scola, 1987). The exact significance is not always clear but it may make contact sports or sports which could jar the neck more dangerous. For this reason, the Special Olympics requires lateral neck X-rays prior to participation. The need for these X-rays, however, is the subject of ongoing research and debate.

Exercise is believed to have many benefits. Although reduction in coronary artery disease and hypertension would not appear to be major benefits in adults with DS (because of the infrequent occurrence of these diseases), exercise probably has several other benefits. Although this topic has not been studied as much in persons with DS, in the general population exercise helps improve the overall sense of well-being, self-esteem, and fitness of those who regularly participate (Simon, 1985). It is an excellent mechanism to help people deal with stress and reduce its effects.

IMMUNIZATIONS

In addition to the preventive measures discussed as part of a healthy life-style, there are several other recommendations to promote health. Immunizations are recommended for all adults. After the usual immunizations of childhood, a diphtheria-tetanus booster is recommended every 10 years. For persons older than 65 and for persons with certain chronic illnesses, an annual influenza (flu) shot is recommended as well as a one-time pneumonia vaccine (some pulmonary and infectious disease specialists are now recommending the pneumonia vaccine every 7 years for those in the high-risk categories). Some investigators have recommended that adults with DS should receive the flu and pneumonia vaccines in their fifties instead of waiting until 65 because of their relatively weaker ability to fight infections. Down syndrome by itself is not one of the conditions that requires a child or younger adult to receive these immunizations; however, those with associated health problems such as congenital heart disease or recurrent pneumonia should receive them. In addition, flu vaccine is recommended annually for people living in residential facilities.

The hepatitis B immunization is recommended for residents of residential facilities. Some studies have found that adults with DS are at greater risk for getting hepatitis B, possibly in workshops or other settings. Although hepatitis B transmission generally occurs through blood (blood transfusions, shared needles) and sexual activity, the hepatitis B virus is actually shed in all body secretions. Thus in any setting where regular contact with an infected person's secretions occurs, or where hygiene may be limited, hepatitis B can be transmitted. The hepatitis B immunization is given in a three-shot series. The second and third doses are given 1 and 6 months after the first. A blood test (hepatitis B surface antibody) should be drawn 1–2 months after the third dose to confirm the effectiveness of the vaccine in providing immunity.

ANTIBIOTIC PROPHYLAXIS

Another preventive measure is antibiotic prophylaxis. Some people with congenital or acquired heart disease need antibiotics to prevent an infection in their heart, before and after going to the dentist (even for a routine cleaning), or when they undergo procedures to their gastrointestinal or urinary tracts. This is usually done with amoxicillin 500-mg tablets: 4 tablets 1 hour before the procedure. For those allergic to amoxicillin (or other penicillins), alternative regimens are recommended.

HEALTH SCREENING

An annual health maintenance evaluation, including a review of the patient's history and a physical exam, will help find problems early in their course and provide an opportunity to review the issues of a healthy life-style. Routine health screening that is recommended for the general population is recommended for adults with DS as well. This includes mammograms, pap smears, screening for colo-rectal cancer, and cholesterol screening. With further study, these recommendations could change depending on the frequency of these diseases in persons with DS.

The history and physical exam should give special attention to problems areas that are more common or present differently in adults with DS than in the general population. The Down Syndrome Medical Check List (Cohen, 1996) recommends a physical exam and thyroid blood tests annually. We recommend lateral neck X-rays in the neutral, flexion, and extension positions, once in the asymptomatic adult, to screen for atlantoaxial instability. If symptoms arise or the screening X-rays are abnormal, then further studies may be indicated. We recommend hearing and vision screening every 1 to 2 years.

THYROID

Hypothyroidism is more common in people with DS (Pueschel and Pezzullo, 1985). Approximately one-third of the people we have seen have hypothyroidism. Symptoms include mental slowness, dry skin, obesity, constipation, and others. Because so many of the symptoms are seen in persons with DS who don't have hypothyroidism, it is very difficult to diagnose from the history and the physical exam.

EYES

Poor visual acuity (eyesight) is a common problem just as it is in the general population. However, the adult with DS may have a difficult time perceiving the problem or communicating it to someone who can help. If work skills or other daily skills deteriorate, the cause could be as simple as a decline in eyesight.

HEARING/EARS

Hearing loss is also more common in adults with DS (Evenhuis et al., 1992). It can be from reversible causes such as ear wax or fluid behind the drum, or it can be permanent and associated with inner ear problems. A person who seems to be losing daily life skills may have a problem with decreased hearing from wax obstruction.

GYNECOLOGIC

General gynecologic care includes daily care issues and evaluation in the physician's office. Education is important for self-care and in preparing the woman for the office evaluation. In the office a slow, gentle approach is often all that is needed although sometimes light sedation is necessary. Modified exams can be done to get a Pap smear and sometimes an ultrasound of the pelvis can be done to provide some information that is not obtained in the exam.

ORTHOPEDIC

In addition to atlantoaxial instability being an issue in exercise (as previously discussed), it must also be considered as part of evaluation prior to any surgery. Some persons with DS who have atlantoaxial instability have received severe neck injuries during surgery when their necks were extended to allow for placing the endotracheal (breathing) tube. The anesthesiologist must make adjustments to prevent this. Even with normal X-rays, special care should be given to the neck of a person with DS during anesthesia.

CHOLESTEROL

The rate of hypercholesterolemia, elevated cholesterol levels in the blood, seems to be similar to that seen in the general population. However, the incidence of coronary artery disease (heart attacks, plaques in the arteries) seems to be uncommon in people with DS. Therefore, if we find someone with high cholesterol we recommend dietary changes but have less tendency to use cholesterol-lowering drugs because the side effects of the medications may actually cause more problems.

HEALTH PROBLEMS WITH A LOWER INCIDENCE

In addition to the lower incidence of coronary artery disease, in adults with DS, there is a lower incidence of hypertension. We have also found a lower incidence of asthma and suicide gestures (despite a similar rate of depression). We have also found that most of our adult patients have fewer problems with constipation and ear infections than children with DS.

HEALTH PROMOTION SUMMARY AND RECOMMENDATIONS

There are a variety of means for supporting health and well being for adults with DS. Dietary and exercise recommendations are similar to those for the general population. These include following a diet with limited fat intake and a diet high in complex carbohydrates. Regular exercise is also recommended, especially because persons with DS tend to burn less calories per day. In addition to the preventive measures discussed as part of a healthy life-style, there are several other recommendations to promote health. Immunizations are recommended for all adults with DS. A diphtheria-tetanus booster is recommended every ten years. For older persons and for persons with certain chronic illnesses, an annual influenza (flu) shot is recommended as well as a one time pneumonia vaccine immunization. In addition, flu vaccine is recommended annually for people living in residential facilities. Immunization for hepatitis B is also strongly recommended for individuals who attend either workshop programs or who live in residential facilities. The use of an antibiotic to prevent infection is also recommended for people with congenital or acquired heart disease before and after going to the dentist or when they undergo procedures to their gastrointestinal or urinary tracts.

As in the general population an annual health maintenance evaluation including a review of the patient's history and a physical exam is recommended. There are several health problems more common in persons with DS that merit special attention including hypothyroidism, hearing, and visual problems and atlantoaxial instability problems

SUMMARY

Our focus has been on a broad range of medical and psychosocial health issues identified during the course of a multidicliplinary clinic serving the needs of more than 500 adults with DS. We hope this accumulated knowledge will be of use to caregivers and professionals in other settings who endeavor to serve the needs of this population.

ACKNOWLEDGMENTS

Work for this chapter was partially funded by the Research and Training Center on Aging with Mental Retardation, Institute on Disability and Human Development, the University of Illinois at Chicago. Funded by the U.S. Department of Education, National Institute on Disability and Rehabilitation Research, Grant No. H133b30069.

REFERENCES

Bandura A (1971): "Social Learning Theory." New York: General Learning Press.

Beck AT (1976): "Cognitive Therapy and Emotional Disorders." New York: International Universities Press.

Berk LE (1994): Why children talk to themselves. Sci Am 271:78–83.

Brattstrom L, England E, Bun A (1987): Does Down syndrome support homocysteine theory of arthersosclerosis? Lancet I:391–397.

Brown MC, Hanley, AT, Nemeth C, Epple W, Bird D, Bontempo T (1986): The developmental disability profile. New York State Office of Mental Retardation and Developmental Disabilities.

Chicoine B, McGuire D (1996): Promoting health in adults with Down syndrome. Document available through the Clearinghouse on Aging and Developmental Disabilites of the RT C on Aging in Persons with Mental Retardation, The Institute on Disability and Human Development, the University of Illinois at Chicago.

Chicoine B, McGuire D, Hebein S, Gilly, D (1995): The development of a clinic for adults with Down syndrome. Ment Retard 32:100–106.

Clegg JA, Standen PJ (1991): Friendships among adults who have developmental disabilities. Am J Ment Retard 95:663–672.

Cohen WI (ed.) (1996): Health care guidelines for individuals with Down syndrome (Down Syndrome Preventive Medical Check List). Down Syndrome Quart 1:1–10.

Dalton, AJ, Crapper-McLachlan DR (1984): Clinical expression of Alzheimer's disease in Down's syndrome. Psychol Clin North Am 9:659–670

Dalton AJ, Seltzer GB, Adlin MS, Wisniewski HM (1994): Association between Alzheimer disease and Down syndrome: clinical observations. In Berg JM, Holland AJ, Karlinsky J. (eds.): "Alzheimer Disease and Down Syndrome." London: Oxford University, pp. 1–24.

Devenny DA, Silverman WP, Hill AL, Jenkins E, Sersen EA, Wisnewshi KE (1996): Normal aging in adults with Down's syndrome: a longitudinal study. J Intellect Dis Res 40:208–221.

Diaz R, Berk LE (1992): "Private Speech from Social Interaction to Self Regulation." Lawrence Erlbaum Associates.

Eyman R, Call T, White J (1991): Life expectancy of persons with Down syndrome. Am J Ment Retard 95:603–612.

Evenhuis HM (1990): The natural history of dementia in Down syndrome. Arch Neurol 47:263–267.

Evenhuis HM, Van Zanten GA, Brocaar MP, Roerdinkholder WHM (1992): Hearing loss in middle-age persons with Down syndrome. Am J Ment Retard 97:47–56.

Gibbons FX (1985): Stigma perception: social comparisons among mentally retarded persons. Am J Ment Defic 90:98–106.

Greenspan S, Grandfield JM (1992): Reconsidering the construct of mental retardation: implications of a model of social competence. Am J Ment Retard 96:442–453.

Greenspan S, Shoultz J (1981): Why mentally retarded adults lose their jobs. Social competence as a factor in work adjustment. Appl Res Ment Retard 2:23–38.

Greenwood RD, Nadas AD (1976): The clinical cause of cardiac disease in Down's syndrome. Pediatrics 58:278–281.

Hasazi SB, Gordon LR, Roe CA, Finck K, Hull M, Salembier G (1985): A statewide follow-up on post high school employment and residential status of students labesed "mentally retarded." Educ Training Ment Retard 14:222–234.

Heller T (1982): Social disruption and residential relocation of mentally retarded children. Am J Ment Defic 87:48–55.

Lai F, Williams RS (1989): A prospective study of Alzheimer disease in Down sundrome individuals. Arch Neurol 46:377–385.

Luke A, Rozien NJ, Sutton M, Schoeller DA (1994): Energy expenditure in children with Down syndrome: correcting metabolic rate for movement. J Pediatr 125:829–838.

Martin JE, Rusch FR, Lagomarcino T, Chadsey-Rusch JR (1986): Comparisions between workers who are nonhandicapped and mentally retarded: why they lose their jobs. Appl Res Ment Retard 7:476–474.

McGuire, D., & Chicoine, B. (1996): Depressive disorders in adults with Down Syndrome. Hab Ment Healthcare Newsl 1:1–7.

Oliver C, Holland AJ (1986): Down syndrome and Alzheimer's disease: a review. Psychol Med 16:307–322.

Pueschel SM, Pezzullo JC (1985): Thyroid dysfunction in Down syndrome. Am J Disease Child 139:636–639.

Pueschel SM, Scola FH (1987): Atlantoaxial instability in individuals with Down syndrome: epidemiologic, radiographic, and clinical studies. Pediatrics 80:555–560.

Reiss S, Benson B (1985): Psychosocial correlates of depression. Am J Ment Defic 89:331–337.

Reiss S, Levitan G, McNally R (1982): Emotionally disturbed mentally retarded people. Am Psychol 37:361–367.

Simon H (1985): Sports medicine. Sci Am, Feb:2–28.

Sovner RS (1986): Limiting factors in the use of DSM-III criteria with mentally ill/mentally retarded persons. Psychopharm Bull 22:1055–1059.

Sovner RS, DesNoyers HA (1993) Commentary: psychotoform psychopathology. Hab Ment Healthcare Newsl 3:126–112.

Sylvester PE (1974). Aortic and pulmonary valve fenestrations as ageing indices in Down's syndrome. J Ment Defic Res 18:367–375.

Vitello B, Spreat S, Behar D (1989) Obsessive-compulsive disorder in mentally retarded adults. J Nerv Ment Dis 177:232–234.

Weyman P, Moon SM, Everson JM, Wood W, Barcus JM (1988): "Transition from School to Work: New Challenges for Youth with Severe Disabilities." Baltimore: Paul Brookes Publishing.

Wisniewski HM, Rabe A (1986). Discrepancy between Alzheimer-type neuropathology and dementia in people with Down syndrome. Ann New York Acad Sci 47:247–259.

Zetlin A, Turner J (1985): Transition from adolescents to adulthood: perspectives of mentally retarded individuals and their families. Am J Ment Defic 89:570–579.

Where Do People Want To Live? Can They Make It Work?: How People with Down Syndrome and Their Families Can Improve Both Housing Options and Housing Choice

Kathleen H. McGinley

Where did you want to live when you reached adulthood? Maybe somewhere near your family or your friends, near your job or near where you were going to school, near a bus or a train route if you didn't have a car, near places to have fun, shop, worship, and just hang out. Then again, maybe you didn't want to live anywhere near your family—maybe you wanted to make a clean break and be on your own. The point is, you had your own opinion and you wanted to make your own choices.

It's likely that you found out—just as most of us do, unless we are independently wealthy—that there are some things that limit your choices. What if you can't afford your own place? What if you find out that if you are going to be able to pay the rent, you have to have a roommate? What if you find out that if you live near your job because you don't have a car, that you aren't close to places to eat, or shop, or go to the movies and you have to depend on someone for a ride? What if you really want to buy that little apartment in midtown? However, you don't have the money for a down payment and with your salary you can't meet the mortgage payments so you have to rent until you save more money or until you get a better job with better pay? Usually when we face these kinds of issues and choices, no matter how angry and frustrated reality may make us initially, we usually realize that we are not the Lone Ranger. We can look around and see that most people we know are in the same boat. So we try to stick it out and follow our best instincts.

However, what if no one lets you make your own choices? What if your family or your friends or people and organizations that are supposed to be "supporting" you

Down Syndrome: A Promising Future, Together, Edited by Terry J. Hassold and David Patterson
ISBN 0-471-29686-4 Copyright © 1998 by Wiley-Liss, Inc.

decide that you can't really make these decisions? What if—instead of trying to help you figure things out—they just go ahead and decide for you because they think they know what is right? In doing this, they may not only make things more frustrating for you, they may also end up going to one of two extremes.

You can end up being either overprotected or pushed into something that you don't want, simply because someone else thinks that is what you should want. Most of us eventually would rebel against these types of shackles. Maybe openly, maybe in some subtle form depending on the power relationship. What we all would be is frustrated because what everyone wants is some type of control over their own life.

Consider the following two true examples. In the first case, the individual was supported and helped to achieve his goal. In the second case, the individual's fate was decided by others. The first is an example of the creative use of housing options and funding sources to ensure that the housing meets the individual's needs and desires. The second is an example of a continued reliance on existing, limited housing options that demand that the person fit the housing—not that the housing fit the person.

- Mr. A. was one of the last individuals to leave an institution in his home state. Advocates wanted to help him buy his own home in the community. Mr. A. had strong opinions of his own. He did not want to leave where he was living and move into the community unless he could live in the house in which he grew up. His mother had moved to a continuing care facility a few years before and the family home, which had been sold once, was back on the market. Mr. A. now owns that home. He bought it with help from a first-time home buyer program. He has several live-in support staff who pay him rent and he is living a full and happy life in a neighborhood with which he had ties.
- Mr. B. lived at home with his parents. Eventually, both parents died and he lived in the family home with his dog. It was determined that the house was in bad shape and that he really shouldn't continue to live there, that he should move into a group home. However, he did not want to do that. One major reason was that he couldn't take his dog. Mr. B was allowed to go with his dog when it was taken to the animal shelter to see that it would not be put to sleep. He is now living in a large, congregate setting. Mr. B's behavior deteriorated—is it any wonder?—so he was placed on medication.

What if a real choice can't be made by anyone because there is nothing to choose from? We all write about and discuss the importance of having control and choice rest with the individual. This is a philosophical underpinning, the importance of which cannot be underestimated. However, too often we ignore the issue of how we can ensure the availability of appropriate options; these options are what "operationalize" true choice making.

PEOPLE WITH DISABILITIES FACE A HOUSING CRISIS

Independence, integration, and productivity are among the most important values and goals shared by people with disabilities, their families, advocates, and service providers. Local, state, and federal housing policies that affect the lives of people with disabilities must therefore reflect these values and be designed to achieve these goals. The shortage of available, affordable, and accessible housing is an increasingly serious problem for people with Down syndrome and other disabilities. This housing shortage has limited people's abilities to have independent and integrated lives in the community, as well as productive employment and full integration into society. Access to decent, safe, affordable housing in the community can be the true cornerstone to independence for people with disabilities.

In virtually every part of the United States, people with Down syndrome and other disabilities face an extreme crisis in the availability of affordable housing that meets their needs and desires. Far too many people with disabilities live in substandard housing or pay 50–75% or more of their limited incomes for rent. Many others live at home with aging parents or are forced to choose between restrictive congregate settings and homelessness. Still others remain in inappropriate institutional settings because there is no affordable housing available in the community. Nationwide, state-based disability-specific waiting lists for so-called "residential services" (housing) in the community are overflowing. Table 1, based on information provided by the National Low Income Housing Coalition in its 1996 report, *Out of Reach: Can America Pay the Rent?,* clearly demonstrates the challenge faced by people with disabilities.

Like all individuals, people with disabilities have a need for decent, safe, affordable, and appropriate housing. Like all individuals, people with disabilities vary in their abilities, interests, desires, and needs over the span of their lifetime. For many people with disabilities, affordable housing simply means access to generic housing or rental assistance within the community. For some other people with disabilities, the need for affordable housing linked with services and supports lasts throughout their lifetime. In September 1996, The Consortium for Citizens with Disabilities (CCD) Housing Task Force and the Technical Assistance Collaborative published a report entitled *Opening Doors: Recommendations for a Federal Housing Policy for People with Disabilities.* In *Opening Doors,* CCD/TAC reported that:

> People with disabilities are currently the population group most in need of federal housing assistance. The U.S. Department of Housing and Urban Development (HUD) *1994 Report to the Congress on Worst Case Housing Needs* states that people with disabilities often have multiple housing problems and are the group most likely to live in severely inadequate housing. Unfortunately, HUD's 1994 report and a subsequent HUD report issued in March of 1996, significantly underestimates the number of people with disabilities who have priority housing needs. Since these HUD reports were issued, the CCD Housing Task Force has estimated that over 1.8 million people with disabilities receiving Supplemental Security Income (SSI) benefits may be in need of federal housing assistance. . . .

In order to afford housing in the community, low-income people with disabilities and advocates have been seeking various forms of federal housing assistance in increasing numbers. Unfortunately, in this era of federal, state, and local budget con-

Table 1. Fair Market Rents, Income, Affordability

	Estimated Fair Market Rents (FMR)		1996 Median Renter Income	Income Needed to Afford FMR		Estimated Percent Unable to Afford		Hourly Wage Needed		Maximum SSI Grant as Percent of FMR	
	One BR	Two BR		One BR	Two BR	One BR	Two BR	One BR	Two BR	One Person	Two Persons
State Median	$437	$543	$24,480	$17,487	$21,718	36%	45%	$8.41	$10.44	115%	172%

National Low Income Housing Coalition, Out of Reach, May 1996.

• Fair Market Rents are the standards established by HUD for use in the Section 8 Certificate and Voucher Program.
• The Median State Fair Market Rent is compiled based on state by state information. Rents vary from a high in Hawaii of 1BR = $826, 2BR = $973 to a low in West Virginia of 1BR = $330, 2BR = $406.
• The needed wage levels cited here are the lowest at which the FMR could be paid at 30% of the individual's income.
• SSI benefit levels in this chart were calculated for elderly individuals living independently based on information in the 1994 Green Book compiled by the House Ways and Means Committee. SSI as a percentage of the FMR varies from state to state also. For example, the maximum SSI payment is only 55% of the 1BR FMR in Hawaii, 74% in New York and New Jersey, and 135% in West Virginia.

straints, affordable housing opportunities for people with disabilities under age 62 are declining, rather than expanding. This is due in part to the implementation of "elderly only" designated housing policies in public and federally assisted housing. *Opening Doors* included data demonstrating that the designation of elderly-only public and assisted housing could lead to loss of access to previously available housing for more than 273,000 people with disabilities.

Alternative housing resources must be provided to compensate for the loss of these units. In addition, demands by people with disabilities for other public and private resources have increased. At the same time, unfortunately, federal funding for housing for individuals with low incomes is at an all time low and pending federal policy changes would allow these scarce resources to be shared with the less needy. Additionally, current efforts at the state and federal level to restructure public welfare and health systems, such as supplementary security income (SSI) and Medicaid, are putting pressure on funding streams on which people with disabilities rely to help provide needed services and supports.

Another problem is the widespread use of disability-specific "residential services" waiting lists. These lists abound because of the wide variety of disability-specific service systems that have developed nationwide. This phenomenon has made it extremely difficult to quantify accurately the extent of housing needs of people with disabilities. It is recognized in the housing industry that good data are the key to making a successful argument for additional resources at the local, state, and national levels. Anecdotal information alone does not begin to describe the magnitude of the need which exists. For example, more than 3 million adults between the ages of 18 and 62 are currently living on SSI benefits, which provides them an income less than 25% of median income. In some states, SSI benefits are as low as 15% of median income. The U.S. Department of Housing and Urban Development (HUD) has documented that more than 70% of households with incomes below 30% of median have priority housing problems. It is a fact of life that people with disabilities make up a large proportion of those with "worst-case" housing needs.

Even when the housing needs of people with disabilities have been accurately estimated—as has happened in a few communities during the preparation of the HUD mandated Consolidated Plan—the affordable housing delivery system has been resistant to expanding housing opportunities for people with disabilities. Among the many reasons for this lack of response are a lack of information and understanding of disability issues, stigma, and housing discrimination, which continues to occur within the affordable housing system.

For too long, people with disabilities and advocates have concentrated most of their activism solely on the "entitlement" funding streams. There has been a long held, and not incorrect belief, that "reforming" the Medicaid program is the answer to the availability of more community-based supports and services. Medicaid reform, however, is only one-half of the equation. If you have Medicaid funds flowing into the community and following the individual, you still have not answered the question of just where that individual will live or how he or she will pay the rent or mortgage.

DISABILITY ADVOCATES MUST LEARN TO PLAY THE "HOUSING GAME"

Given the decline in affordable housing resources and funding for human services, it is critical that people with disabilities, their families, and advocates work with federal, state, and local officials and governments and with others in the community for the development and implementation of comprehensive and consistent housing policies at every level, policies that are responsive to the housing needs and desires of people with disabilities. Otherwise, the housing "safety net" for people with disabilities will increasingly be inappropriate institutionalization or homelessness.

Consider the housing options that, ideally, should be available to all people in the community—options that are responsive to the needs of all people in the community, including those who have very low incomes, those with moderate incomes, those with accessibility requirements, and those with large or small families. Consider how people with disabilities, families, friends, advocates, and other community members can best work together to ensure that the same options are available to all people with disabilities.

- Options available should include affordable and accessible rental housing—apartments, condominium units, houses—open to a person who lives alone, as part of a couple, or with roommates.
- Homeownership should be an option for an individual, a couple, friends, or others who may want to buy a house, a condominium, a cooperative, or manufactured housing.
- Some individuals may choose housing that comes with certain services or supports attached, such as assistance with daily living skills, transportation, or child care.

HOW TO CHANGE THE HOUSING "SYSTEM"

Consider the positive variables that affect choice: geographic location, financial situation now and future potential, long-term aspirations and goals, current and future family status, current and future job aspirations, personal need or desire for certain amenities, transportation, shopping, recreation, family, friends, and pets.

Consider the negative variables that affect choice. Lack of money, range of affordable housing options, accessible housing, ongoing discrimination in the rental and homeownership markets, community resistance, family resistance, and service provider resistance.

The goal of people with disabilities and advocates in relation to developing inclusive housing policies must be to reduce the negative variables so that the positive ones are the ones that actually guide a person's choices in life. In this section, I want to detail ways in which positive variables can be enhanced and negative variables can be defused and/or eliminated so that people with Down syndrome and other disabilities have the opportunity to make real housing choices based on their needs and their hopes.

- The reality is that people with Down syndrome and other disabilities continue to face discrimination in the housing market, in the job market, and in everyday life. NIMBYism—Not in My Back Yard–syndrome is alive and well. In fact, in many parts of the country it is getting worse as communities make the determination that they have done enough for people with so-called "special needs." This is a situation that must be faced head on. Communities and citizens must be educated and concerns must be shared with policymakers. People with disabilities are protected by federal civil rights laws, such as the Fair Housing Amendments Act, the Americans with Disabilities Act, Section 504 of the Rehabilitation Act, and the Individuals with Disabilities Education Act. People with disabilities and their advocates must be educated about these laws and should be willing to work for their effective implementation and enforcement at the local, state, and national levels.

- The reality is that most people with Down syndrome and other disabilities have low or very low incomes. As stated earlier, this makes them perfect candidates for federal, state, and local housing assistance. Unfortunately, as also stated earlier, the assistance available at each of these levels of government has been shrinking, not growing. Housing people with low incomes is not a top national priority. This may not have always been the case, but it has been the case since the early 1980s and in today's balanced budget and welfare reform driven world. Federal housing programs assist a total of more than four million people, and yet this is only a small percentage of those who need help. HUD's *Rental Assistance at a Crossroads: A Report to Congress on Worst Case Housing Needs* reports that 5.3 million households have worst-case housing needs. These households are made of very low income renters who get no federal housing assistance and pay more than one-half of their income for housing, live in severely substandard housing, or both. This is almost 13 million individuals. According to *Out of Reach: Can America Pay the Rent?*, there are nearly 19 million low-income households—households with incomes below 80% of the median income in the United States.

- The reality is that individuals with disabilities, their families, and advocates do not consistently speak about their housing needs with their United States senators and congressmen; HUD officials; state senators or representatives; governor, mayor, city councilman, city manager, county supervisor; or leaders at the local or state housing authority and the state housing finance agency. Making elected (and other) officials aware that people with disabilities and their families are their constituents is an important goal. One of the most positive things that advocates can do is to "put a face" on an issue. The Arc, an association devoted to mental retardation issues, has developed a series of "Personal Profiles" of children or adults with mental retardation from all over the country. These one-page profiles explain the person's situation and detail how that situation has been improved or should be improved by changes in public policy. Issues tackled include education, housing, health care, and employment. In addition, how many times have disability advocates opened a dialogue with generic housing providers, realtors, builders, or generic housing advocacy groups? Unfortunately, in most places, the disability "community" is not doing this, whereas advocates for other equally needy groups are—and the needs of the disabled are not being met. It is true that "the squeaky wheel gets the oil."

- The reality is that if policymakers at all levels don't know that you are out there, they are not going to respond to your needs. If policymakers know you are out there and understand your issue, it is much more likely that they will respond positively. As indicated earlier, data on the housing needs of people with disabilities are not well organized or not available. It is incumbent on individuals with disabilities, families, advocates, and service providers to work to improve this data and then to ensure that it is disseminated. As indicated previously, the CCD/TAC report, *Opening Doors,* included data demonstrating that the designation of elderly-only public and assisted housing could lead to more than 273,000 people with disabilities losing access to housing that was previously available to them. When *Opening Doors* and its numbers were used by responsive members of the U.S. Congress, it led to an appropriation for fiscal year 1997 of $50 million for Section 8 tenant-based rental certificates/vouchers specifically for people with disabilities and designed to attempt to offset this loss. The fiscal year 1998 HUD appropriations bill also includes $40 million for Section 8 tenant-based rental assistance for people with disabilities and $48 million for Section 811 tenant-based rental assistance. In addition, the Government Accounting Office (GAO) has been directed by Congress—at the urging of disability advocates—to undertake a nationwide study of the housing needs of people with disabilities. This will be a major endeavor because the GAO will attempt to count the needs of all people with disabilities, not only a specific segment. This report should be ready in April 1998, in time for the start of the fiscal year 1999 HUD appropriations process. "Personal Profiles" of people with housing needs or housing success stories were also an effective tool during the appropriations battles.
- The reality is that while advocates work to document need in the community, there are a number of other things that should be going on simultaneously. The first is discarding the notion that people with Down syndrome and other disabilities should only be on "special disability-specific" lists, or only on state or local disability agency lists, or only on disability provider lists. There are many types of housing in each community. There is public housing, which in many cases is decent housing. There is federally assisted housing, which is often some of the nicer affordable rental housing in the community.* There is federally funded tenant based rental assistance (Section 8). There are first-time home-

---

*Much of the federally assisted housing in communities that may have previously served both non-elderly people with disabilities and the elderly may now be elderly-only because of changes to federal housing law made in 1992. These changes led to elderly-only public and assisted housing. Housing authorities that designate elderly-only public housing are currently required to file a specific plan with HUD. However, housing legislation currently in the Congress could make it easier for public housing authorities to designate housing. From the beginning, assisted housing providers have faced few demands by HUD. In fact, HUD has no record of what assisted housing has been designated as elderly-only. Therefore, people with disabilities and advocates will be hard pressed to determine just how much assisted housing has been lost in their communities.

buyer programs through the federal or state government or through entities such as Fannie Mae or Freddie Mac. There are federal block grant funds that come to towns and cities, such as HOME or the Community Development Block Grant, that can provide rental and/or homeownership assistance. There are often other state or local housing programs, such as rental assistance or homebuyer programs sponsored by the state housing finance agency. People with disabilities who want and need housing should be on each and every generic waiting list that is available. Only in this way will their needs become familiar with the generic housing community.

• The reality is that you may run into some resistance as you attempt to access these lists. This resistance will be based on a number of factors. It will be based on ignorance of the fact that people with Down syndrome want access to the same housing options as people without disabilities. Efforts will probably be made to direct people with disabilities to "disability" housing. These efforts should be resisted. Although "disability" housing is a viable option, it is not the only option. Resistance will also be based on the rigidity of the bureaucracy that has been built up around housing. Usually the local housing authority is the keeper of the lists for both public housing and Section 8 tenant-based rental assistance. If a housing authority indicates that there are no waiting lists or that the waiting lists are closed, individuals and advocates should question these statements and ask to be notified when the lists open. In addition, people with disabilities and advocates should be prepared to educate the housing authority. Often a housing authority is unaware of housing assistance that is available for people with disabilities. The following examples demonstrate the need for education.

In 1997 and 1998 Congress appropriated a total of $90 million for Section 8 tenant-based rental assistance certificates or vouchers to help offset the loss of public and assisted housing to the elderly. As we entered 1998 approximately 15,000 one-year Section 8 certificates and vouchers (8400 for fiscal year 1997 and approximately 6500 for fiscal year 1998) were available for people with disabilities. Housing authorities applied for only a small number of the 8400 available in 1997 for a number of reasons. Some housing authorities were not aware of their existence. Others were aware of their existence but were turned off by the confusing application process. Even more of a problem are those housing authorities that assert that there is no need for them to apply because there are no people with disabilities on waiting lists. Certain legislative changes were made that should solve the first two problems and make it easier for housing authorities to apply. However, no matter how easy the process, consumers and their advocates still carry the major responsibility of making the housing needs of people with disabilities visible so that the community can respond.

A notice of the availability of 2000 five-year Section 811 certificates or vouchers was published in April 1997 with a two-month application deadline. HUD received applications for almost 20,000 units from approximately 280 of the 2600 housing authorities that administer rental assistance programs. Housing authorities were chosen through a lottery process and in the fall of 1997, 25 housing authorities were awarded a total of 1756 certificates and vouchers. Although the overwhelming response to the notice of these funds helps demonstrate the breadth of the housing needs of people with disabilities, it is obvious—because the majority of housing authorities did not even apply for these funds—that activism by people with disabilities and advocates is critically needed. This activism must be designed to educate the community, the housing authorities, and policymakers. It must be designed to ensure that the extent of the housing needs of people with Down syndrome and other disabilities is clearly demonstrated.

- The reality is, as stated earlier, there are many things that consumers and advocates must be doing at the same time. Placing people on waiting lists is one small but critically important first step. Educating the community about people with Down syndrome and their goals and needs and aspirations is another important first step. However, the most important thing that people with disabilities and their advocates can do is to be a "player." As housing decisions are being made in the community, the range of needs of people with disabilities must be part of the equation. Each community and state that receives housing assistance in the form of block grants is required to submit a "Consolidated Plan" to HUD. In the ConPlan, a community must quantify and prioritize its housing needs, and based on these needs describe how it will use these funds. People with disabilities, families, advocates, and service providers must take advantage of the requirements for community involvement built into the ConPlan process. It is important to remember that housing needs among individuals with low incomes far outstrip the supply of housing assistance that is available in most communities. This means a community must decide among competing demands for limited resources. A primary means of influencing the decision making process is to provide clear and compelling evidence of housing need Developing this evidence will require cooperation among people with all types of disabilities, cognitive, physical, and mental; families, friends, and advocates; a wide range of public sector and private providers of services and supports, and school districts. Examples of sources include the following:

the number of people on waiting lists for community housing options;
the number of people living at home with aging parents;
the number of young adults graduating from school;
the number of people residing in state-operated or private facilities due to the lack of affordable housing in the community;
the number of people who are homeless;
the number of people who are paying over 50% of their income for housing or living in substandard housing; and
the number of people who are currently on subsidized housing waiting lists, such as those for Section 8 rental assistance, public housing, or assisted housing. (*Opening Doors: A Housing Publication for the Disability Community,* Issue 2, Oct. 1997)

Developing these data on housing needs will require gathering more than just numbers of people who need housing. It will also require determining where people want to live and what must be done to makes these desires real. This is a critical step that must be taken to ensure that people's "choices" are real choices. Do some of the people want to live in apartments? Do some want to live together in a house? Do some want to buy their own place? In each and every case, a different type of support is probably needed: affordable rental housing, rental assistance, affordable housing for purchase, down payment assistance, funds for accessibility modifications, housing counseling, and so on. All of this is useful knowledge to bring to the table.

Once the needs of people with disabilities have been determined, what do you do with this information? This is when the groundwork laid through outreach and education for and with local and state policymakers and housing professionals should pay off. This is when the information gathered (and organized in a clear and concise manner) should be taken to the local housing authority, state housing finance agency, and all other entities in a position to help add to the supply of affordable housing in the community. This information must be shared with those developing the state or local ConPlan. With a well prepared case, people with disabilities and their advocates must demand inclusion in the community's plan. This is not a one step process. Beyond demanding inclusion of the needs of people with disabilities, advocates must demand that the ConPlan developed addresses these needs; and they must follow the progress of the plan and monitor that it really does reflect and attempt to address the needs of people with disabilities. If satisfaction is not derived from this process, people with disabilities and their advocates should inform policymakers of their concerns, as well as provide recommendations on how any deficiencies can be rectified. Policymakers to be informed include not just those involved in ConPlan development but those above them at the local, state, and federal levels.

SUMMARY

The ultimate goal of all these activities is to increase the decent, safe, affordable, and accessible housing available to people with disabilities in the community. To accomplish this goal, a number of things must be going on simultaneously. People with disabilities, their families, advocates, and providers of services and supports must work to defuse the negative forces that have limited the housing options of people with disabilities At the same time, policymakers at all levels must be made familiar with the housing needs and desires of people with disabilities. Data must be provided and faces must be attached to these data—who are the people in need? They, too, are important members of the community. Finally, people with disabilities, their families, and advocates must be "players" at the local, state, and federal level. If all these efforts are successful, the probability is very good that the range of housing options in the community can be increased. Success will be characterized by communities that no longer tolerate discrimination and no longer presume that all people with disabilities belong in "disability" housing. Instead, communities' future plans will include the needs of people with disabilities. If rental housing is developed, the needs of people with disabilities will be considered. If homeownership programs are developed, people with disabilities will be part of the whole.

A final reality is that powerful advocacy forces, such as the elderly, have been extremely successful in sending a strong message to policymakers at all levels of government, but especially at the federal level. On the one hand, advocacy by the elderly has consistently led to the defeat of legislative initiatives that would increase their housing costs. On the other hand, their advocacy has also led to continuing high levels of funding for housing of individuals who are elderly and for more restrictive policies, such as elderly-only public and assisted housing or age-restricted housing. These high levels of funding and these discriminatory policies continue to be approved by Congress, even at a time when it is clear elderly individuals are usually not those with the greatest needs.

The message here is that well organized vocal advocacy pays off. The disability community has lagged behind in this area and as a community has been fragmented and, therefore, weakened. People with disabilities and their families should be involved with advocacy groups such as the National Down Syndrome Society and The Arc. These groups that work on behalf of individuals with mental retardation and related disabilities and their families should work with groups that represent individuals with physical or sensory or other types of mental disabilities. It is critical to remember that, when it comes to housing most people with disabilities have something in common. They have low incomes and they need some type of housing assistance. If communities are to change, if state and federal policies are to change, people with all types of disabilities, their family members, advocates, and providers of supports and services must speak with one voice.

APPENDIX 1. ACTION ITEMS

- Get to know who makes the housing decisions at the local, state, and national levels.
- Educate yourself about how the affordable housing system works.
- Identify existing affordable housing in the community and get on every waiting list available.
- Raise concerns about affordable housing now closed to people with disabilities because of "elderly-only" policies.
- Work with other advocates to find out how many people need housing, where people live now, and where they would like to live.
- Educate policymakers and the public about people with Down syndrome and their housing goals.
- Be at the table when housing policy decisions are made.
- Keep an eye on the outcome of these decisions.
- Keep in touch with elected and appointed officials and let them know your concerns.
- Remember, the squeaky wheel gets the oil.

Why is the ConPlan important to the disability community?

The ConPlan outlines how a state or local government will use HUD funds to meet the priority housing needs in its area. The ConPlan also outlines any other funds, such as state and local funds, that will be committed to these priority activities. In addition, any application for HUD discretionary funding (e.g., programs for which nonprofits and government agencies can apply directly to HUD, such as the Section 811 Supportive Housing for Persons with Disabilities program) must receive certification from the jurisdiction that the application is consistent with the housing priorities that are in the ConPlan. The Con Plan determines the use of and/or access to almost all federal housing dollars within a jurisdiction with the exception of Section 8 certificates and vouchers and public housing. If the disability community wants to ensure that a fair share of federal housing dollars are used to meet the needs of individuals with disabilities, it must become actively involved in the development of the ConPlan.

Are there requirements to ensure that the disability community can have an impact on the ConPlan?

There are two ways that the disability community can play a role in the development of the ConPlan:

- *Consultation.* State and local governments are required to consult with private agencies that provide assisted housing, health services, and social services during the preparation of the ConPlan, including agencies that provide services to people with disabilities. Though such consultation is required, HUD does not prescribe at what point in the preparation of the ConPlan this must take place or just what constitutes consultation. Therefore, the disability community will need to work to ensure that this consultation is meaningful to the ConPlan process and takes place early in the planning process. This is the only way that the needs of people with disabilities and housing activities to meet these needs will get included in the plan.

- *Citizen participation.* The ConPlan requires the adoption of a citizen participation plan that sets forth a jurisdictions policies and procedures for citizen participation. It must "provide for and encourage citizens to participate in the development of the ConPlan, and substantial amendments to the ConPlan, and performance reports." Toward this end, a jurisdiction is expected to take whatever actions are appropriate to encourage the participation of all citizens, including individuals with low and moderate incomes, minorities, non-English speaking persons, and people with disabilities. There are minimum requirements that must be in the citizen participation plan. These include providing public notice of the ConPlan process, sponsoring two public hearings, and making the draft ConPlan available for public comments. However, the details and timing of these requirements are left to the locality or state. It is critical that the disability community not only know what must be included in the citizen participation plan, but also play a role in its development to ensure that there is a meaningful and participatory process in place.

What must be included in the ConPlan?

There are six major components: a description of the planning process, housing and homelessness needs assessment, housing market analysis, strategic plan, action plan, and certifications. The disability community must play an active role in the entire process. It must not wait to be asked for housing needs data—this information must be provided early in the planning process to ensure that the nature and extent of the housing needs of people with disabilities are accurately represented. Ongoing active participation is the only way to ensure that the needs of people will be included and that community actions to meet these needs are part of both the community's or state's strategic plan and action plan.

APPENDIX 2. IMPORTANT INDIVIDUALS AND ENTITIES TO KNOW IN THE EFFORT TO INCREASE HOUSING OPTIONS IN THE COMMUNITY

Local Level
Mayor
Members of city/town council
Members of city/town commission
City/town manager
City/town attorney
City/town housing authority (need to
    add information on Section 8)
City/town office of housing and
    community development
Local HUD office
City/town office of planning
City/town office of affordable housing
City/town office of civil rights
City/town office of disability
Members of advisory boards on
    housing, low-income issues,
    homeownership
Board of realtors
Mortgage bankers
Chamber of Commerce
Local association of home builders
Local association of multifamily
    housing managers
Local disability organizations

State Level
State delegates, representatives,
    senators
State attorney
State office of civil rights
State housing finance agency
State office of housing and community
    development
State office of planning
State housing authority
Regional HUD office
State offices of disability
State disability organizations

National Level
Senators
Representatives
U.S. Department of Housing and
    Urban Development
U.S. Justice Department
National disability organizations
National Low Income Housing
    Coalition
National Association of Home
    Builders
National Mortgage Bankers
    Association
Fannie Mae
Freddie Mac
National Home of Your Own Coalition
Enterprise Foundation
White House

REFERENCES

Center for Community Change Through Housing and Supports (1993): A national study of housing affordability for recipients of supplemental security income. J Hosp Commun Psychiatry (May).

Consortium for Citizens with Disabilities Housing Task Force (Washington, DC) and the Technical Assistance Collaborative (Boston, MA) (1996): Opening doors: recommendations for a federal policy to address the housing needs of people with disabilities (Sept.).

National Low Income Housing Coalition (1996): Out of reach: Can America pay the rent? Washington, DC.

Technical Assistance Collaborative (Boston, MA) and Consortium for Citizens with Disabilities Housing Task Force (1997a): Opening doors: a housing publication for the disability community, Issue 1 (May).

Technical Assistance Collaborative (Boston, MA) and Consortium for Citizens with Disabilities Housing Task Force (1997b): Opening doors: a housing publication for the disability community, Issue 2 (Oct.).

Turner L, O'Hara A (1996): The consolidated plan. Boston, MA: Technical Assistance Collaborative.

U.S. Department of Housing and Urban Development, Office of Policy Development and Research (1996): Rental assistance at a crossroads: a report to Congress on worst case housing needs.

IX. The Role of the Family

Family Values

Michael Bérubé

One afternoon I was having a long lunch with a pair of friends who have an adult daughter with a severe disability. That was one of the reasons it was a long lunch: I'd met their daughter the year before, I'd just published *Life As We Know It* about my son James, and we had a lot to talk about. Another reason it was a long lunch is that the girl's mother, a teacher and feminist philosopher, had been taking part in a year-long symposium on the ethics of "selective abortion"—or "preventive" prenatal screening for fetuses with disabilities—and my lunch companions and I had a similar jumble of ambivalent feelings, philosophical positions, hedges, and worries about the subject. But the heart of our conversation, interestingly, had to do with the siblings of our children with disabilities—a young man graduating from college in their case, and a precocious, sensitive 11-year-old in mine. How did *they* feel about being part of the support system for a child with disabilities, and how did they feel about things like abortion and prenatal testing? Did they feel privileged, burdened, neglected? Were they overcompensating or deflecting or acting out or dealing just beautifully, or all of the above in gradual rotation?

At one point during lunch, I started to mention some advice that had been given to Janet and me by our therapist, a woman we began to consult in September of 1996, as James turned five and just before my book about him was to appear. But I wasn't sure whether I should disclose that Janet and I were "in therapy" to a pair of relative strangers. I was in a fashionable New York City restaurant at the time, and I knew from my 20 years as a New Yorker that in such situations one is more likely to feel

When Jamie Bérubé was born in 1991, his parents knew little about Down syndrome. As they sought to understand exactly what Down syndrome is, they learned not only about the current medical and social treatment of developmental disabilities, but also the history of how society has treated children like Jamie. Michael Bérubé published the compelling story of his attempt to make the world more accepting of his son, Jamie, in 1996 in *Life As We Know It: A Father, a Family, and an Exceptional Child*. Bérubé follows up his critically acclaimed work with this chapter. Michael Bérubé is an English professor at the University of Illinois at Urbana-Champaign.

Down Syndrome: A Promising Future, Together, Edited by Terry J. Hassold and David Patterson
ISBN 0-471-29686-4   Copyright © 1998 by Wiley-Liss, Inc.

conversationally squeamish about the fact that one is *not* seeing a therapist, but still, I paused uncomfortably before saying that my wife and I had started therapy a few months earlier in order to deal with some of the accumulated stress of raising James—as well as some of our underacknowledged grief about him, which had begun to warp our otherwise rich and deeply textured marriage. The moment I mentioned therapy, however, my companions stared at me in alarm. *Oh, no,* I thought. *They're weirded out. Just what I was afraid of. They think we can't handle it, we're not strong enough. They think we're traitors to the cause. They think. . . .*

"Michael," said my philosopher friend, "Jamie is how old now?"

"Five and a half." Her eyes widened still further.

"Five and a half," shaking her head slowly. *"And you and Janet went five years without therapy?!?"*

Well, I laughed in relief, at the time. But before long, I had begun to wonder yet again: Janet and I always worry about whether we're doing enough for James, and we always weigh ourselves in the scales and find ourselves wanting. But in all our worries about James, and all our ancillary worries about Nick, had we forgotten to worry about ourselves?

The point of this anecdote is not to advocate therapy for all couples who have children with disabilities, though my sense is that in many cases it sure wouldn't hurt. The point is that the family dynamics of families with such children are more complicated than most of us can reasonably keep track of, let alone calibrate and control in an emotionally harmonious and mindful way. But the irony is that I was unaware of some of the most important of those dynamics even when, in 1995–1996, I thought I was writing about them. This essay, then, is about some of the stuff I hadn't known to think about when I thought I was thinking about James and his family. It's also something of an update on James' relation to his brother Nick, and the extent to which his desire to emulate Nick contributes to his cognitive, motor, and social development. And it's also a reminder—to myself as well as to other parents—that whatever we try to do for ourselves and our families, checking on the emotional status of our fellow family members is something we can never do too much of.

I thought that by writing *Life As We Know It,* I was doing what I could for James. I think of myself as a writer and a teacher, and I'm accordingly torn between the conviction that my work makes a difference in people's lives and the fear that I'm utterly useless in the world. My first book sold 600 copies, mainly to university libraries, and is now useful primarily for killing large crawling insects. But my book on Jamie, I thought, might actually matter to people—Jamie not least among them. Since his birth I'd been struck by the relative invisibility of people with developmental disabilities in the general culture, an invisibility that is being remedied only slowly and fitfully. I wrote the book during a scary political time during which anti-government conservatives were crusading against the Americans with Disabilities Act and even talking about refusing to reauthorize the Individuals with Disabilities Education Act, so I worked with a sense of urgency that's probably pretty clear on every other page of the manuscript. And when, in the fall of 1996, I prepared for a national book tour in the middle of an election season, my hopes were as high as they could be. I worked on crafting my message into media-friendly sound bites such as "we don't know what 'normal' is until we try inclusion first"; I chose passages for public readings of the book; I made up interview questions and answers for my "media packet." And whenever I felt that twinge that we weren't doing enough for Jamie, say, when I agonized that he still couldn't put on a pair of socks by himself, I could look at my book and say, "but at least I'm doing *this*. . . ."

How convenient this turned out to be for me: I could displace my personal worries onto my professional work, and my professional work would actually help to assuage my worries. Only too late did it occur to me that Janet didn't have the same mechanism. We'd talked about co-authoring the book, and of course she worked on it with me at every stage, but still, it didn't "solve" things for her the way it was doing for me. In an unexpected way, then, *Life As We Know It* became one more thing we had to figure out. Needless to say, that particular difficulty is specific to my family and my family alone. But what *isn't* specific to us is the emotional dilemma underlying our different reactions to the book: each of us, as it turned out, was silently trying to live up to (what we thought was) the other one's expectations, thinking all the while that we shouldn't confess to our feelings of failure or foreboding lest we damage the other's emotional equilibrium. So Janet wasn't allowing herself to speak freely because she feared, as she put it, taking the wind out of my sails; meanwhile, I was doing all I could just to match her incredible competence and compassion as a parent. Something like an emotional version of the famous O. Henry short story, "The Gift of the Magi."

Of course, it could be much, much worse. We were caught in a strange cycle in which each of us admired the other's ability to cope, so much so that we sometimes just weren't coping. But many parents go through more difficult cycles than this; they withdraw, they become depressed or angry, they go into massive denial, they experience the entire range of mental and physical states to which we mortals have access whether we want to or not. There's a recent novel written by a brilliant writer who just happens to be a good friend—*Galatea 2.2*, by Richard Powers—and in it there's a family that looks a lot like mine: two children, the older one based on Nick and the younger one based on Jamie, and a single mother whose resemblance to Janet is remarkable. In *Galatea 2.2*, the father of this family has abandoned his wife and children because he couldn't deal with the disparity between his "gifted" child and his child with Down syndrome. When I finished thanking Rick for rendering this flattering portrait of me (and informing him that there's no significant increase in the divorce rate for parents with "disabled" children), I decided to take his book as something of a reminder that there are *many* ways in which one can express one's feelings of inadequacy as a parent, and that it's probably best to try to feel inadequate—because one can never fully insulate oneself from feeling inadequate—in the least destructive way possible.

Easier said than done? Yes, but that's precisely my point. As long as Janet and I were talking only to each other about Jamie, there was no way for us to break the cycle we were in. We couldn't work this one out by ourselves, because *we* were actually part of the problem. It was impossible, we've learned, to calibrate our feelings about ourselves and each other as parents of James without the help of a third party— and we strongly suspect that we're not alone in this respect. The third party doesn't have to be a therapist; he or she can be a close friend, a member of the extended family, a minister, or a mentor. But when two parents are orbiting each other, as couples usually are, it's hard for either parent to get a good idea of who's doing what or why. Motion is relative, after all, and sometimes, if you want to figure out what's going on, you need the perspective of someone who's not in your orbital path, and can see your world from a relatively stable frame of reference.

In physics, it's fairly easy to predict orbits when you're dealing with only two objects. For low speeds, Newton's laws work just fine. *Three* objects orbiting each other, however, will produce mechanical mayhem: it's called the "*n*-body problem," and nobody can figure it out. Nobody even wants to try. Fortunately, however, the third body in *our* system—Nick—isn't worried about how well he's doing. He's doing very well, thank you. He has an identity as Jamie's brother, but he also has a life of his own: plenty of playmates; a fondness for computer games; a deep fascination with history, geography, and the configuration of the world; and a very interesting, gradually emerging aesthetic sense that he applies to music, movies, clothes, and buildings. Adolescence, I know, is right around the corner. I can't wait for him to meet other siblings like himself, though, because he's never exchanged notes with another child who has a brother or sister with Down syndrome. Right now, he's serving James as a guide, a shepherd, and a role model, and he seems pretty comfortable in all three roles, each of which I'll explain briefly.

Nick as role model: this is probably the most predictable identity for an older brother, regardless of whether the younger sibling has Down syndrome. But because Jamie is Jamie, there's not a lot of competition between Jamie and Nick. Certainly Jamie draws parental attention away from Nick, but that's not always a bad thing; and certainly Jamie sometimes angers or upsets Nick, but it would be odd to expect otherwise. Every once in a while, on the rare occasion when Jamie demolishes one of Nick's elaborate Lego structures or exits Nick's computer game, I have to console Nick; but I always remember to remind him, "Jamie didn't mess up your stuff because he's your little brother with Down syndrome—he messed up your stuff because he's your little brother. All little brothers are required by law to mess up their big brothers' stuff a certain number of times per year, and Jamie's just abiding by the rules." In partial compensation, James admires Nick completely and emulates him in everything, from basketball to tae kwon do to drawing to climbing trees. Few things motivate Jamie so emphatically as the desire to *be like Nick* (it's our own personal family ad campaign), and Janet and I are not shy about exploiting this to full effect. We've dutifully pointed out that Nick eats lettuce to get strong, and that Nick puts on his own pants; this past spring, as we got Jamie ready to start kindergarten in the fall, we noted that he took real delight in the thought that he would be going to *a big school like Nick.*

Nick as guide and shepherd: we've always been amazed by how watchful, how observant Nick is. Nick cautions Jamie—sometimes gently, sometimes sternly, as circumstances dictate—not to put balloons in his mouth, not to run unescorted through the parking lot, not to growl gutturally when he asks for things. Nick is *solicitous,* and just by being Nick he shows Jamie how to be solicitous too. Best of all, Nick shows other children, by example, how to deal with Jamie: how to listen to him, how to play with him, how to shoot baskets or work the video games, how to include him in the gang. For the most part, Nick does this simply by treating Jamie like a nice little brother, thereby letting all the other kids know that there's nothing "special" they have to do in order to play or talk with James—just listen carefully, and treat him as you would any younger child who needs the basket moved a little lower or the video game set a little easier.

How different our family would be if our *first* child had Down syndrome and our second did not; how different it would be if Jamie had two, three, four siblings, or none. Every family configuration produces different dynamics, and every family configuration is bewilderingly complex. The more I talk with other parents of children with disabilities, the more I realize how many subtle differences underlie our similarities, and vice versa. Some parents need help with the child who keeps throwing car keys down the toilet; some parents need help with the nondisabled sibling who feels burdened; some parents need help with feelings of failure; some need help with feelings of denial. Sometimes the children are far apart in age, sometimes less than a year apart; sometimes the child with a disability is the oldest, watching his or her siblings grow up more quickly; sometimes the youngest, getting more developmentally remote from siblings each year; sometimes there's more than one child with a disability, or more than one disability. . . . And sometimes I think the only advice that's equally applicable to all of us is the advice that we should seek advice.

But whenever I think this way, I remember something Jamie has taught me over the past year. He rarely calls himself "Jamie" any more, by the way—he usually points to himself and says "James," as in, "How 'bout James and daddy hockey," which means he'd like to accompany me to my roller hockey league and (ahem) play with the big boys. (Once someone at a conference showed him a copy of *Life As We Know It* and asked him if he knew what the book was "about." To the astonishment of his listeners, James called the book "we know it," nodded, pointed to himself, and said, "James Bérubé.") It was during the spring of 1997, Jamie's last season at First United Methodist daycare before he would start kindergarten in 1997–1998, and the occasion was a classroom game in which each of the children told their teachers what they wanted to be when they grew up. From every child except James, the list of occupations bore out the Lily Tomlin joke that if we'd all grown up to be what we said we wanted to be at the age of five, we'd live in a world populated by cowboys, firefighters, and ballerinas. When the class got to James, though, the teachers weren't even sure that my little boy would understand the question, let alone come up with an intelligible answer. Still, they politely asked him, last among the preschool kids, "And what would you like to be when *you* grow up, James?"

Later that day, Janet and I were told that James had answered the question immediately, and with just one word.

Big.

To their credit, James' teachers were duly astonished: not only had James understood the question, he'd come up with an answer that changed everyone else's understanding of what the question meant. All of a sudden, in other words, that stock query, *what would like to be when you grow up,* a question no adult expects a five-year-old to answer seriously, had some real substance to it. For what had Jamie said, by saying "big"? That he wants to grow up. That he wants to be healthy. Perhaps even that he wants people to treat him well. In his odd way, Jamie had readjusted his classmates' and teachers' understanding of the parameters of the question. And that's not just my interpretation; that was *their* interpretation. Janet's interpretation (and, henceforth, mine) is this: precisely because Jamie answered the question so literally, people saw him differently. In saying he wanted to grow up to be big, James was no longer the "special needs" child; on the contrary, he became the *normal* child, the universal generic Child. Think about it for a moment. What Jamie said is something almost *all* children can say or sign or hope, whether they were born in Australia or Algeria or Albania or Alabama. Janet and I have seen such moments before, moments in which Jamie is not only irreducibly and idiosyncratically Jamie but also, somehow, representative of children everywhere. And in such moments we realize how Jamie has helped us to see that all children have fundamental needs that we share in common as humans. Of course, some children have "special" needs, and we wouldn't deny it for an instant; James himself needed a good deal of physical therapy, occupational therapy, and (most obviously) speech therapy just to get to the point at which he could tell adults he wanted to be big when he grows up. But the general lesson, I hope, should be clear—that whatever our differences and whatever our family dynamics, it's our job to help make a world in which all our children can grow up to be "big."

The Future: The Life Planning Approach

Richard W. Fee

If you ask parents what they want for their child with Down syndrome in the future, they will generally tell you that they want him or her to lead as normal a life as possible. When you pursue it a little further and ask them to tell you how their child will be able to maintain this meaningful and, hopefully, comfortable standard of living without them, you get some very conflicting answers. One mother commented that this would not happen as people with Down Syndrome always die young. Another said that she went to bed every night with the prayer that she would live one day longer than her child. The good and bad news is that persons with Down syndrome are living longer due to advances in medical science and sadly, families are not preparing for their offspring to outlive them.

Families need to plan for both the short and long term. Planning must be done whether the parents are young or old for the simple reason that a long and healthy life is not guaranteed to anyone. Too many families with young children justify lack of planning as unnecessary because they are young, healthy, and will live forever. A quick glance at any newspaper will show that many young couples die unexpectedly in car crashes leaving young children at home and at the mercy of a very impersonal social service system. How many of these children have disabilities that make them harder to adopt or even to be taken in by loving relatives? It should be noted that the use of the words "child" or "children" does not have any deep philosophical or politically correct implications. Most families of adult children in their 50s still consider them "their children."

The question that every family must answer within their own hearts, and probably on a daily basis, is "Will our child be able to enjoy a meaningful life-style without us?" And "without us" implies more than simply dying. The American Association for Retired Persons estimates that approximately 60–70% of people will have go into a nursing home before they die, that their average stay will be 2 years, and they will exhaust their own personal resources within 1 year. Therefore, we have to assume that some parents will be incapacitated in nursing homes, wishing they had put everything into place.

Down Syndrome: A Promising Future, Together, Edited by Terry J. Hassold and David Patterson
ISBN 0-471-29686-4   Copyright © 1998 by Wiley-Liss, Inc.

The reasons for developing and implementing a well thought out plan of action or Life Plan are very logical and convincing. We need to do the following:

1. Leave clear instructions to those who follow on what you want for the future.
2. Protect your child's government benefits—poor planning can lose them. Your tax dollars are there for those who can't help themselves, including your child.
3. Provide supplemental income based on real needs, not emotions.
4. Guarantee that someone will be there to look after your child, an advocate or guardian.
5. Make sure that future resources will be managed properly.
6. Determine final arrangements, including ensuring that your child will have a proper and dignified funeral—remember, you won't be here to plan things.
7. Set up an environment where the remaining family members can work together. Make it easy for them to support your plan.

When families finally do overcome some of the emotional barriers preventing planning, such as facing their own mortality, and actually take the first step, they tend to approach it from the traditional legal or financial viewpoint. We'd better leave some money for our child. We need to find a lawyer to write a will. We assume that money and a legal document are the only things that need to be done. Although this traditional approach is better than nothing, it is really not a plan that will help your child live a safe and comfortable life.

We need to make a paradigm shift in our thinking about this topic. Our focus must go from solutions (will, money) to the issue at hand, the person. How can you give a possible solution (money, will), if you don't even know the problem? Concentrate on the quality of life of the individual. Where do you want your child to live? What about employment, social relationships, religious experiences, and so on? Sit with your child if possible (depending on age, level of functioning) and discuss with him or her "their" desires. Determine a basic goal that summarizes your feelings. It can be a simple goal: We want Mary to live in a semi-independent living situation (shared apartment) near family members, work in a sheltered workshop, attend church regularly, and so forth. *Once you settle on this underlying goal or Life Plan, you can refine it and then begin to find individualized solutions.*

We tend to overemphasize the ability of total strangers or government representatives (case managers) to make wise personal choices for us. A lawyer may be able to draft a nice will and trust, but he probably is not able to advise you on where your child should live. Even your favorite teacher who worked with your child for a year in high school cannot give you advice on the right type of government benefits. These responsibilities fall on your shoulders. Families are in a unique position because they have this life-span perspective. Professionals come, test, do short term interventions, give opinions, and leave. The family is always there. You have known your child through the peaks and valleys. You have a better idea of what your child wants and is able to do than most professionals who see him or her for short periods. The bottom line is that we have to stop devaluing the role of the family. The family has to make the tough life planning decisions and then seek professionals such as attorneys and financial planners to help them to refine and implement the plan.

Over the years we have tried to develop a step by step guide for life planning. Although the actual number of steps have varied, the following major groups provide a good simple guide for families.

PREPARE A LIFE PLAN

Step 1: Determine What You Want for the Future

In your preliminary thinking, come up with a basic goal with your child. For example, you want your child to live in as independent a setting as possible. Once you have established this underlying goal, you can begin to fill in the details. As you plan you need to look at the following key areas:

Residence
Education
Employment
Social
Religion
Medical care
Guardianship or advocacy—who should be there to assist or supervise
Financial Life-style—comfortable or rich

There may be other areas that are unique to your family. Many of these are interrated. Your would prefer that your child attend the local synagogue or church, but this means he will have to live in a local group home, which is your second choice. It is important to realize that you don't know how long your plan will need to last. Your child may be 40 years old at your death and still live another 40 years. How do you build in this important contingency? Start by listing as many options as you can under each heading. For instance, when you look at a future residence list four or five options in priority order. Your first choice may be for your child to live in his/her own apartment with a roommate, second choice to live with a sister, third choice to live with a brother, and finally, if there are no other relatives, to live in a group home. No matter where he/she lives, he/she should have his/her own room and some degree of privacy. It is essential to build in these options because we may need a long period of time. Our choices may not be always available. For example, the brother may be in the middle of a divorce and cannot take him/her in at that time.

One of the major benefits of this system of life planning is that the number of surprises to both your child and the relatives will be greatly reduced. No one should attend a reading of your Last Will and Testament and learn for the first time that they now have responsibility for your child.

Step 2: Choose a Guardian or Advocate

Many persons with disabilities function quite well by themselves. They are able to make their own decisions concerning finances or just make good sound choices in life—medical, housing, employment, and so on. However, there are many persons who do need some type of assistance. Families generally provide this type of assistance just being around the person. Up until age 18, parents have legal guardianship of the person. They have the legal right to make these decisions on behalf of the person. Now the second the person turns 18, whether or not they have a disability, they are adults. They are emancipated, free! No one can make decisions on their behalf unless . . . unless a court intervenes and appoints another person or agency to do so.

There are at least four ways in which persons with Down syndrome make decisions:

1. *Independently* just like everyone else.
2. *Advocate assistance:* A person or agency serves as a "friend" and helps person, such as with taxes. The advocate does not have any legal rights to make decisions for the person.
3. *Guardianship/conservatorship (CA), tutorship (LA):* someone petitions a court to be appointed the legal guardian for the person. Generally, the basic rights are taken away and given to the guardian.
4. *Limited guardianship/conservatorship/tutorship:* in this situation, the court does not take away the rights, but gives another person legal authority to make decisions in certain areas.

The legal system considers these rights to include the right to do the following:

Handle finances
Choose residence
Choose employment
Choose education
Engage in social and sexual relations
Marry
Make medical decisions

The decision whether or not to request legal guardianship (full or limited) is a very tough one because parents want all their children including those with disabilities to function independently. Yet parents also know their children better than the so-called expert. They sometimes err on the side of being very protective and do not want "strangers" making decisions for their child. If their child needs guardianship or some advocacy they want to do it until they pass away. Many people believe that no one should make these decisions regardless of the severity of the disability. The bottom line is that IF a person cannot make those decisions than someone else will. Parents want to retain this power. This is a major point of dissension between persons with disabilities, their parents, and advocacy organizations.

Families need to make a decision as to advocacy versus guardianship in the quiet of their home, not sitting in the lawyer's office with the $200-per-hour clock running. The decision needs to be made based on the strengths of the individual. There is no disgrace in setting up a system of assistance. Let's face it, we all need help with taxes, maybe even balancing the checkbook. Your child may also need this simple assistance. Or if you think he or she may be taken advantage of by others then there may be a need for full time court appointed help to handle all of the finances.

Once YOU (and your child) have made the decision, you will need to consult a qualified attorney to assist you. Again, remember the attorney can give you the pros and cons, but this is *your* family member. You must set up a plan that BOTH you and your loved one can accept.

What about the future? Just as you have done with the life planning choices, you have to build in lots of options. Your elderly aunt may be a great choice to serve as an advocate or guardian, but she may outlive you by one day. Put her down as a first choice and then look at four, five, even ten other choices. Sometimes your first choice is willing but unable at the time of the emergency (e.g., in the middle of a divorce, moving to Alaska). Some families have only one or two choices. If you are fortunate enough to have an "advocacy" group in your area, you may want to contract them for this long-term service. Ask your local support group for the names of potential advocacy groups.

Step 3: Put it in Writing

If you play the party game of "pass the message," you know that the first person whispers the "message" in the ear of the next person. The message may go through five or six people. The joke is how garbled the message is when the last person hears it. When we pass the message of how we want our child to be treated in the future to a number of people, the results may sound humorous, but are probably tragic for your child. And surprisingly, this is how most planning is done. The mother tells the oldest daughter a few personal things about the sibling with Down Syndrome and hopes she "passes the message."

Once you have made your life planning decisions and have decided on who will assist you in carrying out your plan—advocate or guardian—take some time to write down your wishes and desires. We use the term "Letter of Intent" when we discuss this type of report because you are telling your posterity and the courts what your "intentions" are for your child.

The Letter of Intent should be very simple. Take out a clean sheet of paper or open up a new file in your favorite word processing program. Start at the beginning with one thing in mind: providing enough information so that anyone who has to become your child's care-provider in the future will be able to provide quality care.

Here are some general guidelines:

1. Handwritten, typed, or on a computer program, your choice.
2. First paragraph: write something about your family, for example, names of parents and siblings, and information about where the family has lived.
3. Then cover each of the main areas of the Life Plan stated above (residence, education, etc.). Here is a nice concise way to convey the information. Write the heading, for example, Residence. In the first paragraph, write where your child has lived in the past. In the next paragraph, describe your child's present residential setting. And finally, in the last paragraph, list your preferences in priority order for the future: 1. With sister, Mary. 2. With brother, Harry, and so on.
4. After you have completed all of the above areas, SIGN and DATE it.

5. Make copies and give them to everyone who is involved with your child's future. I can assure you that this may be the first time that the siblings really understand what you have done in the past and the seriousness of their future commitment. Put a copy in your house where people can find it, in case of an illness or accident.

In this letter, you have the opportunity to explain why you have made certain decisions. You also can give crucial information about sleeping and eating habits, favorite activities, and little things that upset or please your child.

The Letter of Intent is a never-ending story. It is something that you write and continually update. For instance, in one section, you have listed current medication. Medication changes and when it does, you only have to redo that section (good reason for computer), and then sign and date it again. Circle your calendar and on that date, make sure you take out the Letter of Intent and make all of the changes.

I am sometimes accused of overemphasizing the importance of the Letter of Intent. I am guilty. I truly believe that few people will read wills and trusts when they are trying to figure out how to take care of your child. They want to do the best they can, but they need the kind of information that only you know and can provide.

Let me summarize the importance of this letter. This may sound a little morbid. Tomorrow at 1 PM, while you are shopping at the mall, you suffer a heart attack. As the sole care provider for your 45-year-old son who lives with you, you keep a little card in your wallet letting people know your son is at home and will need help. The police show up at the door with a social worker. What should they do? If you have left a Letter of Intent in an easily found place, the social worker will pick it and quickly note the following:

> *In the case of such an emergency, my son should go to stay with his sister, Mary. Please make sure he takes his medication at the appropriate time. He has a tendency to seizure when he becomes stressed despite the medication. Make sure you send over some of his favorite clothes.* (This carefully planned transition process beats the standard practice of taking your child to the nearest foster home or police station. Write it TODAY.)

DEVELOP A FINANCIAL PLAN

Step 4: Look at Financial Reality

All parents want the very best for their children. Your plan may call for a Helen Keller model of care, where your child will always have an Ann Sullivan Macy there to help. Although Helen was bright and articulate she still needed Ann Sullivan Macy to assist her. Initially, her family covered the expenses of this arrangement and later on Helen generated sufficient income to maintain it. We know that more than 97% of all persons with developmental disabilities rely solely on government assistance to sustain themselves. And the word *is* "sustain"; maybe the word "exist" is more accurate, for the typical government package is roughly two-thirds of the poverty level today.

We know that unless families are there to supplement or add to this basic benefit package than the person is condemned to a life of poverty. Some parents say, "Well, my child will live in a nice government group home." Yes, Medicaid does pay for most of it and yes, the group home will even provide some "spending" money for personal needs (toothpaste, clothing, etc.). This spending money is roughly $30 a month. Even a wise shopper at the Salvation Army can scarcely buy sufficient clothing and still go out to McDonalds once a month or year.

Although the families are still around, they generally provide that little extra to help the person enjoy a comfortable life-style. We have found that most families of adults with disabilities give consciously, or usually unconsciously, about $150–200 per month. It is not a great deal but it is very important.

After the parents and other family members depart the scene, where does this "difference" come from? Like Blanche in a "Street Car Named Desire," will your child then be dependent on the kindness of strangers?

Families need to address this problem head on. Sit down and add up all of your current expenses. Look at the future expenses, the things that you cover—housing, advocacy, telephone bills, and so on. Consult the *NICHCY News Digest on Estate Planning* (Fee, 1997) for a worksheet that will help you determine your future expenses.

Of course, identifying the costs does not mean much unless you determine a realistic method of funding the future expenses. Do not be surprised that the average savings required will be in the $400,000–500,000 range. It may seem like a lot of money (except to the government), but your child will need to live off the interest for a long time.

Your first inclination when you see this large amount is either to get new batteries for the calculator or to fire your financial advisor. Don't do either one. Take a few days to let it sink in and then begin to look for the resources you will need.

The good news is that there are many different methods that the average family can use including the following:

1. *Government benefits:* determine the base amount. This becomes the foundation for your plan.
2. *Life insurance* on one or both parents. Other relatives can certainly take out policies on themselves.
3. *Savings:* unless you already have major assets, you will need to save something regularly.
4. *Investments:* have special investment programs specifically for your child, separate from your main estate.
5. *Retirement plans:* some retirement plans allow you to list your children with disabilities as beneficiaries. The U.S. Military has an excellent plan.
6. *Other:* a house you wish to leave, relatives who have tax problems who need to gift money each year, and so on.

Financial planning in this area must consider both the short term and long term. There will be a need for cash should you become disabled yourself or if you must go into a nursing home. The money you have set aside for your child may be needed for your own care. As you will recall, the average stay in a nursing home prior to death is about 2 years. A good rule of thumb is to have two to three years of supplemental funds in a savings account (or invested elsewhere) where someone can get to it easily.

A Certificate of Deposit may be great in your overall planning except it may not be easily converted into cash in an emergency. The long-term planning is a little harder because you are trying to build a larger fund. Many people take out a low cost life insurance policy. You can use term insurance while you build up your investment portfolio or use a universal or whole life policy that can be paid up (universal technically cannot be paid up). Then you know that no matter what happens to you or your investment strategy, your child will be guaranteed a large fund at a very low cost. One word of caution: because assets in your child's name may disqualify him or her from government benefits, do not name your child as the beneficiary of any policy. We discuss how to do this in the legal section below.

You really should use a skilled financial planner to assist you. Some people enjoy playing in the stock market; however, the risks you take to increase your own retirement should not be considered when you must provide some real financial security for your child with a disability. As with all types of planning, ask your friends and local agencies for recommendations. Look for professionals with the professional designations (ChLAP, CFP, or ChFC) after their names. And just as importantly, make sure they know something about persons with disabilities. Without being too unkind, there are many unscrupulous people in this field who take advantage of families in great emotional need. Do not trust anyone without checking them out. You can't bet your child's future on great sales techniques.

DEVELOP A LEGAL PLAN
Step 5: Write Will and Trust

In this section, there is some information concerning the legal aspects of life planning. In no way is it meant to eliminate the need for consultation with a skilled lawyer. In fact, the only way to do the planning properly is with sound legal advice. With this major disclaimer that this is not legal advice, let's begin.

If you ask parents who went though the planning process 10 years ago what they did to plan they probably will tell you that they found a good lawyer. The lawyer listened for a few hours and then gave them a wonderful Last Will and Testament. If you probe a little more and ask for specifics you would get a few interesting answers.

The lawyer told us to:

1. Exclude all of the other kids and leave everything to our son with the disability because he would really need the money.
2. Ask someone we could trust such as a relative to manage the money for us.
3. Obtain guardianship when our child turned 18 and name someone who would take over in the future.
4. Stop worrying too much about the future; it is too hard to predict so don't worry about residential care, medical care, and so on. A relative or social agency would look after our child.

On the surface this sounds like excellent advice: leave some money and because we can't predict the future, hope for the best. Was the lawyer being overly callous, naïve? Probably not. Ignorant of the unique needs of persons with Down syndrome and modern-day social services and benefits? Definitely! You have to remember that the average lawyer is like the average person on the street—he or she is totally ignorant of the needs of persons with disability. In fact, their only perception of a person with Down syndrome might be based on a television program. And while we all love Chris Burke, we know that he is not a typical person with Down syndrome.

Today, when you go to a qualified and experienced attorney, you will probably receive the following kind of advice:

1. Do not leave any money directly to your child. He or she may be disqualified from receiving government benefits. You must state in your will that you do not want anything to go to your child—yes, that is called "disinheriting" him or her.

2. You should set up a Special Needs Trust (SNT). Your will should direct your assets (or percentage—let's leave something for the other siblings to keep them happy) to the SNT.

3. The SNT should be a living or intervivos trust. Some attorney may tell you to include a testamentary trust in your will which means the trust will not start until after your will is probated. Most experts in this field will tell you to set it up now because you want to use it to save some money to meet emergency needs (nursing home, money while your will is being probated, 6 months to 6 years). A living SNT also can now be funded by relatives who want to remember your child in their wills.

4. If you don't trust your relatives with small loans then don't make them the trustee (manager) of your child's trust, which may be a half a million dollars. They may decide to manage the trust from the Bahamas.

5. As long as you are alive and healthy, manage the trust yourself. Upon your death or in the event you have to go into a nursing home, name a bank or trust company to manage the funds. There will be peace of mind in knowing that the money will be handled in a prudent manner. There used to be concerns that a bank might charge high fees, be very impersonal, or not even want to handle the trust. There are ways to overcome these very real problems. First, if your trust account is more than $250,000 (after your death), the bank fees are very reasonable and well worth it in terms of safety and security. Second, always name a relative or a local charity as a co-trustee. The co-trustee who has a personal interest in the child will advise the bank on how to spend the money. For instance, the co-trustee could be a representative of the local Down syndrome group. He or she may notice during a visit to your child in his group home that he could use a new TV or maybe a visit to his sister upstate. The co-trustee would go to the bank and work with them to arrange the financial details.

6. Advocate or guardian (conservator/tutor)—decide now! If you really want to be the guardian, go through the court proceeding now. And while you are going through the process of becoming the guardian, look around for two or

more potential guardians. Most states will allow you to nominate successor guardians in your petition. Why? Okay, back to the nursing home scenario. If you go into the nursing home, who will have authority to look after your child? The social service agency, the ones that visit every 18–24 months (and it is always a different social worker because of the low pay and high case loads)? If you become incapacitated, the court approved successor trustee can take over for you. Some attorneys will also advise you to list some potential guardians in your will. There is no guarantee that these people will be approved by the court later, but at least the court has some idea of quality people you trusted. What if you don't believe in guardianship? You still want someone to advise or advocate for your child. Today, there are many local charities that have set up advocacy services. You need to sign up for their services now. They will develop a file. There may be a small charge to establish the account. And even if they are a nonprofit service, they will charge for the service. Most will visit your child on a regular basis, apply for government benefits, and fight the good fight. All of them will require some proof that you have funded the future service. Some will ask to be named beneficiaries in your will, life insurance policies, and so on. When selecting a service, look at their record of service. This is a relatively new type of service with a very high turnover. Ask them what their contingency plans are if they can no longer afford to run the service. They will not be offended. Though we all expect to live forever, we know that bad economic times, rapid inflation, and so on can destroy even the best program. Some advocacy groups handle advocacy and trusts whereas others only do the advocacy and refer you to a bank for trust management. Having a large, strong bank manage assets in a Special Needs Trust with clear instructions to employ an advocacy service seems to be a pretty safe bet.

Finding a qualified attorney is just as difficult as finding other qualified professionals. Again, rely on the judgment of good friends and local agencies, but keep in mind some of the options presented above. Every situation will be different so your attorney may have other options for you.

IMPLEMENTING YOUR PLAN

Step 6: Let Others Know

This may sound like just good common sense, but many families fail to do it. Once you have developed a sound Life Plan, written your initial Letter of Intent, worked out the finances, and completed all of the legal documentation, do not—repeat, do not—lock it up in your safety deposit box to await your demise. Call a meeting of all those involved, those who have agreed to be the advocates, guardians, trustees, and so forth. Share with them your plan. Tell them where you keep your plan. Discuss the reasoning behind certain components.

Then place the original plan and documents in your safety deposit box. Purchase a low cost three ring binder with a large number of plastic inserts. Put in it copies of all of your documents and anything else you feel future care providers will need such as copies of social security cards, health insurance cards, Individualized Education Plans, and medical records. Keep the binder in a place where you know people will be able to find it in an emergency. I have found that in a crisis situation, people tend to look for financial records and checkbooks. Some good advice is to put the planning binder under the checkbook. People will find it. Placing the binder there also serves another purpose in that you see it every time you go to write a check. This constant visual check can give you a sense of well-being, knowing that you have got things in place, and it can also remind you to update it regularly. As new government records, medical records, and other items are mailed to you, you have one place to keep them.

Planning for the future of a loved one with Down syndrome is not easy. No matter how well you plan you will always feel that there is something else you should have done. If you can go through the above steps in a fairly detailed manner, you will have done an excellent job. Instead of a couple of legal documents sitting in the safety deposit box with a Certificate of Deposit, you will have a well thought out plan that will give future care providers the inside track on providing the best possible care for your loved one. Life planning works.

REFERENCES

Fee RW, Russell ML, Grant AE, Joseph SM (1995): "Planning for the Future—Providing a Meaningful Life for a Child with a Disability After Your Death," 3rd ed. Evanston, IL: American Publishing Company.

Fee RW (1997a): The letter of intent. NICHY News Digest—Estate Planning, pp. 11–15.

Fee RW (1997b): The special needs trust. NICHY News Digest—Estate Planning, pp. 6–11.

"The Life Planning Newsletter," CMS Publications, 110 E. 13th Street, #2E, New York, NY 10003 ($24.95/year).

Listening to and Learning from Young Adults with Down Syndrome and Their Siblings

Judy S. Itzkowitz

This chapter, somewhat different from the other chapters compiled for this book, is my personal reflection about what I have learned from the individuals who live with Down syndrome and those individuals who we label as "siblings," who also live with Down syndrome. These reflections are based upon my own personal experiences with young adults with Down syndrome and my private practice as an educational consultant.

As I have had the privilege to get to know individuals with Down syndrome, their brothers and sisters, their parents, grandparents, aunts and uncles, and cousins, I have seen very clearly that each member of a family makes a unique contribution to that entire family system. Sometimes the contribution is obvious, sometimes more subtle. It is through the voices of family members, communicated through words and through behavior, that learning occurs. The lessons articulated below are a result of the opportunities I have had to listen to parents and young people who have such intimate experiences with Down syndrome, both individuals with Down syndrome and their siblings. I thank them for sharing their lives and learning with me; this chapter is dedicated to those gracious families who have allowed me to listen and to learn from them.

THE LESSON OF LISTENING

What can be learned from listening to the young adults with Down syndrome and their brothers and sisters is really at the heart of this chapter. Clearly, their words and voices teach us about our role as a family member, professional, friend, ally, and advocate. Each individual has his or her own personal experience with Down syndrome; these experiences provide the person and those who care about

Down Syndrome: A Promising Future, Together, Edited by Terry J. Hassold and David Patterson
ISBN 0-471-29686-4 Copyright © 1998 by Wiley-Liss, Inc.

the person with opportunities for intimate learning. The voices of those young adults with Down syndrome must be heard; their needs, desires, thoughts, reactions, fears, concerns, problems, and joys teach us how we can be supportive to the person who was once a child and is now becoming a young adult. Open discussions about the person's full range of life experiences and his or her reactions to these situations are critical to supporting the person with Down syndrome in being equipped to respond to the challenges and joys inherent in life (e.g., experiencing joy as a member of the high school basketball team; being in the same classes as peers without disabilities; participating in the science competition; graduating from high school with the friends with whom they have gone to school; having a circle of friends to depend on; feeling lonely about not having a close friend, being asked to the prom, talking on the phone with friends, or being invited over to a friend's house; feeling frustrated when people do not understand their communication; feeling frustrated that some activities take more effort to learn than their peers; responding to teasing or unkind words). Siblings remind us how important it is for parents to really listen to their unique concerns, experiences, needs, and ideas. Concerns about understanding their sibling's condition, their fears and concerns about their sibling and their parents, their sense of joy and pride with their sibling's accomplishments, and their hopes and dreams for themselves and their sibling with Down syndrome are just a few of the issues that siblings need to be able to discuss. So many times, siblings themselves have invaluable ideas about solving problems and addressing concerns.

The skill of listening is about hearing not only the words that are spoken but the affect and the underlying message of the person's communication. Listening involves hearing the person's story through his or her own eyes, rather than through one's own personal filters. As Covey (1989) writes, "Seek first to understand, then to be understood" (p. 235). Do we truly listen and really hear even when the message is one that is uncomfortable for us? Do we listen to and value the contribution that individuals with Down syndrome and their siblings make or are we concerned with our own personal agenda? As we truly listen, we learn about the person's intimate feelings and experiences thereby supporting siblings and young adults with Down syndrome through their own personal journeys in life. Equally important is listening to the behavior and actions of the person; many times individuals "speak" through their actions, especially those individuals who engage in challenging behavior—it is our responsibility to figure out the meaning of the communication.

THE LESSON OF ASKING DIFFICULT QUESTIONS, HEARING DIFFICULT ANSWERS, AND HAVING DIFFICULT CONVERSATIONS

With listening comes the opportunity to engage in conversations that are sometimes challenging. Perhaps it is the conversation with your son about puberty or with your daughter about what her dreams are for the future. Maybe it is the conversation about understanding Down syndrome, developmental disabilities, or mental retardation—supporting the person with Down syndrome in better understanding their own strengths and needs. Whatever the content of the discussion, open and honest conversations support families in maintaining the health and well-being of each member of the family and the family as a whole. Empirical research has suggested that families who communicate effectively are more resilient to life's challenges. These families solve problems, make decisions, and resolve conflicts. They express feelings, even when the feelings are labeled by society as negative and seem to be unjustified. Actually, all feelings are valid; they have a purpose or outcome. It is especially important that each member of the family develop competence as an effective communicator. This skill development is imperative for the young adult who happens to have Down syndrome so that the person can express opinions, dreams, feelings, reactions, thoughts, and so on in his or her own voice; this minimizes the dependence on other people around them to speak for them, to interpret what is being said, and to advocate for them. It is critical for all young people, with and without Down syndrome, to express feelings, needs, hopes, dreams, and desires so that they are understood.

Although discussions can be confronting and challenging, they can serve to unite families and support family members in honestly articulating who they truly are, what they value, what they dream about, and what they fear. These "heart-opening" conversations, open, honest, and candid, provide family members with opportunities for learning and growth in the context of each family. Some of the topics that are sometimes difficult for discussion include the future (e.g., where the individual with Down syndrome will live as parents get older, the preference that the person with Down syndrome has for where he/she will live, what happens when individuals with Down syndrome graduate from high school with no, few, or dissatisfying options for employment and a career), when a person's experiences are different from his or her dreams, and what happens when the expectations associated with becoming an adult are different for the adult with Down syndrome (e.g., other people are graduating from high school and beginning college, dating, getting married). Other conversations that are emotional for family members but so very important to have include the specifics associated with Down syndrome, the label of mental retardation, adolescence and becoming a teenager, sexuality, dating, adulthood, life-style, careers and employment, residential options (a home of their own), relationships and friendships, medical decisions, and aging. For siblings, discussions about their brother or sister with Down syndrome, the cause of the disability, whether the disability is inherited, their role with their sibling with Down syndrome, how friends respond to their brother or sister, feeling that they are responsible for their sibling's disability, dealing with their parents' feelings, recognizing their parents' stress, participating in child-rearing activities, talking with and interacting with friends, coping with their friends' reactions to their brother or sister with Down syndrome, dealing with teasing, dating, going to school with their brother or sister with special needs and other school-related issues, coping with community awareness and acceptance, decisions about guardianship, and figuring out their current and future relationship with their sibling with Down syndrome, including how to support their sibling when parents are unable to fulfill this role, are difficult topics for conversation yet these topics must be discussed. These conversations must start when children are young so that they realize they have permission to initiate conversations on varied (and sometimes emotional) topics. As with any discussions, information is supplied that is appropriate to the age and maturity of the child. Questions asked are those questions answered. If children want more information, they will ask additional questions for clarification. Through these discussions, young people learn the skills to communicate ideas, feelings, experiences, needs, dreams, and concerns effectively.

THE LESSON OF RELATIONSHIPS (WITH YOURSELF AND OTHERS), CONNECTIONS, AND BELONGING

All individuals within the family benefit from close personal relationships in and outside of the family unit. "Developing friendships is not something that comes easily or naturally to most of us, children or adults. Most people simply have trouble connecting with other people. . . . Yet, it is our friendships and relationships that are our only real hope, our guideline to being true members of our community. It is friendships that protect us from vulnerability and ensure that our lives are rich and full" (Strully and Strully, 1989, pp. 61). Relationship building is a lifelong process (Perske, 1988). There are challenges inherent in initiating, fostering, and maintaining friendships, yet the benefits are obvious.

As you support your own children (whatever their ages) in developing friendships, consider your responses to these questions.

- Can you articulate the reasons why people would want to be friends with your children?
- Can you see the gifts, talents, and strengths that your sons and daughters possess? Do you acknowledge these talents and gifts? How do you help others see those gifts? How do you support your children in seeing their own unique gifts?
- Do you really believe that other people would want to be a friend with your son or daughter?
- How committed are you to making friendships a priority? Have you made friendships a priority for all your children?
- Have you been reflective about the way you personally develop friendships?
- Are you a model with respect to developing and fostering friendships in your own life?
- Have you taken the time to teach, support, and foster skills that help to build friendships?
- Have you thought about the activities other young people your child's age do; their style of clothing, their music?
- Have you thought about where other young people this age like to go and what activities they are involved in?
- Are you aware of your child's choices in friends? Do you know your child's friends?
- Have you thought of activities that will encourage young people to want to be together?
- Have you made your home a "magnet" where young people like to "hang out"?

- Have you considered unobtrusive, respectful ways to assist your son or daughter to participate in activities with his or her peers?
- Have you communicated to professionals the importance you place on friendships and relationships for your child?
- Does your son or daughter with Down syndrome have goals and objectives in their educational plan that facilitate friendships? teach skills that result with friendships?
- Do you have open and honest discussions about friendships within the context of your family?
- Are you perseverant? If something does not work, do you try again and again?
- Do you know the times to "push" and struggle, and the times to "let go?"
- Do you encourage your children to be as independent and competent as possible? Do you support them in asking for help if needed? Do you reach out and ask for help?
- Do you provide your son or daughter with opportunities to learn about him/herself as a person including his/her strengths, limitations, and disability?
- Do you talk with individuals in your community to support them in better understanding your children and their experiences?
- Do you really believe from the depths of your soul that genuine friendships are possible for young people with and without disabilities?

As a parent, you are your child's best advocate and "public relations agent," if you are unable to see your child as someone with whom other people would want to be friends, how can other people see your child as a potential friend?

The support system developed by each family member is a key to the resiliency of a family in the face of crisis or challenge. Asking questions about how families can foster these relationships is critical. As parents, it is essential that you create your own circle of support—a group of individuals who support you, as a parent, with dealing with the day-to-day challenges and opportunities. By creating your own circle of support, you are modeling for your children the process of creating and maintaining circles of friends/support. It is important that each member of your family have a circle of support and friends who genuinely care about and value the individual for their strengths, gifts, and abilities. A circle of friends or a circle of support is a network that allows for the genuine involvement of children in a friendship, caring, and support role with their peers (Forest and Lusthaus, 1989; Snow, 1989). A circle provides a nurturing, supportive, and reinforcing climate to assist a person in becoming part of his or her class, school, and community. O'Brien describes circles of support as "dream catchers"; bringing together people who genuinely care about an individual to support the individual in articulating and making their dreams come alive. Circles start around two people who are in a strong relationship with each other and who want to see change. The purpose and direction of the circle are defined by the person's dreams or goals. The question that must be asked constantly is, "What do you really want?" Circles can become a safe place for people to share their dreams and visions with others. The person who is the focus of the circle will change in direct relationship to the honesty and commitment of the circle membership. If the circle is too small, everyone will feel the pressure. If the circle is too big, people may quit because they do not have enough to do. When a person requests what he or she really wants, the circle members feel needed and all of the people in the circle feel empowered—they see that they make a difference.

THE LESSON OF "FAILURE IS FEEDBACK"

In thinking about communication, it is important to recognize that breakdowns in communication are inevitable. When a breakdown occurs, it is helpful to view this as an opportunity for learning and feedback rather than a failure. There is no failure, only feedback.

THE LESSON OF DREAMING

So many times families are told to be realistic. However, the way that systems and services have changed for individuals with Down syndrome and their family members is through the visions generated by families themselves. One of the greatest gifts family members can give to each other is the permission to dream, to articulate their dreams to others, and to provide each other with support to make those dreams happen. Futures planning or person-centered planning [e.g., McGill Action Planning System (MAPS) and Planning Alternative Tomorrows with Hope (PATH) (Forest and Pearpoint, 1992; Giangreco et al., 1998; Mount, 1991, 1995; Pearpoint et al., 1993; Smull et al., 1996)] are techniques that support individuals in "dream catching," articulating dreams and planning to bring dreams alive. These processes support individuals in seeing people as whole, in acknowledging that the person and those who love the person with Down syndrome are the best experts and authorities—they know the person the best. None of us knows whether our dreams will come true; but those dreams provide us with the momentum to take action and to take risks as we work in the direction of our dreams. With any dream comes the risk of disappointment, of anxiety, of some fear; in the words of Helen Keller, "Security is mostly a superstition. It does not exist in nature, nor do the children of men and women as a whole experience it. Avoiding danger is no safer in the long run than outright exposure. Life is either a daring adventure or nothing."

Too often, when a person meets someone with Down syndrome, all they see is the Down syndrome. Person-centered planning supports people in seeing the positive characteristics, attributes, and gifts of the person. This process of futures planning helps to identify the preferences and desires of the person. It is a process that believes that all people have important gifts to contribute; it is up to each of us to uncover and discover these gifts and support people in sharing their gifts with others.

THE LESSON OF COMPETENCE, INDEPENDENCE, AND INTERDEPENDENCE

When someone has a disability, it is easy to focus on the disability rather than the ability of the person. Highlighting people's competencies, strengths, and gifts rather than their deficits or disabilities is integral to supporting people in becoming as competent as possible and in having access to the same opportunities as people without noticeable labels. The futures planning processes described above support people in recognizing and valuing these strengths and abilities. Encouraging participation, independence, and interdependence along with supporting young people in participating in extracurricular activities and in the community (e.g., church, synagogue, sports, music and dance lessons, scouting, swimming or horseback riding lessons, neighborhood gatherings) is paramount. Individuals with and without Down syndrome need to have opportunities to gain skills that will prepare them to be contributing members of their respective communities and be as independent as possible, yet learn to be part of the larger community. Supporting individuals to ask for help, to offer assistance, and to say "yes" and "no" based upon their preferences, dreams, and desires are skills that will prepare people for being part of and living in the community.

THE LESSON OF PERSISTENCE

Life is full of gifts and challenges. However, regardless of these gifts and challenges, persistence is a characteristic that supports each human being in "climbing the mountain," "getting through the valley," and "surviving the changes of the weather." In considering how people become successful, the key is persistence. Thomas Edison conducted 2000 experiments prior to the invention of the light bulb; John Grisham (the author of *The Client, The Chamber, A Time to Kill*) submitted manuscripts to publishers numerous times prior to his success. Abraham Lincoln was defeated numerous times throughout his life prior to being elected President—he ran for state legislature and lost; he wanted to go to law school but was rejected; his business went into bankruptcy; he was engaged to be married and his fiancée died; he was defeated in his attempt to become speaker of the state legislator; he lost his bid for Congress; he lost his bid for United States Senate. . . . Each of these individuals was persistent; they kept their dreams in focus, dealt with the rejection and disappointment, and continued to persevere in spite of the "defeats." Helping children to deal with disappointment, rejection, and perceived "failure" are important lessons; actually, if we can help people to view "mistakes" as valuable feedback integral to the learning process, then we can support people in persevering in the face of the obstacles they may encounter. As we are persistent, we also reflect on our actions and determine what to do differently; as the adage goes, "If you always do what you've always done, you'll always get what you always got. If what you are doing is not working, do something else!"

THE LESSON OF ASSERTIVENESS: ASKING FOR WHAT YOU WANT

No person, even those individuals who know us well, can read our minds. Supporting our children in being assertive (rather than aggressive) is an important skill to master. Assertiveness is speaking up for your own rights without stepping on the rights of others, being able to communicate what I think or feel without discounting the ideas and opinions of others. These skills take a lifetime to master. However, in order to make your own dreams come true, each of us must be skilled at advocating for ourselves and the people we care about.

THE LESSON OF RESPECT AND DIGNITY

Each person deserves to be treated in a respectful and dignified manner. As President Kennedy (1963) said, "Every American ought to have the right to be treated as he would wish to be treated, as one would wish his children to be treated." When we treat the people we care about in a respectful and dignified manner, they learn how they want to be treated and how to treat others.

THE LESSON OF TAKING CARE OF YOURSELF

One of the greatest gifts we can offer to the people we care about is showing them the importance of taking care of ourselves. The ability to experience balance in our lives, to do what brings us joy and satisfaction, and to take time for ourselves enables each of us to be able to do what we need for ourselves, our families, and the people we care about. Showing your sons and daughters the lifelong contribution that occurs in the quality of your life by taking care of yourself can only serve to support them to do the same in their own lives, whether it means taking time for a walk, a bath, to read a book, to go for a run, or to go golfing.

THE LESSON OF ATTITUDE

Carlos Casteneda wrote, "The trick is in what one emphasizes. We either make ourselves miserable or we make ourselves strong. The amount of work is the same." In each moment of life, we have a choice point about how to respond to the circumstances of our life. We can choose joy or sorrow, ease or struggle; in any circumstance, the choice is a personal one: the glass is half empty or half full. Frankl (1963), a concentration camp survivor, wrote in his book:

> We who lived in concentration camps can remember the men who walked through the huts comforting others, giving away their last piece of bread. They may have been few in number, but they offer sufficient proof that everything can be taken from a man but one thing: the last of the human freedoms—to choose one's attitude in any given set of circumstances, to choose one's own way.
>
> And there were always choices to make. Every day, every hour, offered the opportunity to make a decision, a decision which determined whether you would or would not submit to those powers which threatened to rob you of your very self, your inner freedom; which determined whether or not you would become the plaything of circumstance, renouncing freedom and dignity to become molded into the form of the typical inmate. . . .
>
> It becomes clear that the sort of person the prisoner became was the result of an inner decision, and not the result of camp influences alone. Fundamentally, therefore, any man can, even under such circumstances, decide what shall become of him—mentally and spiritually (p. 75).

Although the human journey is not a simple one, it can be full of joy, unexpected surprises, challenges, and opportunities. As we walk with siblings and young adults with

Down syndrome through their journeys in life, each of us, parent, relative, professional, advocate, friend, can support the person in taking actions that will bring the person closer to his or her dreams.

REFERENCES

Covey S (1989): "The Seven Habits of Highly Effective People." New York: Simon & Schuster.

Forest M, Lusthaus E (1989): Promoting educational quality for all students. In Stainback S, Stainback W, Forest M (eds.): "Educating All Students in the Mainstream of Regular Education." Baltimore, MD: Brookes, pp. 43–57.

Forest M, Pearpoint J (1992): Putting all kids on the MAP. Educational Leadership 50:26–31.

Frankl V (1984): "Man's Search for Meaning: An Introduction to Logotherapy," 3rd ed. New York: Simon & Schuster.

Giangreco MF, Cloninger CJ, Iverson VS (1998): "COACH. Choosing outcomes and Accommodations for Children. A Guide to Educational Planning for Students with Disabilities." Baltimore, MD: Brookes.

Mount B (1991): "Person-centered Development. A Journey in Learning to Listen to People with Disabilities." Manchester, CT: Communitas.

Mount B (1995): "Capacity Works. Finding Windows for Change Using Personal Futures Planning." Manchester, CT: Communitas.

Pearpoint J, O'Brien J, Forest M (1993): PATH. A workbook for planning positive possible futures. Planning alternative tomorrows with hope for schools, organizations, businesses, families. Toronto, Canada: Inclusion Press.

Perske R (1988): "Circle of Friends." Nashville, TN: Abingdon Press.

Smull MW, Sanderson H, Harrison SB (1996): Reviewing essential lifestyle plans: Criteria for best plans. College Park, MD: University of Maryland.

Snow JA (1989): Systems of support. A new vision. In Stainback S, Stainback W, Forest M (eds.): "Educating All Students in the Mainstream of Regular Education." Baltimore, MD: Brookes, pp. 221–231.

Strully JL, Strully CF (1989): Friendships as an educational goal. In Stainback S, Stainback W, Forest M (eds.): "Educating All Students in the Mainstream of Regular Education." Baltimore, MD: Brookes, pp. 59–68.

Early Intervention in Down Syndrome:
Brain Development and Aging

Ira T. Lott

NEUROBIOLOGICAL ISSUES IN EARLY INTERVENTION

There is a large collection of experimental literature detailing the relationship between sensory experience and the interactions of nerve cells through synaptogenesis. The relationship of these experiential studies to the sensory stimulation exposures in human early intervention is uncertain but the animal models provide a number of interesting observations. Innocenti et al (1995) review studies that suggest that axons in the corpus callosum synchronize activity within the cerebral hemispheres in ways relevant to the binding of perceptual features. In development, transient and widespread arbors of callosal axons in white matter and deep cortical layers seem to provide the basis for plasticity resulting from visual experience. In the visual cortex of the kitten, dendritic growth and branching of nerve cells occurs during a period of overlapping synaptogenesis and this process is sensitive to visual experience (Zec and Tieman, 1994). In a brain injury model in which there is a lesion placed in the forelimb area of sensorimotor cortex in rats, there is use-dependent overgrowth of layer V pyramidal cell dendrities in the cortex of the noninjured hemisphere (Kozlowski et al., 1996). Moreover, if use of the nonimpaired limb is prevented, there is severe impairment of dendritic growth as well as chronic behavioral deficits. The authors suggest that these results show that behavioral experience after brain injury may enhance neural growth and that the region surrounding the injury may be vulnerable to behavioral pressure during the early post-lesion period. In a review of some experimental studies on the psychobiology of brain elasticity, Rozenzweig and Bennett (1996) note that Hebb first hypothesized in 1949 that experience induced plasticity of the nervous system. Subsequently it was determined that training or differential experience would induce neurochemical changes in the cerebral cortex including increased cortical thickness, enhanced sized of synaptic contacts, and increased number of dendritic spines and

Down Syndrome: A Promising Future, Together, Edited by Terry J. Hassold and David Patterson
ISBN 0-471-29686-4 Copyright © 1998 by Wiley-Liss, Inc.

branching. The results of enriched early experience were similar to those following formal training of the laboratory animal. The authors point out that research on use-induced plasticity is being applied to promote child development, successful aging, and the recovery from brain injury.

GENERAL PEDIATRIC STUDIES ON EARLY INTERVENTION

There are a number of clinical studies that have examined early intervention regimens in cohorts of children not having Down syndrome and it seems worth examining some of these studies as background for the more specialized observations. In highly stimulating home environments, children of very low birth weight have been found to catch up on measures of cognitive delay (Weiglas-Kuperus et al., 1993). When a mother-focused Newborn Intensive Care Unit program was instituted, a more optimal performance was seen on the Bayley Scales of Infant Development (Parker et al., 1992). Early home intervention stimulation programs have been shown to reduce developmental delays experience by low-income urban infants with nonorganic failure to thrive (Black et al., 1995). When an early intervention program emphasized maternal techniques to maintain the infants' attention and directiveness, a positive relationship was seen in expressive language skills in the high-risk infant at 12 months of age (Smith et al., 1996). In an update following a 30-year literature review, (Ramey and Ramey, 1994) children of low-IQ mothers responded positively to intensive high-quality early intervention. The sensitive period for the relationship of growth to mental development not unexpectedly seems to be between birth and 15 months of age (Skuse et al., 1994). In an early intervention study aimed at parents, Parush and Hahn-Markowitz (1997) provided a primary prevention program to increase mothers' sensitivity to the child's special needs and determined that enhanced knowledge beyond that of a control group was sustained for up to 2 years. Home-based early intervention counseling in high-risk families has been associated with improved mental health in adolescents (Aronen and Kurkela, 1996). Sounding a note of caution, Fewell and Glick (1996) reported the results of intensive early intervention in 44 children and found no overall gains in actual versus predicted post-test scores. Findings by subgroup revealed that in cognition, gross-motor, and fine-motor domains, the group with less severe impairments made more progress. The results were interpreted in light of constraints imposed by current measurement tools. McCarton et al. (1996) reported that a multisite randomized clinical trial of low-birth-weight infants to evaluate the efficacy of combining developmental and support services along with pediatric follow-up demonstrated only modest success. The authors indicated that future research endeavors should investigate the type, duration, critical age onset, and intensity of the intervention as well as which subgroups of low-birth-weight infants might benefit from such programs.

EARLY INTERVENTION PROGRAMS IN DOWN SYNDROME

The reader is referred to the recent review of the effectiveness of early intervention for children with Down syndrome (DS) by Hines and Bennett (1996). As pointed out in this review, a number of workers have cited a decline in intellectual quotients with age in DS from the first year until late childhood. There are some medical characteristics of children with DS that may contribute to this deceleration in development. These include hypotonia and congenital cardiac defects. Ear infections and structural craniofacial abnormalities also contribute to the difficulty in expressive language, although there appear to be intrinsic central processing difficulties that are to be part of the syndrome. Even social development, which has been long recognized as a relative strength in the behavioral repertoire of infants with DS, appears to undergo a different developmental sequence from that of typically developing children.

It is against this background that studies on early intervention in DS must be evaluated. Hines and Bennett reviewed approximately 20 studies in which early intervention was assessed in children with DS. Virtually all the studies showed some benefit, even if objective testing failed to demonstrate a difference from control groups. For example, in their review of recent intervention studies (since 1981), some children with DS who received early intervention had higher scores on measures of intellectual/adaptive functioning and did not show the typical decline referred to above. In other studies, higher scores in reading and numerical skills accompanied early intervention. Many children with DS met the program objectives in a quicker and more robust manner than children without this stimulation. But, as the authors point out, there are significant limitations to our ability to interpret these studies. There seems to be no common design strategy from one study to another. Although there is a significant biologic homogeneity in DS, individual children with the syndrome differ widely in potential and in regard to medical complications. Parental involvement in the program is a variable that is difficult to control. The criteria for control groups are ambiguous. Developmental progress may occur in areas not measured by standardized tests, such as family and sibling adjustment, and there are no robust long-term IQ advantages.

Nonetheless, the results to date appear to be promising enough to continue early intervention strategies and to move toward larger population studies in DS that can attempt to control for some of these variables. It is hoped that more convincing answers about the timing of intervention will be generated with carefully designed research.

EARLY INTERVENTION, SYNAPTOGENESIS, AND AGING—SPECULATION

Experiential factors are critical in the development of communication among nerve cells (synaptogenesis). Synaptic formation differs appreciably among brain regions in the developing infant (Volpe, 1995). In the medulla, dendritic spines reach a peak at 34–36 weeks gestation, whereas in the visual cortex, the most rapid period of synaptogenesis is between two and four months post-term. In the latter structure, this is a critical time for the development of function. Plasticity in the developing nervous system is also influenced by synapse elimination, which generally occurs at later stages of infancy and childhood. In children with developmental delays including Down syndrome, there are diminished numbers of dendritic spines and synapses (Petit et al., 1984; Ross et al., 1984; Becker et al., 1986, 1991; Takashima et al., 1989; Wisniewski 1990). There is some recent evidence that processes such as synaptogenesis and dendritic spine development may be relevant as protective factors for the onset of Alzheimer disease. Mori et al. (1997) have shown by use of high-resolution magnetic resonance imaging that premorbid brain volume may be a determinate of reserves against the intellectual decline in Alzheimer disease. Albert et al. (1995) has shown that education is a direct predictor of cognitive change over a two-and-a-half year study period in the normal population. As measured by the mini-mental status examination, cognitive function declines most steeply as a function of age in those without a bachelor's degree in a population of older women (Butler et al., 1996). In a population of African-Americans, there was a potential protective role of education against the development of dementia (Callahan et al., 1996).

Although speculative in nature, one might hypothesize that the role of education and early stimulation of brain development provides a robust synaptic circuitry that in older age may be preventive against the onset of dementia. Early intervention may be one means of cognitive enhancement that will unite the processes of development and aging.

SUMMARY

In this brief review, data relative to early intervention in Down syndrome is presented. The results of early enriched experience in a laboratory setting in animals suggest that dendritic growth and branching is sensitive to early experiential input. In the general pediatric population, early intervention programs have shown to have at least short-term effects in high-risk families associated with pre-term birth, low socioeconomic status of the mother, and growth failure in the child. The evaluation of early intervention in Down syndrome is made difficult by a number of base-line variables including hypotonia, congenital cardiac defects, and structural craniofacial abnormalities. Although there are no robust long-term IQ advantages, there are, nevertheless, considerable short-term gains facilitated by early intervention in DS. Early intervention research is quite difficult and it is hoped that future studies will control some of the variables that complicate our interpretation of existing data. Recent findings from the Alzheimer disease literature suggest that education may have protective effects toward the onset of dementia. Early intervention and its potential effect on synaptic development may contribute to a neuronal network that is more recalcitrant to the onset of clinical dementia in Down syndrome at older ages.

REFERENCES

Albert MS, Jones K, Savage CR, et al. (1995): Predictors of cognitive change in older persons: MacArthur studies of successful aging. Psychol Aging 10(4):578–589.

Aronen ET, Kurkela SA (1996): Long-term effects of an early home-based intervention. J Am Acad Child Adolesc Psychiatry 35(12):1665–1672.

Becker L, Mito T, Takashima S, et al. (1991): Growth and development of the brain in Down syndrome. In: "The Morphogenesis of Down Syndrome." New York: Wiley-Liss.

Becker LE, Armstrong DI, Chan F (1986): Dendritic atrophy in children with Down's syndrome. Ann Neurol 20:520–526.

Black MM, Dubowitz H, Hutcheson J, Berenson-Howard J, Starr RH, Jr (1995): A randomized clinical trial of home intervention for children with failure to thrive. Pediatrics 95(6):807–814.

Butler SM, Ashford JW, Snowdon DA (1996): Age, education, and changes in the Mini-Mental State Exam scores of older women: findings from the Nun Study. J Am Geriatr Soc 44(6):675–681.

Callahan CM, Hall KS, Hui SL, Musick BS, Unverzagt FW, Hendrie HC (1996): Relationship of age, education and occupation with dementia among a community based of African-Americans. Arch Neurol 53(2):134–140.

Fewell RR, Glick MP (1996): Program evaluation findings of an intersive program. Am J Ment Retard 101(3):233–243.

Hines S, Bennett F (1996): Effectiveness of early intervention for children with Down syndrome. Ment Retard Devel Disabilities 2:96–101.

Innocenti GM, Aggoun-Zouaoui D, Lehmann P (1995): Cellular aspects of callosal connections and their development. Neuropsychologia 33(8):961–987.

Kozlowski DA, James DC, Shallert T (1996): Use-dependent exaggeration of neuronal injury after unilateral sensorimotor cortex lesions. J Neurosci 16(15):4776–4786.

McCarton CM, Wallace IF, Bennet FC (1996): Early Intervention for low birthweight premature infants: what can we achieve? Ann Med 28(3):221–225.

Mori E, Hirono N, Yamashita H, et al. (1997): Premorbid brain size as a determinant of reserve capacity against intellectual decline in Alzheimer's disease. Am J Psychiatr 154(1):18–24.

Parker SJ, Zahr LK, Cole JG, Brecht ML (1992): Outcome after developmental intervention in the neonatal intensive care unit for mothers of preterm infants with low socioeconomic status. J Pediatr 120(5):780–785.

Parush S, Hahn-Markowitz J (1997): The efficacy of an early prevention program facilitated by occupational therapists: a follow-up study. Am J Occup Ther 51(4):247–251.

Petit TL, LeBoutillier JC, Alfano DP, et al. (1984): Synaptic development in the human fetus: a morphometric analysis of normal and Down's syndrome neocortex. Exp Neurol 83:13–23.

Ramey CT, Ramey SL (1994): Which children benefit the most from early intervention? Pediatrics 94(6 pt 2): 1064–1066.

Rosenzweig MR, Bennett EL (1996): Psychobiology of plasticity: effects of training and experience on brain and behavior. Behav Brain Res 78(1):57–65.

Ross MH, Galburda AM, Kemper TL (1984): Down syndrome: is there a decreased population of neurons? Neurology 34:909–916.

Skuse D; Pickles A, Wolke D, Reilly S (1994): Postnatal growth and mental development: evidence for a "sensitive period." J Child Psychol Psychiatr Allied Disciplines 35(3):521–545.

Smith KE, Landry SH, Swank PR, Baldwin CD, Denson SE, Wildin S (1996): The relation of medical risk and maternal situation with preterm infants' development of cognitive and daily living skills. J Child Psychol Psychiatr Allied Disciplines 37(7):855–864.

Takashima S, Ieshima A, Nakamura H, et al. (1989): Dendrites, dementia and the Down syndrome. Brain Dev 11:131–133.

Volpe JJ (1995): "Neurology of the Newborn," 3rd ed. Philadelphia: WB Saunders, pp. 73–75.

Weiglas-Kuperus N, Baerts W, Smrkovsky M, Sauer PJ (1993): Effects of biological and social factors on the cognitive development of very low birthweight children. Pediatrics 92(5):658–665.

Wisniewski KE (1990): Down syndrome children often have brain with maturation delay, retardation of growth and cortical dysgenesis. Am J Med Genet Suppl 7:274–281.

Zec N, Tieman SB (1994): Development of the dendritic fields of layer 3 pyramidal cells in the kitten's visual cortex. J Comp Neurol 339(2):288–300.

X. Perspectives: Young Adults with Down Syndrome Speak Out

Love yourself, Love your neighbor

Brenda Lynn Bargmann

I am very happy to have been asked to write about my experiences. I was discriminated against after I was born. The doctor wanted my parents to leave me in the hospital, to be placed in an institution. Thank God they said, "No way!" They loved and accepted me just as I was. Because of that, I live a fairly normal life.

While I was in school, some children were cruel. They called me names and made fun of me. It hurt a lot. My mom said to ignore their words and pray for them. That advice helped me to overcome rejection.

I graduated from Chaparral High School in 1983. The psychologist tried to discourage me from enrolling there but we persisted. They never had a student with Down syndrome before, even though they had a "special ed" class. I tried to enroll in the drama class, but was rejected. After a few weeks, the psychologist apologized to my parents and said I did very well. In 1993, I took three courses at Scottsdale Community College and earned an "A" in two of them.

After graduation, I got a job at the Radisson Hotel. I was put in charge of the employee's cafeteria. I was there four years. I am now working at the Days Inn in Scottsdale. I have been there for ten years.

I love to travel. While in school, we moved five times in three years. We lived in Texas, Ohio, Oregon, and Arizona. We also went on a pilgrimage to Italy, Israel, and Venezuela.

I participated in Special Olympics for three years and won 17 medals, for track, swimming, bowling, ice-skating, and race walking. I was nominated the "Most Inspirational Athlete" in 1990. I play the piano and the synthesizer. I belong to a dance group. We dance in various churches.

I have been a Eucharistic Minister in my church for eight years. My pastor was not too sure about my being one, but the lady in charge had faith in my abilities, and gave me the opportunity. I am a core member of an international group called "Faith and Light," who serve mentally challenged people. I belong to "Women's Aglow," a Christian organization.

Down Syndrome: A Promising Future, Together, Edited by Terry J. Hassold and David Patterson
ISBN 0-471-29686-4   Copyright © 1998 by Wiley-Liss, Inc.

I was honored to give the invocation for a baseball Hall of Famer's banquet for two years. This was a benefit for a Down syndrome group called "Sharing." I have been a voter for 12 years and have helped in a political campaign.

For many years, I kept after my mom to teach me how to drive a car. She kept saying, "Next year." Then I met a very special person to whom I shall always be grateful. She said, "I will teach you how to drive." Last November, I received my driver's license on my first try. I was so happy and excited! Three weeks ago, I was given a Pontiac station wagon by a friend. Mom won't let me drive it alone yet, but "Look out, here I come!"

One of the most exciting things I have done for the past four years is speaking in public schools for an awareness program called "Everyone Counts." It is my way of showing the children that we have values too. That we do many of the things they do and they should not discriminate against us, or anyone with a disability. Their response has been great. They ask questions, and say things like, "I wish I had the courage to stand in front of the class and do what you are doing." I have received many beautiful letters from them. *New Times,* a Phoenix newspaper, did a cover story about the school program.

My goals are to love and help anyone I can, to pray for people, to continue to give my testimony in schools, and to use my gift of dancing before the Lord. I also would like to take some computer classes.

I love and accept myself just as I am and I love you too.

Believe in Yourself

Chris Burke

My name is Chris Burke and I am pleased to contribute to this book. We have come together on this project to inform one another, to educate one another, to gain from one another, and to pass this knowledge on to you! I have always wanted to help every challenged person to achieve his or her goal in life.

When I graduated from school in 1986, I had two goals in life: (1) to help people with disabilities and (2) to be an actor. I'm happy to say I accomplished both goals.

First, I worked at a school for the multi-handicapped in New York City. I loved all the children and had fun helping them. Then, I did become an actor—I loved playing Corky in ABC-TV's *Life Goes On* for four years. It was the greatest! I have also appeared in a few other television shows, such as *Promised Land, Touched by an Angel, The Commish, Heaven and Hell, Desperate,* and *Jonathan, The Boy Nobody Wanted.* I really enjoy acting and hope more opportunities come along.

When *Life Goes On* ended, some people thought I would be lost, but instead, I have gone on to do many more interesting things, such as working for the National Down Syndrome Society. I am the proud editor-in-chief of *News & Views,* a magazine for and about young people with Down Syndrome and their siblings. I hope all of you have seen it and are subscribers. I also am the Goodwill Ambassador for the Society, so I talk to other young people with Down Syndrome to encourage them to do the very best they can, because there are lots of things that people with Down Syndrome *can* do.

In addition to talking to young people, I speak to parents and teachers and legislators. I tell legislators how important it is to support services for children so they can grow up to be independent and good citizens. In between all of this, I entertain with my two friends, Joe and John DeMasi. We have recorded two albums so far and a third one is in the works. We are on the road quite a bit but we have a lot of fun!

Sometimes I wonder how all these experiences came about. *Well,* for one thing I have never minded getting up early and doing for myself—such as making up my room, fixing breakfast, and preparing my lunch. I started doing this when I attended

Down Syndrome: A Promising Future, Together, Edited by Terry J. Hassold and David Patterson
ISBN 0-471-29686-4   Copyright © 1998 by Wiley-Liss, Inc.

day camp many years ago and continue doing it today. It makes me feel self-confident and independent to do for myself. So I highly recommend it to all!

Then, when I got an idea about something I wanted to do, I *really* pursued it. *For acting*—I volunteered for every show or play that was held at school, at day camp, or in our Boy Scout troop. I watched my favorite stars on television and studied them very carefully, so I could learn how to show emotions without even speaking. And I attended special classes for improvisation before and after I graduated from school. It prepared me for the roles I played. I had no trouble as a teacher's aide, because when I was at The Don Guanella School during the school year and at day camp during the summer months, I always volunteered to help the counselors with the younger children. It was so much fun to interact with them and it eased the work load for the counselors. And I learned a great deal!

When I was a student, I loved writing for our school newspaper so I became a reporter. I even wrote a letter to President Reagan telling him about our school, and he wrote back to me. It was all printed in the paper. So that prepared me for my job with the National Down Syndrome Society.

And now the music—I wasn't born with a great singing voice but I have never stopped trying to improve on my limitations. I guess you can say my love of music comes through and it seems to be working. Determination is the key to success.

So the message I want to leave with you is: believe in yourself, work hard, and never give up, so all your dreams can come true!

Perspectives on Education

Jason Kingsley

My name is Jason Kingsley. I would like to tell you about the education I've had. I am very lucky. When I was born 22 years ago, the obstetrician said to my parents that I should not have any education at all. I would never learn anything, or accomplish anything. He said it would be a waste of time to try to teach me anything.

I am very lucky because my parents didn't listen to that obstetrician. They made sure I got the best education that I needed. I started infant stimulation when I was only 10 days old! In the days that I was in school—preschool, elementary school, middle school, and high school—nobody knew much about inclusion. It was not popular as it is now. I was in separate special education classes for people with learning disabilities. Those kids were so smart and were good role models for me. I had to work hard to keep up, but it worked out fine.

In New York State we have six Regents Competency Tests. They are in reading, writing, science, mathematics, American history, and two years of world history. Some of the things on the test we haven't even covered yet. These tests are three hours long, and they are very sad and miserable. But I am proud to tell you that I passed all six of my RCT exams. Because I passed all those tests, when I graduated in 1994 I got a regular full academic diploma—not a special ed IEP diploma, but the same diploma everybody else in the school got!

I didn't experience inclusion in my classes. The only real inclusion I had in high school was when I joined the drama club, Wig & Whiskers. In the drama club, I was right in with everybody else. I did all the same things everybody did. In the spring musicals every year, I was the prop manager. I worked on sets, I was part of the chorus, and I even had some small speaking parts on stage. Every year in our talent shows, I would recite Shel Silverstein poems. They are very funny, and they were a big hit every year.

Even though I had some special needs, everyone was nice to me and accepted me. I went to all the cast parties and I made a lot of friends. Some of them I still see. But I didn't have very many other friends from Lakeland High School, because as soon as

Down Syndrome: A Promising Future, Together, Edited by Terry J. Hassold and David Patterson
ISBN 0-471-29686-4   Copyright © 1998 by Wiley-Liss, Inc.

school was over, I had to take the bus back home. So I couldn't hang around and do stuff with kids after school like most kids do. And when I went home, I didn't know anybody in my own town. So socializing was always a big problem. My Mom and Dad started some teen parties to get teenagers with Down syndrome together once a month. Those parties were fun, but it's not the same as having friends in school and your home town.

I am sorry I didn't have inclusion when I was in school. To get my good education, because they didn't have any good classes in my neighborhood, I had to travel on a bus to a faraway district. So I didn't know anybody in my own home town. If I could go back in time and do it again, I would prefer to go to school in my own town so I could have gotten to know some local kids. But I did get a good education in the Lakeland district and I have accomplished many good things. I have acted on television. I have given speeches all over the country. And I guess you know I have written a book with my friend and co-author, Mitchell Levitz. It's called *Count Us In: Growing Up with Down Syndrome*. I am happy to tell you our book sold out the entire hardcover edition. It is in its fourth printing in paperback, and it just came out in Japanese. Now I am attending Maplebrook School in Amenia, New York. This is a postsecondary transitional program that helps you learn independent living skills and vocational experiences. This is still not inclusion. It is a special school for young adults with learning disabilities, but it is teaching me all the things I need to know to live on my own in the future.

This summer I am working in the office of the Westchester Council for the Arts. I will be doing clerical work for them. And, I will be taking public transportation to get there. I will be making $125 a week. That's a lot of money.

After I graduate from the Apartment Living Program at Maplebrook School, I plan to get a job, and find a place to live on my own. Then maybe some day I will get married and start my history of being a family, just like my Mom and Dad.

Inclusion: Our Human Right

Mitchell Levitz

Parents were told by their pediatricians that their child will never live a normal life and that he should be put into an institution. Doctors did not really know anything about disabilities and especially about Down syndrome. It is your job as parents to tell the doctors they are NOT the experts, and that WE are the experts.

My parents have always been very active in my life and education. They brought me home from the hospital and gave me every opportunity there was. They wanted me to be in the community with other children. You know what I think? The doctors never thought my parents would have the courage to take advantage of the opportunities to show that there are people out there who care.

People do care! They care about what happens to our children and they want the best! Think about what happened in the Oklahoma bombing. Think about the 80 children who died because of terrorism. Let me tell you something, it is a nightmare for parents to live with what happened that day.

Now think about what happened in the early 1970s when parents were told to lock their children up in an institution and forget them. You know what, that is not the answer, to put children in institutions. That is no answer at all. The answer is to give them an opportunity—give them a life. It is people like Chris Burke who set that example by having the courage to go on television and show people like us, the young adults that will be the leaders in the future. It is our job to say yes, we can live the dreams we have and take advantage of the opportunities before us. It is our basic human right. We should be treated with dignity and respect and we cannot let others deny us.

And you know what Congress is doing now. They are saying wait a minute here, IDEA (Individuals with Disabilities Education Act) is important but we don't have the funding for the program. Let me tell the members of Congress that we want them to work with us for the common good of all Americans. One way to do that is for us to work together as a TEAM—because Together Everyone Achieves More. TEAM

Down Syndrome: A Promising Future, Together, Edited by Terry J. Hassold and David Patterson
ISBN 0-471-29686-4   Copyright © 1998 by Wiley-Liss, Inc.

makes good business sense! We need to work hard together, to work hard to show people how capable we are. People like us can prove to the world that we can do it.

Think about people like Sandra Jensen who had a hard young life and needed an organ transplant to live. The hospital and the doctors said wait a minute, we can't give her an organ because she has Down syndrome. Let me tell you something, it's the person that counts, not the fact that they have Down syndrome. Everyone is entitled to an organ transplant and should NOT be denied because they have Down syndrome.

It is people like Martin Luther King who said we have a "dream." Our dream is to fight for inclusion for all and to make it work. It will work because we want to be treated with dignity and respect and that is important to us. That is why we must tell the members of Congress to take a better look at IDEA and to start working for the common good of the American people.

We need people to focus on our abilities and capabilities. We need to work together as a TEAM. That is what the organization I work for, Capabilities Unlimited, does. We believe by working together as a TEAM we can make a difference.

In conclusion, I am the Editor-in-Chief of a newsletter called the Community Advocacy Press. It is a newsletter written by people with disabilities about issues important to us. I'll bet that the doctors never would have thought that we would be able to write and publish a newsletter. I'll also bet the doctors never thought our parents and families would support us to be leaders in our community. That is why people like us want to make a difference and that is why I say "inclusion for all."

Mia, A Proud Researcher

Mia Peterson

My name is Mia Peterson. I am 22 years old and I work at HyVee Grocery Store and Deli in Webster City, Iowa. I really like this job, because I enjoy people, and I see lots of them every day. I have been appointed to the Iowa Governor's Council on Developmental Disabilities by Governor Terry Branstad.

I would like to talk to you about a research project I'm working on about communications and learning language, and how I first got started. It all started when I was co-editor of a newsletter called *DS Headline News*. There was a conference call of editors one day, and I was assigned to interview and write a story about Dr. Laura Meyers, a very nice person, who is a linguist and has a Ph.D. I called her, and she told me about an idea she had about doing a research project on communications. She wanted someone with Down syndrome to be her researcher. She also thought it would be cool to give a workshop at a Down syndrome convention. I got really interested and said, "I want to be that researcher!" And I am.

My first workshop was at the National Down Syndrome Society's conference in Phoenix, AZ. I felt so important and proud! I'm really being heard! This research project is important. I have learned from Laura how to make up a grant application, and I wrote it with a little assistance and support. With all that assistance and support I got funded by the Enoch Gelbard Foundation. This project is so important because it asks questions that are important for professionals on communications to know the answers to. By asking them directly, I am learning about how people with Down syndrome learn to communicate. Most research is done by professionals. My research is being done by me, with Dr. Meyers helping me write about what I learn. This research study is all about the way people with Down syndrome learn how to use language best. I am using a survey to ask people what has helped them the most. It asks questions such as "What was it like when you were a little kid?" and then "What is it like now?" Here is a sample question: "What was it like when you were a little kid in understanding family and friends? Was it the worst, hard, easy, or the best?" My answer would be "the best," because those were the people who taught me when I was

Down Syndrome: A Promising Future, Together, Edited by Terry J. Hassold and David Patterson
ISBN 0-471-29686-4   Copyright © 1998 by Wiley-Liss, Inc.

little and had to learn to communicate and talk. I had to understand them, and they had to understand me.

Now I am working with a different newsletter called *The Community Advocacy Press*. I work with Essie Pederson. She is the director of a business called Capabilities Unlimited. Judy Roth, Tia Nelis, and Mitchell Levitz work with us too. They are great people to work with! I'm still working on my research project with Dr. Meyers.

Finally, I am an advocate for people with Down syndrome by working on this important project. I am also being heard for myself! My advice for all of you is to speak up for yourselves and not let others speak for you.

We Are All Special

Christi Todd

I want you to look at the person to your right and to your left. Each of you is special, and each of you is special in different ways.

My name is Christi Todd. I have curly blonde hair and I am 4 feet 9 inches tall. I keep my room clean and I attend church. I also have Down syndrome, and that's okay.

Having Down syndrome may mean I have to work harder to prove I can do something. So, I do work harder and I can do many things.

I want to tell you how God has blessed my life. When I was born in 1968, the doctors told my parents that my life would not have much value because I was born with Down syndrome. They said that I might not talk, I would not walk before age 3, and the average life for children born with Down syndrome was only 12 years. They also said I could never attend public school and an institution would be an appropriate place for me.

Fortunately, my parents did not listen to the doctors and in June of 1990 I graduated from Shadow Mt. High School in Scottsdale, Arizona. Since then I have taken classes at Paradise Valley Community College.

My education began when I was 2 ½ years old. My parents found a preschool run by a group of caring parents. This gave me an opportunity at an early age to develop good speech. This early intervention gave me a head start in learning. I was able to move to a public school when I was 5 years old. A wonderful woman in our classroom spent extra time with me, and taught me to read! I read so well that soon I was able to move to a regular second-grade class for reading. God has given my life great value. My parents cared about me and gave me a chance to accomplish something. My teachers cared and taught me many things.

When I was 10, my teacher Cynthia Strum, in her free time, taught me gymnastics and introduced me to Special Olympics. Who would ever think that a little girl with Down syndrome, who is deaf in one ear, could ever possibly do a cartwheel on a 4-inch balance beam? Well, I can!

Down Syndrome: A Promising Future, Together, Edited by Terry J. Hassold and David Patterson
ISBN 0-471-29686-4   Copyright © 1998 by Wiley-Liss, Inc.

I was able to participate in my high school gymnastics program and I actually assisted my classmates with their routines. It made me feel great!

Gymnastics is my favorite sport, but I have also competed in swimming, diving, basketball, and bowling. I've even tried a little golf. I am currently learning to ride horses. I love riding horses. It's a lot like being on the balance beam, except the horse moves and hopefully I do not! Special Olympics has had a tremendous influence on my life. Special Olympics has given me the opportunity to train and compete and prove to my family and friends what I can do. This makes them proud of me and I am proud of myself. Hopes and dreams can be shattered when mental retardation hits a family. Everyone is affected. But through Special Olympics, people are given the opportunity to get off the sidelines and participate in life. Many people can become contributing members of society rather than a burden.

My successes in Special Olympics have encouraged me to work hard at school and my job as a courtesy clerk for Abco. I have been with Abco over seven years and I enjoy talking to people every day. And I think they enjoy talking to me too.

My public speaking and the many friends in high school who accepted me, caused me to be invited to speak at my graduation from Shadow Mt. High School. I encouraged my fellow 500 graduating classmates to work hard and reach for the stars, to make a positive difference for the future. I challenge you to do the same in your life. Think about how God has blessed you and how you can share that blessing with someone else.

In my travels, I have had the great pleasure of meeting many celebrities including Michael Landon. I have also been in a made-for-TV movie with Randy Travis, Barbara Mandrell, Danny DeVito, Arnold Schwarzenegger, John Kennedy, Jr., Maria Shriver, and others. And yes, Danny DeVito really is that short. He is one of the few people who make me feel tall!

One of the many blessings I have been given was the recognition for my volunteer work for Special Olympics. The Hon Kachina Award I received was given to me by the Jefferson Foundation. It was a tremendous honor to be included with 11 wonderful people from Arizona. I was the one of the 12 chosen to go to Washington, DC to receive an additional honor presented in the Supreme Court of the United States.

As I said earlier, I have had to work hard. There have been many challenges in my life but as I have succeeded, I feel much taller than my 4 feet 9 inches. I would say to you, keep a positive attitude. Don't let anyone discourage you. Trust in the Lord in all things. You may have to work hard, but don't ever give up. Always remember that you are important. You are special in your own unique way. And one of the best ways to feel good about yourself is to share yourself with someone else.

Index